# Demystifying COVID-19: Understanding the Disease, Its Diagnosis and Treatment

Authored by

**Ozgur KARCIOGLU**
*Department of Emergency Medicine*
*University of Health Sciences*
*Istanbul Education and Research Hospital*
*Fatih, Istanbul, Turkey*

***Selman YENIOCAK***
*Department of Emergency Medicine,*
*University of Health Sciences,*
*Haseki Education and Research Hospital,*
*Fatih, Istanbul, Turkey*

&

***Mandana HOSSEINZADEH***
*Department of Emergency Medicine*
*Cerkezkoy Community Hospital*
*Tekirdağ, Turkey*

**Demystifying COVID-19: Understanding the Disease, Its Diagnosis and Treatment**

Authors: Ozgur KARCIOGLU, Selman YENIOCAK & Mandana HOSSEINZADEH

ISBN (Online): 978-1-68108-778-8

ISBN (Print): 978-1-68108-779-5

ISBN (Paperback): 978-1-68108-780-1

**Bentham Science Publishers Ltd.**
Executive Suite Y - 2
PO Box 7917, Saif Zone
Sharjah, U.A.E.
Email: subscriptions@benthamscience.net

BENTHAM SCIENCE

# CONTENTS

# PREFACE

For nearly a year, our lives have changed like never before. After attacking Iran and Italy, the center of the pandemic that started in China moved to Europe and the Americas. This pandemic, which healthcare professionals and other organizations all over the world have tried to overcome, will be on our agenda in the coming months and maybe years.

In order to overcome the pandemic with minimal losses, the scientific community, healthcare facilities, professional organizations, chambers, and state institutions should work in coordination and unison. The healthcare system of some countries has passed the exam since the beginning of the epidemic and has tried to do its best to mitigate the catastrophe in a very efficient organization with all medical branches, nurses, and adjunctive health services.

Herein, we have written a book to provide scientific support to these efforts as a whole, to help the public, our patients, and their relatives, and to shed light on future strategies in this manner. In this book, we tried to explain many basic points from case examples to the main principles we follow in diagnosis and treatment, real scenarios in the course of the disease, issues that need attention in specific groups, i.e., those with comorbidities, the elderly, newborns, children, and pregnant women. The spread of the disease in the world and its future predictions also found a place. We also welcome your criticism.

We should all realize that COVID-19 is not the last pandemic. It is obvious that there will be new generations and our long years to spend with masks, sanitizers, and hand disinfectants. It is important in the long run to encourage selective admissions to health institutions and not let the hospitals be overwhelmed by the disastrous situation.

The education of pre-school and school children and women plays a key role in increasing family awareness. Concretizing the virus infection, which is an abstract danger, at a level that will change the lives of people will require serious pedagogical effort and organizational skills. Non-governmental organizations should try to plan in the long term in cooperation with the government and professional chambers.

Our wish is that this book will help both our patients and their relatives, as well as healthcare professionals, who sustain health with their efforts day and night.

Wishing a healthy society and a healthy global future.

## CONSENT FOR PUBLICATION

Not applicable.

## CONFLICT OF INTEREST

The author declares no conflict of interest, financial or otherwise.

## ACKNOWLEDGEMENTS

Declared none.

**Ozgur KARCIOGLU**
Department of Emergency Medicine
University of Health Sciences
Istanbul Education and Research Hospital
Fatih, Istanbul
Turkey
okarcioglu@gmail.coms

# CHAPTER 1

# Contagion of the Pandemics: The Situation in the World

**Abstract:** There are nearly 30 million confirmed cases of COVID-19 in almost all countries and regions worldwide, and more than 900,000 deaths as of September 2020. Almost all of the cases are over 30 years old, and deaths are mostly over 50 years old. The rate of fatality varies greatly by population and geography. Males are represented slightly more than females in confirmed patients in many series, but male predominance is more remarkable in deaths. While there is an increasing trend in deaths since the beginning of March, there is a plateau and a slight downslope after mid-April.

Provided with the progress of the disease in the world, it is seen that the number of cases continues to rise and break records, but deaths do not increase in the same way. Although many countries have a drive for a premature 'normalization', an immature decision of normalization has caused a surge of newly diagnosed cases and deaths in many countries.

**Keywords:** ACE2 receptors, COVID-19, Epidemic, Growth factor, Normalization, Outbreak, Pandemic, SARS-CoV-2.

The final scene in 2011 thriller "Contagion" depicts the imaginary "MEV-1" virus sourced from a pig that ingested a banana dropped by an infected bat. The animal was fleeing from its palm tree destroyed in the China jungle. The pig is then cooked by a chef who shakes unwashed hands with Gwyneth Paltrow, thus transmitting the virus to her. From now on, she is the "index case," to spread the disease to other people (Fig. **1**).

**Ozgur KARCIOGLU, Selman YENIOCAK and Mandana HOSSEINZADEH**

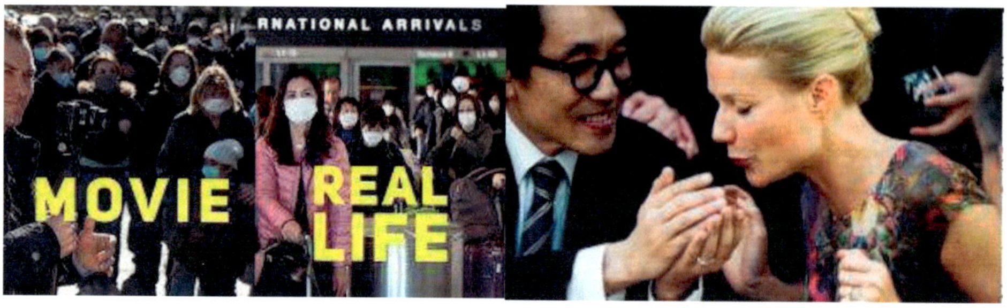


**Fig. (1).** 2011 movie "Contagion" appears to foresee the pandemics in 2020.

The most common disease of humanity in the world is upper respiratory tract infections (URTI). Among them, the majority are precipitated by viruses. Coronavirus family (CoV) is one of the viruses that have caused viral URTI complaints and symptoms for decades. 'Coronavirus disease' (COVID-19), on the other hand, is triggered by one of the sub-strains known as the beta-CoV group and has caused damage and deaths primarily in the Far East since December 2019, and then almost all over the world.

The Spanish flu killed three times more people than WW1 in 1918-1920 pandemics (Fig. **2**).

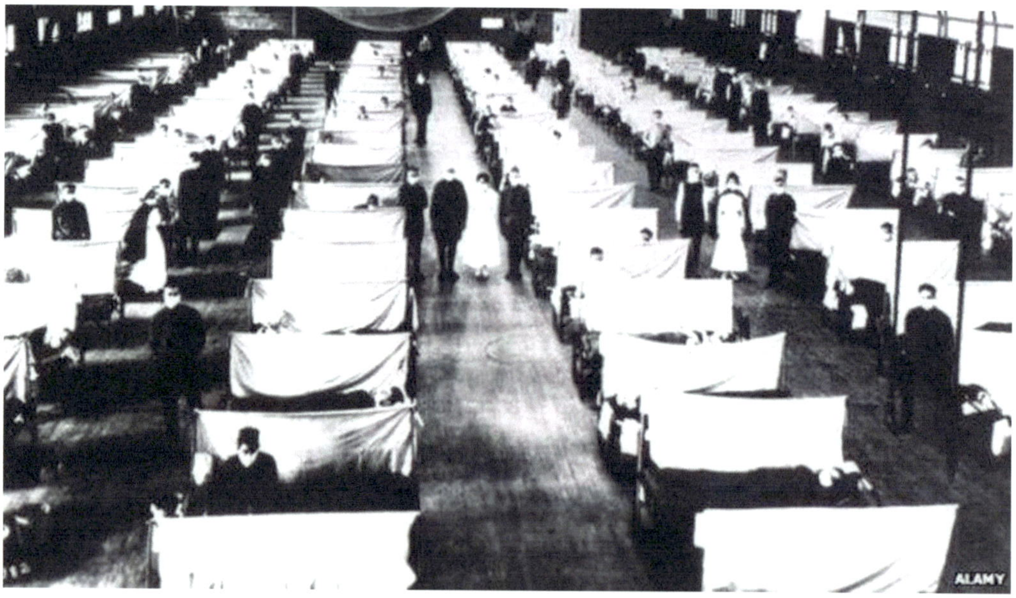


**Fig. (2).** The picture demonstrates a public building that was turned into a hospital to cope with the enormous patient load in the era of The Spanish flu.

**Terminology:** "Fatality" is the ratio of deaths in all patients confirmed to have the disease, while "mortality" is the rate of death among patients whose files have been closed (recovered or died). For example, "COVID-19 fatality approached 6.5% in April 2020, whilst the mortality rate was around 18%".

**Pearl: The most important distinguishing feature of COVID-19 is its ease of spread from person to person, along with its virulance virulence and fatality rate. Since March 2020, COVID-19 has caused more damage and death than SARS and MERS diseases combined (Table 1).**

**Table 1. Comparison of the characteristics of large-scale epidemics and pandemics in different time periods around the world.**

| Year | Region | Disease | Case Fatality Rate |
|---|---|---|---|
| **1918–20** | Almost all the world | Influenza pandemics, 'Spanish flu' | 0.2%-0.5% |
| **1984** | Africa-Macaque monkeys; then almost all the world | HIV-AIDS | 3.9% (person/year) (Lau, 2012) |
| **2002 – 2003** | Civet cats or raccoon dogs; Far East | Severe Acute Respiratory Syndrome (SARS) | **10%** |
| **2009-10** | Mexico; then almost all the world | H1N1 (Swine flu) | 0.1%-0.2% |
| **Almost every year (1999-2015 in the study by Iuliano, 2018)** | 33 countries with large populations (57% of the world population) and high mortality rate | Seasonal influenza | 0·1 to 6·4 / 100 000 (<65 years of age) 3 to 223/ 100 000 (>65 years of age) |
| **2012** | Saudi Arabia and the Middle East | Middle East Respiratory Syndrome (MERS) | 30%-35% |
| **2019-21** | China; then almost all the world | COVID-19 | 2%-14% (varies by country) |

There are numerous subtypes of influenza A virus, and only a few strains precipitate disease in human beings (Table **2**).

"COVID-19" can affect all mammals, not just humans, but one-to-one transmission between humans and other mammals (*e.g.,* pets) is very rare or nonexistent. According to the data of reputable organizations such as CDC and WHO, there are nearly 30 million confirmed cases in almost all countries and regions in the world, and more than 900,000 deaths have been reported globally as of September 2020. The steady and rapid increase in the number of cases within several months explains that COVID has turned into a pandemic that threatens the whole world.

Since the first months of the pandemic, it was very easy for us to monitor the whole world, thanks to several reliable websites that have provided data flow. Through sites such as Worldometer, ourworldindata, https://gisanddata.maps .arcgis.com/, many detailed variables can be monitored and interpreted on a global scale in almost real-time.

**Table 2. The influenza A virus subtypes that cause disease in humans.**

| |
|---|
| **H1N1:** It caused "Spanish Flu" in 1918 and "swine flu" epidemics in 2009, still inflicting sickness and death around the world. |
| **H2N2:** 'Asian flu' in the 1950s |
| **H3N2:** "Hong Kong flu" in the 1960s |
| **H5N1:** It caused a global influenza pandemic threat in the mid-2000s. Its lethality is high, but its contagiousness is low. |
| **H7N9:** It is a subtype of Influenza A viruses that frequently cause new epidemics in the Far East (2013, 2014, 2016). |
| **H7N7:** Causes diseases with its zoonotic potential. |
| **H1N2:** Causes endemic disease in humans and swine. |

## FATALITY AND MORTALITY DIFFERENCES BETWEEN COUNTRIES

Considering the worldwide data, the fatality rate jumped to 7-8% in the first months of the pandemic in COVID-19 cases. In June and July 2020, this rate has gradually decreased to 4%. However, the mortality rate varies considerably around the world. While there are about 9 to 14% deaths in Sweden, Italy and Spain, France in May-June; two countries of Europe, Belgium and England have reached the highest fatality rate with 14 to 24%. The fatality rate not exceeding 4-5% in Northern and Central Europe (Germany, Norway, Finland, Switzerland, Czechia, Austria) draws attention. On the flip side, Mexico, and South American countries such as Brazil, Peru, Argentina, Chile, and Colombia had a boost in the numbers (both cases and deaths) along with Russia and India between May and August. Interestingly, these developing countries have almost uniformly announced considerably low case fatality rates, mostly between 1% and 3%, which has also sparked suspicions in the rest of the world. This remarkable difference is due to the differences in the organization of health services and the developed social state.

## WHICH COUNTRIES HAVE THE HIGHEST NUMBER OF CASES?

The four countries where the total number of cases are boosted in the last months (May-September 2020) are USA, Brazil, India, and Russia. While most of the cases were found in China and the Far East in the first months of the epidemic; after March 2020, the majority of the cases was shifted to Europe and then USA.

There were 3 M cases at the end of April, 6 M at the end of May, 10 M at the end of June and 25.5 M at the end of August in the world. 74% of total cases are closed / completed cases. 4% of this group of patients (closed cases) died and 96% recovered.

The number of cases, which rapidly increased to 80,000 in the January-March period in China, then suddenly braked and left the championship to other countries. This 'braking' phenomenon also raises questions in regard to reliability of data registries, as it is hard for a country of 1.5 billion of people to halt the pandemics so sharply. As of July, around 1/4 of the cases lived in the USA and only 0.3% of them remained in China.

Distribution of cases across countries changed over time. China's dominance was erased after April 2020 and the figures in European countries and Iran, USA, India, Brazil supervened (Graph **1**).

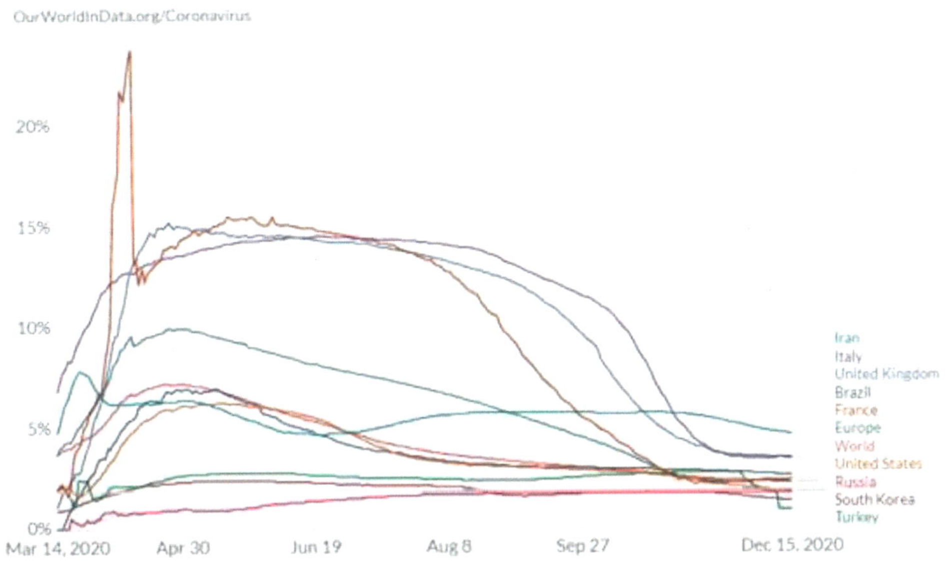


**Graph. (1).** Case fatality rates in December 2020, according to a website accepted among the reliable databases. After the first peak in April and May 2020, numbers of diagnosed cases soared and accordingly, the case fatality rates decreased steadily in most regions. (URL: https://ourworldindata.org/grapher/coronavirus-cfr?cou ntry=ITA~KOR~OWID_WRL~TUR~BRA~Europe~ USA~GBR~RUS~Low%20income~Lower%20middle%20income ~IRN~High%20income~FRA)

Provided with the progress in the world, it is seen that the number of cases continues to rise and break records, but deaths do not increase in the same way. This has highlighted the idea that the virulence or killing power of the virus is somewhat attenuated. As a result, normalization efforts have become evident in Northern European countries, including the USA, where the highest number of cases are found, and partially in the Far East and the Middle East (Graph **2**).

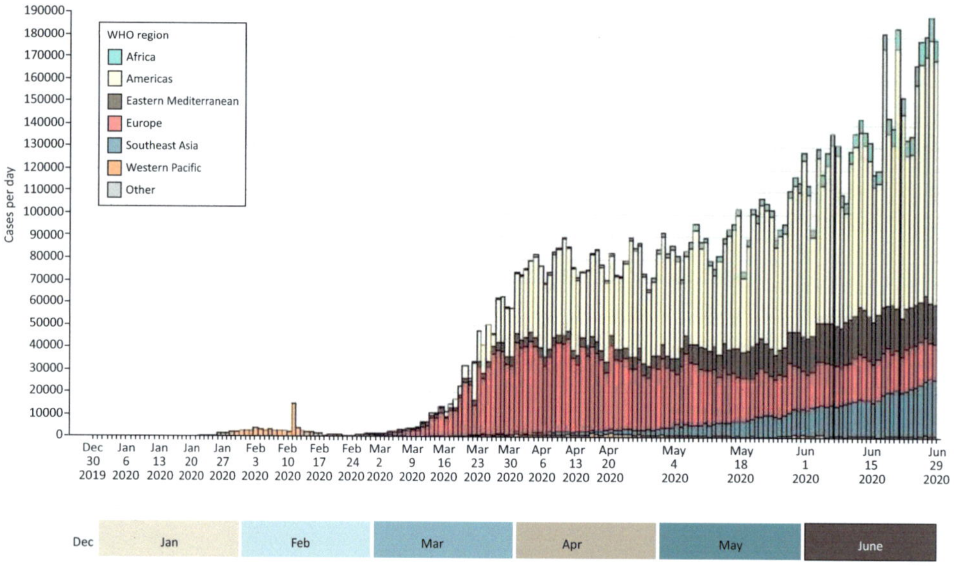


**Graph. (2).** After the announcement of the first case, the shares of continents and regions in the cases changed significantly until June. While America's share increased in the summer months, Europe's share decreased.

**Which factors affect mortality and case fatality rate (CFR)?** The highest death rates in May-July are in England, Belgium, and France, with 14 to 24%. The rate of fatality in the USA was 5%, but in New York, it was 11%.

## TO NORMALIZE OR NOT TO NORMALIZE, IT IS THE MAIN QUESTION!

**Pearl: The most important driving force beneath 'normalization' is that the return of the economy to the 'good old days' is preferred by both the policies in power (*i.e.*, government) and the majority of the people to the continuation of strict measures.**

Strict measures are mostly unwanted because of socioeconomic requirements to make a living and raising the quality of life for the labor and middle classes, white and blue collar people, especially in the developing countries. The question "*should we die of starvation, not from the corona?*", which a Turkish transportation worker who violated the curfews in May 2020, told the cameras is the crystallized form of this situation.

1. **The number of tests performed and its rate in the population:** If tests are performed in a widespread fashion; younger, healthier, asymptomatic people are also caught, thus the number of cases increases and CFR decreases.
2. **Demographic characteristics:** CFR is expected to decrease in countries with a younger population.
3. **Characteristics of the health system:** CFR may increase if there is an overcapacity in hospitals. Deaths can also be high in systems that do not have the habit of responding to such emergency situations (*e.g.,* some European countries).
4. **Additional factors** such as climate characteristics, war, and famine, which break the country's socioeconomic resistance during the pandemic, may affect CFR.

Iran, which is one of the countries that resembles Turkey the most socioculturally, has encountered a rapidly increasing number of cases and deaths in recent months after the rapid normalization efforts. Iran may be the country closest to the "second wave" term, which is always used incorrectly (). However, it cannot be claimed that the first wave is over in any country with many cases in the world. New Zealand and Thailand are probably the countries which deserves to use the term correctly for themselves.

Number of deaths recorded for each day in the world disclosed an increasing trend in deaths since the beginning of March, there is a plateau and a slightly downslope after mid-April. The stable fluctuating trend is stabilized in summer, while an ascent is notable in October and November.

The "growth factor" of the epidemic: When China is excluded, it is seen that the "growth factor" of the epidemic has changed favorably, from large fluctuations in February to small oscillations as of the end of March through July 2020.

Number of tests applied on the suspected cases or with screening purposes also affect the number of cases detected

## Situation in Turkey

Mainly from the second week of March in Istanbul Turkey PCR (+) cases were reported. It is thought that both the road entrances from Iran, which has a wide border with the eastern cities of Turkey, and the arrivals to Istanbul and Izmir from European countries such as Italy. Increasing number of cases were observed in the first weeks after March 11, when the first case was announced. While fatality rates and the number of new cases is expected to decrease with compliance with the isolation and physical distance rules, there was an upward trend in the end of summer and autumn months.

The PCR tests were made available in the mid-March which was associated with a rapid rise in the numbers. After efforts towards an early 'normalization' in the summer, both daily new cases and the death toll escalated in the fall.

## *Age-Related Data*

Most of the confirmed cases are over 50 years old, and the mean age is mostly between 49-56 in most series from different regions. In some patient series in China, the average age was reported to be 50 and the proportion of women was higher (Qian J, 2020, Qian GQ, 2020). In a large South Korean study, the majority of the cases (62.7%) were female, while 60% of the deaths were male (Shim, 2020). Cases over the age of 80 constitute 2.7% of the whole sample and 23.8% of deaths.

Mean age of COVID cases is 40 in S. Korea, 54 in Iran, and 64 in Italy, due to differences in the population structure of countries and health systems. Only 12% of those admitted to the ICU in Italy are under the age of 50 (Table **3**). (WHO, 3 May 2020). A significant increase in death rate is noted with the advancing age.

**Table 3. Distribution of cases and deaths recorded by the CDC in the USA by age groups as of the end of June 2020. While significant number of patients are detected among the young adults, mortality rates appear to boost with age especially after sixties (Wiersinga, 2020).**

| Age | Number of Cases | Number of Deaths | Rate of Deaths per 1000 Cases |
|---|---|---|---|
| **<18** | 116.176 | 50 | 0.4b |
| **18-29** | 339.125 | 385 | 1.1 |
| **30-39** | 328.249 | 1137 | 3.5 |
| **40-49** | 325.190 | 2804 | 8.6 |
| **50-64** | 482.338 | 14.316 | 29.7 |
| **65-74** | 185.942 | 19.520 | 105.0 |
| **75-84** | 116.937 | 24.621 | 210.5 |
| **≥85** | 98382 | 29999 | 304.9 |

38% of the COVID-19 cases hospitalized in the USA are between the ages of 20 and 54. On the other hand, data regarding patients being followed up in ICU is as follows:

- 12% of them are 20-44 years old,
- 36% is between the ages of 45-64.

Less than 1% of hospitalized COVID-19 cases are children and adolescents aged 18 and under.

The median age of the deceased is significantly higher than the survivors

Comparison of those diagnosed and died in Italy until April revealed that the median age of diagnosed cases is 62, while the median of those who died is 80. (Palmieri L,*et al.*, 2020, Istituto Superiore Sanità, 2020, Lippi, 2020).

**Relationship of Age Groups and Gender**

Distributions by age groups of those diagnosed and those who died in Italy until April were studied. Since the 60's, both diagnosis and deaths increase significantly, while there is generally a male predominance, the weight of women stands out in diagnosis and death after the age of 90.

**Headlines for a Summary**

- Almost all of the cases are over 30 years old and deaths are mostly over 50 years old.
- The rate of fatality varies greatly by population and geography. It is around 8% between the ages of 70-79 and 15% between the ages of 80-89.
- 87% of the patients are between the ages of 30 and 79.
- 80% of deaths are over 65 years old.
- The percentage of males in confirmed patients is between 50-60% in different series (Li LQ, 2020 ), but male predominance is more remarkable in deaths.
- The mortality rate among confirmed cases in males was 4.7% for males and 2.8% for females. In S. Korea, it has been revealed that the crude death rate is 1.1% for men, 0.4% for women, and the male mortality rate increases with age. (Shim, 2020 ).
- Being over the age of 65 is a leading risk factor for both death and development of ARDS (Wu, JAMA, 2020 ).

The epidemic curves in Wuhan City also followed different curves in accord with the onset of symptoms or by the dates of diagnoses (Fig. **3**).

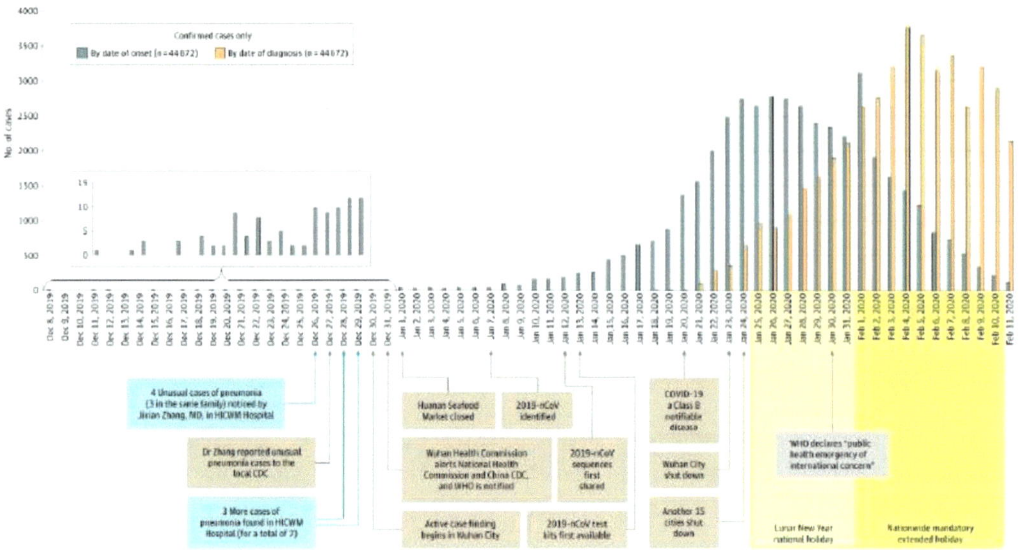


**Fig. (3).** Epidemic Curve of the Confirmed Cases of Coronavirus Disease 2019 (COVID-19). Daily numbers of confirmed cases are plotted by date of onset of symptoms (blue) and by date of diagnosis (orange). Because, on retrospective investigation, so few cases experienced illness in December, these cases are shown in the inset. The difference between the cases by date of symptom onset curve (blue) and the cases by date of diagnosis curve (orange) illustrates lag time between the start of illness and diagnosis of COVID-19 by viral nucleic acid testing. The graph's x-axis (dates from December 8, 2019, to February 11, 2020) is also used as a timeline of major milestones in the epidemic response. The first few cases of pneumonia of unknown etiology are shown in blue boxes on December 26 (n = 4) and 28-29 (n = 3). (Adapted from Wu, JAMA, 2020).

## CONTAGIOUSNESS OF CORONAVIRUS

In various studies, the infectious power of COVID-19 or the "new case production rate" has been calculated to be between 2 and 3, on average around 2.3 (Imai *et al.*, 2020), (Kucharski *et al.*, 2020) (Wu JT, 2020; Leung, 2020).

## IN WHAT WAYS IS CORONAVIRUS TRANSMITTED?

Since coronaviruses are very small, they can spread between individuals by hanging in the air for up to 3 hours through droplets containing viruses *via* sneezing and coughing. This is the most important point in the transformation of CoVID-19 into an epidemic. In addition, it can also be important that people who touch surfaces or things touched by patients afterwards bring their hands to their face and eyes, handshake with other people,*etc*. Close contact from 1.8-2 meters (6 feet) is usually required for the virus to be transmitted from person to person. However, in new publications, this distance can be up to 4.5 meters especially if one sneezes or coughs. Also, fecal-oral transmission has been reported in some cases.

Contagiousness is in question 2 to 3 days before the symptom onset. Asymptomatic / presymptomatic people can also transmit the disease. It has been reported that transmission from presymptomatic patients is proved up to 48% to 62% of the cases (Ganyani, 2020).

## Where is The Contamination Happening?

It is known that most of the transmission occur by sneezing and/or coughing or close contact of sick individuals in the community. On the other hand, a study on patients hospitalized with COVID-19 pneumonia in China revealed that a significant 41% of the infections are in-hospital (nosocomial) contamination (Wang, 2020). In this series, one out of every four cases were admitted to the ICU and the mortality was 4.3%.

## Is It Airborne?

Both yes and no. It is known that the virus, is transmitted by procedures such as intubation and bronchoscopy, which cause overt contagion of the virus into the air, which is called 'aerosolization'. However, only a small number of cases have been shown to be contaminated with particles suspended in the air through breathing. It is known that the virus can remain viable in the air for around 3 hours. For this reason, it should not be forgotten that even two people having a conversation at close range for more than a few minutes in closed, poorly ventilated environments may allow disease transmission.

## Air Conditioning + 1 Patient = 10 Patients: Who is Guilty?

Although the main mode of transmission is *via* droplets from the airways of the patients some other ways are in question for spreading COVID-19. Here, we present a case scenario of spreading the disease with a suspected interference of air conditioning in a closed space. This contamination in the restaurant caused 10 people to be inflicted with COVID-19. The key factor is the path and direction of the airflow.

Regular cleaning and disinfection of air conditioners is vital since both SARS-Cov and Legionella bacteria can colonize and grow in the humid environment inside the air conditioners.

**Case study:** Family A travelled from Wuhan to Guangzhou on January 23, 2020 and had dinner at the restaurant on January 24. We wanted to examine the history that resulted in the illness of 10 people from three families in the form of filing or contact follow-up.

'Restaurant X' (RX) is a class A facility located in a luxurious 5-storey building with air conditioning in central Guangzhou. Each floor has separate air conditioning without any windows. The dining hall on the 3rd floor is 145 m2 and the distance between the tables is around 1 meter. The 53 minutes of the time that families A and B spent there, and 73 minutes of A and C coincide. There is an air conditioner on the table of the C family that takes the ambient air from inside to outside and gives the cold air inside (Fig. **4**).

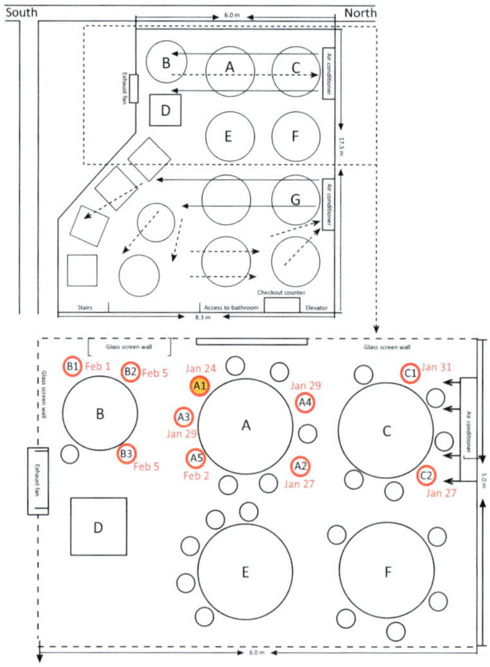


**Fig. (4).** Diagram showing the seating arrangement of the tables and people subject to the COVID-19 spread from the air conditioner in the restaurant in Guangzhou. All the people in the red circle have the disease. The painted in yellow is the case that we call "index-case" and allows other people to be found by contact follow-up because it is diagnosed in the hospital (Lu, 2020).

On January 24, 2020, RX had 83 customers and 8 employees. 10 out of 83 customers caught COVID-19. Seventy-three people were quarantined for 14 days. PCR results from these people and the swabs taken from the air conditioners were negative.

After all, since air conditioners turned out to be negative, the most likely route of spread is the droplets from the airways of the infected person, even asymptomatic. In other words, although the A1 index case is asymptomatic, it has spread the virus with air conditioning. All three members of family B were directly infected through A1. However, there is a small possibility that B2 and B3 are infected through B1. Two members of the C family were directly infected with B1. Again, a small possibility may have been infected while C1 was caring for C2 after January 27th. The patients' clinical and laboratory characteristics were summarized in Table **4A** and **4B**.

**Table 4A. Clinical characteristics of the family clusters infected with COVID-19 (Adapted from Lu, 2020).**

| Variable | Family A | | | | | Family B | | | Family C | |
|---|---|---|---|---|---|---|---|---|---|---|
| Relationship | Patient A1 (Index case) | Patient A2 | Patient A3 | Patient A4 | Patient A5 | Patient B1 | Patient B2 | Patient B3 | Patient C1 | Patient C2 |
| Age (years) | 63 | 60 | 62 | 34 | 63 | 44 | 20 | 53 | 54 | 82 |
| Sex | Female | Female | Female | Female | Male | Female | Female | Male | Female | Female |
| Occupation | Retiree | Retiree | Retiree | Staff | Retiree | Cook | Student | self-em-ployed | Civil servant | Retiree |
| Chronic medical illness | Hyper-tension, hyper-lipidemia | None | None | None | Hypertension | None | None | None | None | None |
| interval between admission to hospital and symptom onset (days) | 1 | 0 | 0 | 0 | 0 | 3 | 3 | 1 | 1 | 9 |
| **Presenting Symptoms and Signs** | | | | | | | | | | |
| Time of onset | Jan. 24 | Jan. 27 | Jan. 29 | Jan. 29 | Feb. 2 | Feb. 1 | Feb. 3 | Feb. 5 | Jan. 31 | Jan. 27 |
| Fever | + | + | + | + | + | + | + | - | + | + |
| Cough | + | - | - | - | - | + | + | - | + | - |
| Running nose | - | - | - | - | - | - | - | - | - | + |
| Polypnea | - | - | - | - | - | - | + | + | - | - |
| Head pain | - | - | - | - | - | - | - | + | - | - |
| Chest pain | - | - | - | - | - | - | - | + | - | - |
| Diarrhea | - | - | - | - | - | - | + | - | - | - |

We know that large droplets (> 5 micrometers, mm) stay in the air for a very short time and fall to the ground. In the RX, the strong air stream may have moved the droplets from all tables to each other. Particles below 5 mcm can be easily transported to distances more than 1 m and can be suspended in the air for hours (Fernstrom, 2013). Such contaminations have also been reported in SARS and MERS (Lee 2013, Kim 2016).

Interestingly, none of the staff or other customers have been infected. This situation is atypical for aerosol transmission. Still, it suggests that the droplets follow the path of the air stream and cannot travel to distant tables.

**Table 4B. Laboratory characteristics of the family clusters infected with COVID-19 (Adapted from Lu, 2020).**

| Variable | Family A | | | | | Family B | | | Family C | |
|---|---|---|---|---|---|---|---|---|---|---|
| Body temperature (°C) | 37.80 | 37.80 | 37.30 | 37.70 | 37.80 | 38.40 | 38.60 | - | 39.90 | 37.8 |
| leukocyte count (×109 cells per L) | 4.08 | 4.79 | 4.76 | 5.19 | 6.51 | 3.52 | 6.39 | 6.53 | 5.40 | 4.7 |
| Lymphocyte count (×109 cells per L) | 0.93 | 1.05 | 1.77 | 1.28 | 2,74 | 1.13 | 1.36 | 1.96 | 1.49 | 0.7 |
| Lymphocyte% | 33.10 | 21.90 | 37.20 | 24.70 | 42.10 | 32.10 | 21.30 | 3.88 | 27.60 | 15.50 |
| Neutrophil count (×109 cells per L) | 1.60 | 3.34 | 2.58 | 2.92 | 2.80 | 2.09 | 4.02 | 30.00 | 3.64 | 3.6 |
| Neutrophil % | 56.9 | 69.80 | 54.40 | 56.20 | 43.00 | 59.40 | 62.90 | 59.40 | 67.40 | 74.90 |

In brief, this contamination in the restaurant caused 10 people to be inflicted with COVID-19 due to air conditioning. The key factor is the path and direction of the airflow. Our recommendation is to scan clients of restaurants by measuring temperature, increase the distance between tables and improve ventilation inside.

## How is The Air Conditioner Cleaned?

Regular cleaning and disinfection of air conditioners is vital since both SARS-Cov and Legionella bacteria can colonize and grow in the humid environment inside the air conditioners. You can call the manufacturer's service for the cleaning of your air conditioner. Or you can do this in a practical way yourself.

## How Should We Clean Our Air Conditioner?

- Open the cover of your air conditioner.
- Carefully unscrew the filter and wash it with clean, cold water without using chemical agents.
- Let the filter dry in the sun or in a suitable environment.
- While the filter is drying, gently sweep the inside of the air conditioner by attaching the brush attachment to the vacuum cleaner, set at medium intensity.
- Replace the dried filter properly.

## CONCLUSION

The steady and rapid increase in the number of cases within several months explains that COVID-19 has turned into a pandemic that threatens the whole world. The disease was viewed as a 'Chinese plague' initially in December 2019 and January 2020, but after March 2020, the center of the pandemic has shifted to Europe and America. It is remarkable that the number of cases continues to rise and break records, but deaths do not increase in the same way. Therefore, many governments pushed for a premature 'normalization' that is preferred by both the policies in power (*i.e.*, government) and the majority of the people to the continuation of strict measures. However, an immature decision of normalization has caused a surge of both *de novo* cases and death in many parts of the world. A rational and scientific basis of these measures and critical decisions will prevent both new surges of the disease and also future pandemics.

## REFERENCES

Fernstrom, A & Goldblatt, M (2013) Aerobiology and its role in the transmission of infectious diseases. *J Pathogens,* 2013, 493960.
[http://dx.doi.org/10.1155/2013/493960] [PMID: 23365758]

Ganyani, T, Kremer, C & Chen, D (2020) Estimating the generation interval for coronavirus disease (COVID-19) based on symptom onset data. *Euro Surveill,* 25

https://gisanddata.maps.arcgis.com/apps/opsdashboard/index.html#/bda7594740fd40299423467b48e9ecf6

Imai, N, Gaythorpe, KAM, Abbott, S, Bhatia, S, van Elsland, S, Prem, K, Liu, Y & Ferguson, NM (2020) Adoption and impact of non-pharmaceutical interventions for COVID-19. *Wellcome Open Res,* 5, 59.
[http://dx.doi.org/10.12688/wellcomeopenres.15808.1] [PMID: 32529040]

Istituto Superiore di Sanità (2020) *Characteristics of COVID-19 patients dying in Italy Report based on available data on.*https://www.epicentro.iss.it/coronavirus/

Iuliano, AD, Roguski, KM, Chang, HH, Muscatello, DJ, Palekar, R, Tempia, S, Cohen, C, Gran, JM, Schanzer, D, Cowling, BJ, Wu, P, Kyncl, J, Ang, LW, Park, M, Redlberger-Fritz, M, Yu, H, Espenhain, L, Krishnan, A, Emukule, G, van Asten, L, Pereira da Silva, S, Aungkulanon, S, Buchholz, U, Widdowson, MA & Bresee, JS Global Seasonal Influenza-associated Mortality Collaborator Network (2018) Estimates of global seasonal influenza-associated respiratory mortality: a modelling study. *Lancet,* 391, 1285-300.
[http://dx.doi.org/10.1016/S0140-6736(17)33293-2] [PMID: 29248255]

Kim, SH, Chang, SY, Sung, M, Park, JH, Bin Kim, H, Lee, H, Choi, JP, Choi, WS & Min, JY (2016) Extensive viable Middle East respiratory syndrome (MERS) coronavirus contamination in air and surrounding environment in MERS isolation wards. *Clin Infect Dis,* 63, 363-9.
[http://dx.doi.org/10.1093/cid/ciw239] [PMID: 27090992]

Kucharski, AJ, Russell, TW, Diamond, C, Liu, Y, Edmunds, J, Funk, S & Eggo, RM Centre for Mathematical Modelling of Infectious Diseases COVID-19 working group (2020) Early dynamics of transmission and control of COVID-19: a mathematical modelling study. *Lancet Infect Dis,* 20, 553-8. [published correction appears in Lancet Infect Dis. 2020 Mar 25;].
[http://dx.doi.org/10.1016/S1473-3099(20)30144-4] [PMID: 32171059]

Lee, N, Hui, D, Wu, A, Chan, P, Cameron, P, Joynt, GM, Ahuja, A, Yung, MY, Leung, CB, To, KF, Lui, SF, Szeto, CC, Chung, S & Sung, JJ (2003) A major outbreak of severe acute respiratory syndrome in Hong Kong. *N Engl J Med,* 348, 1986-94.
[http://dx.doi.org/10.1056/NEJMoa030685] [PMID: 12682352]

Leung, C (2020) Clinical features of deaths in the novel coronavirus epidemic in China. *Rev Med Virol,* 30, e2103.
[http://dx.doi.org/10.1002/rmv.2103] [PMID: 32175637]

Li, LQ, Huang, T, Wang, YQ, Wang, ZP, Liang, Y, Huang, TB, Zhang, HY, Sun, W & Wang, Y (2020) COVID-19 patients' clinical characteristics, discharge rate, and fatality rate of meta-analysis. *J Med Virol,* 92, 577-83.

[http://dx.doi.org/10.1002/jmv.25757] [PMID: 32162702]

Lippi, G, Mattiuzzi, C, Sanchis-Gomar, F & Henry, BM (2020) Clinical and demographic characteristics of patients dying from COVID-19 in Italy *vs* China. *J Med Virol,* 92, 1759-60.
[http://dx.doi.org/10.1002/jmv.25860] [PMID: 32275075]

Lu, J, Gu, J, Li, K, Xu, C, Su, W, Lai, Z, Zhou, D, Yu, C, Xu, B & Yang, Z (2020) COVID-19 Outbreak Associated with Air Conditioning in Restaurant, Guangzhou, China, 2020. *Emerg Infect Dis,* 26, 1628-31.
[http://dx.doi.org/10.3201/eid2607.200764] [PMID: 32240078]

Palmieri, L, Vanacore, N, Donfrancesco, C, Lo Noce, C, Canevelli, M, Punzo, O, Raparelli, V, Pezzotti, P, Riccardo, F, Bella, A, Fabiani, M, D'Ancona, FP, Vaianella, L, Tiple, D, Colaizzo, E, Palmer, K, Rezza, G, Piccioli, A, Brusaferro, S & Onder, G Italian National Institute of Health COVID-19 Mortality Group (2020) Clinical characteristics of hospitalized individuals dying with covid-19 by age group in italy. *J Gerontol A Biol Sci Med Sci,* 75, 1796-800.
[http://dx.doi.org/10.1093/gerona/glaa146] [PMID: 32506122]

Qian, GQ, Yang, NB, Ding, F, Ma, AHY, Wang, ZY, Shen, YF, Shi, CW, Lian, X, Chu, JG, Chen, L, Wang, ZY, Ren, DW, Li, GX, Chen, XQ, Shen, HJ & Chen, XM (2020) Epidemiologic and clinical characteristics of 91 hospitalized patients with COVID-19 in Zhejiang, China: a retrospective, multi-centre case series. *QJM,* 113, 474-81.
[http://dx.doi.org/10.1093/qjmed/hcaa089] [PMID: 32181807]

Qian, J, Zhao, L, Ye, RZ, Li, XJ & Liu, YL (2020) Age-dependent gender differences of COVID-19 in mainland China: comparative study. *Clin Infect Dis* [published online ahead of print, 2020 May 30].

Shim, E, Mizumoto, K, Choi, W & Chowell, G (2020) Estimating the risk of covid-19 death during the course of the outbreak in korea, february-may 2020. *J Clin Med,* 9, 1641.
[http://dx.doi.org/10.3390/jcm9061641] [PMID: 32485871]

Wang, D, Hu, B, Hu, C, Zhu, F, Liu, X, Zhang, J, Wang, B, Xiang, H, Cheng, Z, Xiong, Y, Zhao, Y, Li, Y, Wang, X & Peng, Z (2020) Clinical characteristics of 138 hospitalized patients with 2019 novel coronavirus-infected pneumonia in wuhan, china. *JAMA,* 323, 1061-9. [published online ahead of print, 2020 Feb 7].
[http://dx.doi.org/10.1001/jama.2020.1585] [PMID: 32031570]

Wiersinga, WJ, Rhodes, A, Cheng, AC, Peacock, SJ & Prescott, HC (2020) Pathophysiology, transmission, diagnosis, and treatment of coronavirus disease 2019 (covid-19): a review. *JAMA,* 324, 782-93.
[http://dx.doi.org/10.1001/jama.2020.12839] [PMID: 32648899]

Wu, JT, Leung, K, Bushman, M, Kishore, N, Niehus, R, de Salazar, PM, Cowling, BJ, Lipsitch, M & Leung, GM (2020) Estimating clinical severity of COVID-19 from the transmission dynamics in Wuhan, China. *Nat Med,* 26, 506-10. [published correction appears in Nat Med. 2020 Jul;26(7):1149-1150].
[http://dx.doi.org/10.1038/s41591-020-0822-7] [PMID: 32284616]

Wu, Z & McGoogan, JM (2020) Characteristics of and important lessons from the coronavirus disease 2019 (covid-19) outbreak in china: summary of a report of 72 314 cases from the chinese center for disease control and prevention. *JAMA,* 323, 1239-42.
[http://dx.doi.org/10.1001/jama.2020.2648] [PMID: 32091533]

# CHAPTER 2

# How Can a Country Defeat COVID-19? Value of R0, Rt and Re

**Abstract:** Eradication of a disease is a very difficult and multi-factorial, multi-faceted question. The prevalence of COVID-19 in the regions around the country, the intensity of the population's relationship with other countries, age distribution, and other demographic factors affect the magnitude of the impact of the disease on a population. In addition, the virulence of the virus, the immunity level of the population, measures taken for immunization, availability of necessary drugs, the capacity of the health sector to mitigate the pandemic will affect the damage on the society as a whole. The tests applied to identify the cases, filing, and surveillance are effective factors in the response of the state's health organization to this disease.

**Keywords:** COVID-19, Growth factor, Outbreak, Pandemic, Re, Ro, Rt, Surveillance, Virulence.

Eradication of disease in such a large population is a very difficult multi-factorial and multi-faceted question. The prevalence of COVID-19 in the regions around the country, the intensity of the population's relationship with other countries (with commerce, tourism, *etc.*), age, and other demographic factors affect the magnitude of the impact of the disease on a population. For example, the rapid increase in the number of cases in February and March in Iran and Italy is considered to affect the number of cases in Turkey at the end of March. However , this is not the only factor. Many factors such as the virulence of the virus, the immunity level of the population in general, organization of immunization efforts, and ability to minimize the damage through drugs, the capacity of the health sector to mitigate the tsunami of patients will definitely impact how much the community is damaged by the disease. The tests applied to identify the cases, filing, and surveillance are effective factors in the response of the state's health organization to this disease (Table **1**).

All these concepts are collected in the term of surveillance. Surveillance is the process of timely and systematic collection and processing of data and the evaluation of the findings obtained to provide rapid feedback to the units in need. Technological advances, the magnitude of the population, and the disease itself

**Ozgur KARCIOGLU, Selman YENIOCAK and Mandana HOSSEINZADEH**

will directly affect the success of these efforts. For example, Taiwan, South Korea, Israel, and New Zealand achieved great jobs in this manner, with their smaller populations and technologically advanced industries.

**Table 1. Factors affecting the country's struggle to overcome the pandemic are listed below**

| |
|---|
| **1. Virulence:** The degree of damage caused by a microbe to the host **tissues** or the severity of the disease it inflicts. Virulence may also be defined as the measurable value of the agent's ability to cause disease. The **pathogenicity** of an organism – which is defined as the ability to cause disease - is determined by its virulence factors. |
| **2. Detection of the cases:** Recognition of the patients by applying tests to people as indicated, including asymptomatic ones in some situations. |
| **3. Isolation:** Isolating diagnosed and suspicious cases from disease-naive people. |
| **4. Filing/Filiation:** In medicine, it refers to the connection of things resulting from one another or contact tracing. To open a file for the case whose diagnosis has been confirmed, to examine the case in detail with all his/her contacts, to monitor their condition by phone or home visits, to ensure that they take their medications, to ensure rapid intervention in the development of complications. Filing is a prerequisite for revealing the contacts described in the next item. |
| **5. Person with a contact:** An individual who has had an epidemiological relationship with an infected person, animal, or environment leading to the possibility of acquiring and spreading that infection. |
| **6. Contact tracing/ follow-up:** Efforts to identify individuals who have somehow contacted diagnosed and suspicious cases, monitor them with certain rules, and provide testing. In this way, contacts can be recognized and become aware of their situation. Asymptomatic contacts are also tested and diagnosed. Those determined to be in contact are either quarantined or isolated themselves. |
| **7. Preventing arrivals from abroad:** Either completely stopping the arrivals to the country by sea, land, and air or allowing them to enter after certain procedures (such as quarantine or testing). |

## WHAT ARE R0, RT, AND RE?

**R0:** "R0" or "R zero" represents the startout time of the infection or epidemics. These numbers are derived from the term "basic reproductive number" which describes the average number of people infected by a single infected person. Therefore, if R0 <1, an epidemic will not occur at all. The number R0 is not a universal absolute number (constant). It will vary from region to region and over time. Screening and quarantine measures directly affect R0 (Table **2**).

**Table 2. Estimated R0 and "herd immunity threshold" (HIT) values for the most common infectious diseases (Adapted from Li 2020, Riou, 2020)**

| Disease | Way of Spread/ Contagiousness | $R_0$ | HIT (%) |
|---|---|---|---|
| Measles | Air/respiratory | 12–18 | 92–95 |
| Diphtheria | Saliva | 6–7 | 83–86 |
| Polio | Fecal-oral | 5–7 | 80–86 |
| Ebola | Bodily fluids | 1.5–2.5 | 33–60 |
| Whooping cough | Air/droplets | 12–17 | 92–94 |
| Rubella | Air/droplets | 6–7 | 83–86 |
| Smallpox | Air/droplets | 5–7 | 80–86 |
| Influenza | Air/droplets | 1.5–1.8 | 33–44 |
| Parotitis (Mumps) | Air/droplets | 4–7 | 75–86 |
| SARS (2002-2003) | Air/droplets | 2–5 | 50–80 |
| COVID-19 | Air/droplets | 1.4–3.9 | 29–74 |

When it comes to change over time, effective numbers, "Re" or "Rt" come to the fore. This means the actual transmission or spreading rate of the virus per time unit. For example, while Rt was above 2 in Wuhan in December 2019 and January 2020, closure and contact tracing decreased to below 1 and around 0.3 in March 2020 and after, with the strict implementation of measures such as quarantine. It is up for debate what will happen to Rt as the restrictions have been removed.

As can be understood from here, Rt allows us to track which effective measures are taken in a country, community, or group and which direction the disease evolves.

Number of tests done in a country directly affects the number of cases diagnoses and isolated, For example, South Korea has achieved great success by performing tests to many people, including asymptomatic ones, from the outbreak of the pandemics, isolation of suspicious cases while monitoring contacts.

## INCUBATION PERIOD

The time until the symptoms and signs appear after the patient is infected with the virus is called the incubation or incubation period. The most important point is that the patient becomes contagious and spreads the disease to the environment during this period. There are publications that give a precise limit of 2-14 days for incubation, but comprehensive publications on COVID-19 have shown that the average duration is 5 days, and complaints and symptoms develop within 11.5 days (Lauer, 2020). For this reason, it is thought that when the quarantine is mandated for 14 days, the findings will almost definitely be seen in suspicious cases.

## PRINCIPLES OF SURVEILLANCE AND STRUGGLE WITH THE PANDEMIC: HOW COUNTRIES DIFFER FROM EACH OTHER?

**Pearl: The most basic mistake that can be made may be the admission of patients and patients whose general condition deteriorated to the hospital and use hospitals to respond to this , in short, "meeting the tsunami of the pandemic in hospitals".**

In fact, it is the very effective conduct of filings and screenings, strict quarantine and isolation practices, and minimization of mass mobility with curfew and similar measures. Of note, not every measure would fit into every country or population. Every country will tailor these measures in accord with its cultural heritage, technological advances, and social relationships. For example, many Far East countries did not undertake curfew or restrictions of human mobility, while Middle East or North African countries referred to such strict measures instead of technological applications such as face recognition. In this context, it is also important to be able to monitor tests and suspicious cases in a transparent and open manner.

## HOW EFFECTIVE IS HOME STAY, SOCIAL / INDIVIDUAL ISOLATION IN PREVENTING THE SPREAD OF COVID-19?

According to the Seattle Disease Modeling Institute, COVID-19 infection is known to double in 6-9 hours when no intervention is done. (IDM Coronavirus InfoHub: URL: https://docs.google.com/document/d/ 1UZ4eyAqaNnmO4kYKF-Z9-HWA0y0wyR30RRAT-_Wxi9c/preview)

An analysis has been made on how isolation affects the number of cases and deaths against virus spread. Accordingly, the total number of cases, which is 100 today, is proportional to the percentages of staying home and the rate of COVID-19 spread within two weeks:

a. 25000 cases and 500 deaths with 0% homestay
b. 5,000 cases and 100 deaths with 25% homestay
c. 2000 cases and 40 deaths with 50% homestay
d. 200 cases and 4 deaths with 75% homestay
e. are expected. In other words,
f. Total case and death rates can be reduced by 99.2% with 75% staying at home,
g. reduced by 92% with 50% staying at home,
h. reduced by 80% with 25% staying home

Fig. (**1**) shows the potential impact of effectivity conferred to measures including social / individual isolation in preventing the upsurge of the number of cases with COVID-19 in a given population.

## BELGIUM HAS A VERY DIFFERENT CASE SITUATION

When two calculations are undertaken with different points of view, Belgium is among the countries with the highest deaths toll. It is both the country with the highest number of deaths compared to the population, and the country with the highest death rate among those who have the disease, which we call the case-fatality rate (CFR). When the reason for these situations is investigated, a very interesting fact emerges: It was seen that more than half of the 10 thousand people who lost their lives in the country with a population of approximately 11 million 500 thousand died in nursing homes. The essential detail is that it is remarkable that the elderly who died in nursing homes with signs and symptoms suggestive of COVID-19 and rapidly deteriorated were recorded as death due to COVID-19, regardless of the availability of test results. The fact that higher mortality rates are recorded in the country where diagnosis and treatment are carried out respecting the clinical and radiological (mostly tomographic) findings, and regardless of the tests, suggests that this is actually the right thing and that other countries underestimate numbers and indirectly, the disease.Relatively high case fatality rate in Belgium stems from differing methods of data recording.

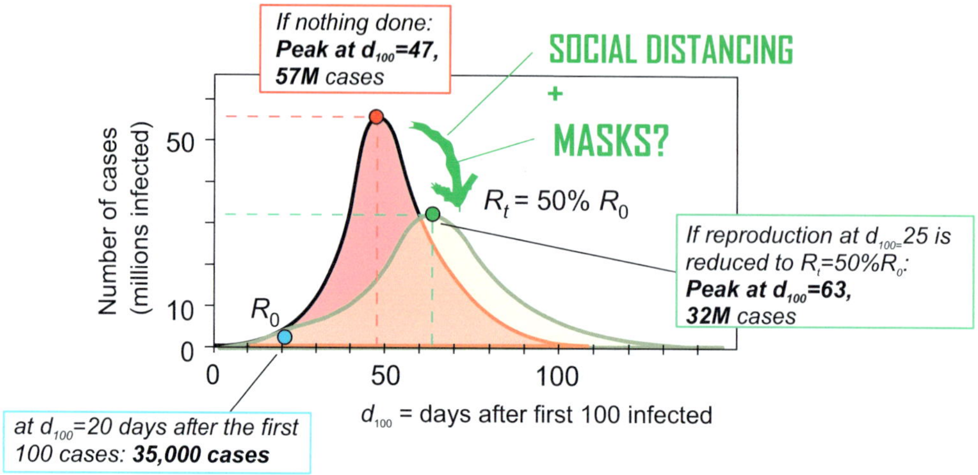


**Fig. (1).** With the strict use of personal protective equipment and the implementation of individual isolation / curfew, the spread of the pandemics will take place over a longer time and sudden loads on the health system can be tolerated over time.

Increases in case numbers, Rt values may differ substantially between countries and even among regions within a country, depending on the practical implications of the measures, geographical and cultural variations, *etc.*

Change in the number of cases within days in 7 countries revelas that although data security is questioned in China, which has taken strict measures, the number of cases has entered a horizontal trend. However, the upward trend continues in countries such as Germany, Spain, and Italy. The steep rise is worrying in the USA, which was too late to take action and is in disputes within the country.

When we combine different scenarios related to the epidemic, it can be seen that all of them predicted it could be eradicated in the end of 2021 at the earliest (Fig. **2**).

COVID-19 also offered a great opportunity to observe the impact of processes in controlling the epidemic; for example, 'lock-down': Fig. (**3**) gives a rough estimate of the short and long-term potential effects of lock-down.

Peak levels can be seen a few weeks after the total closure, which means that the highest level of precautions can be taken. If the precautions are continued in the strictest way possible after the peak level is seen and the cases start to decrease, the pandemic can be mitigated, and numbers are minimized.

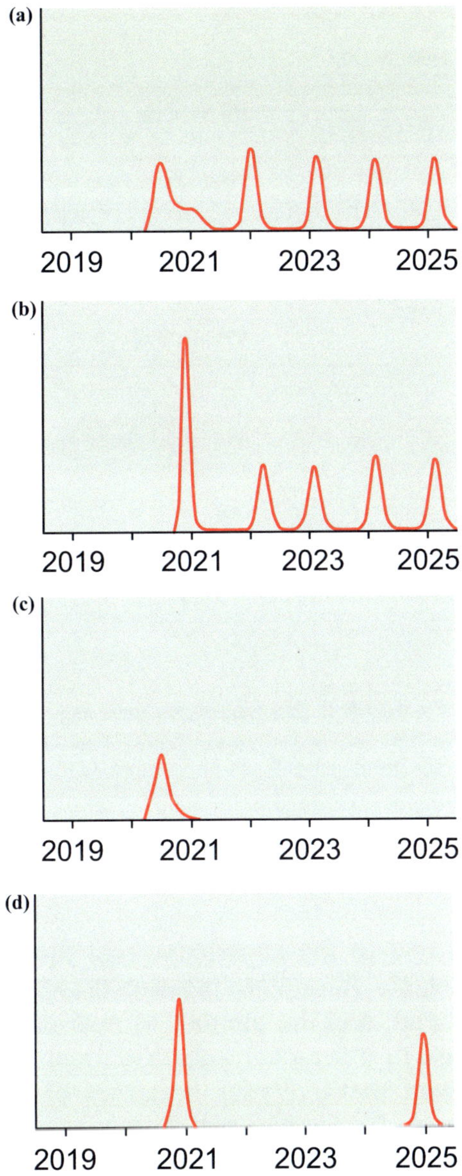


**Fig. (2).** Similar to the swine flu experience in 2009, it is a realistic forecast that it continues with seasonal "small" peaks in the next years (a), with the largest peak in 2020 (scenario b). Scenario c is the most optimistic scenario, which is hard to see come true. Scenario d estimates it will become negligible for some time and then appear again as a real outbreak after several years.

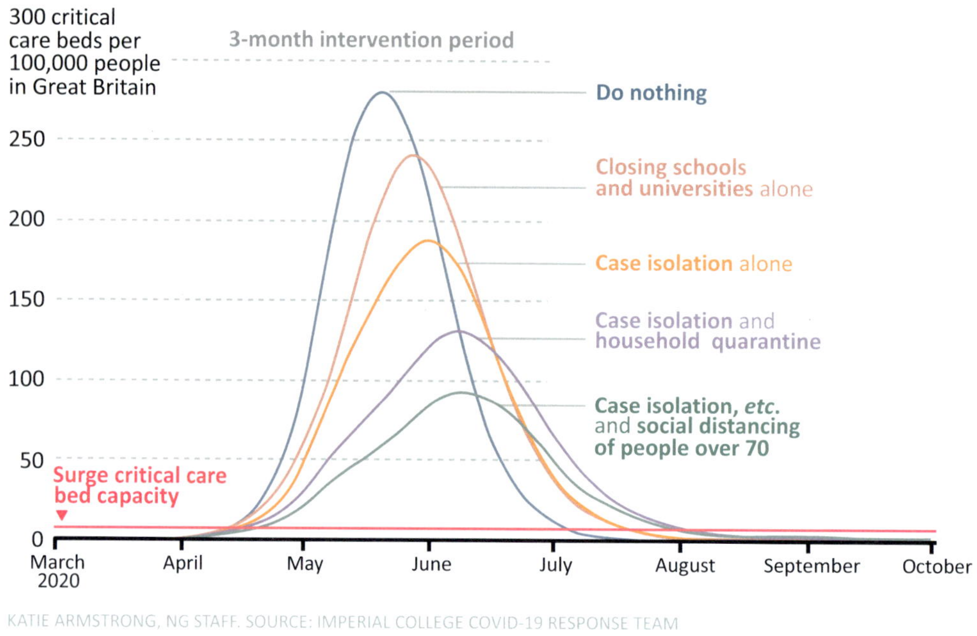


**Fig. (3).** Estimates of the curves of the number of cases that the epidemic will follow and the measures to be taken in the rise of the pandemic on March 20 in the UK (URL: https://www.nationalgeographic.com/science/2020/03/uk-backed-off-on-herd-immunity-to-beat-coronavirus-we-need-it/). If nothing is done, all ICU capacity will have to be allocated to COVID-19-related patients at the peak of the epidemic.

## HERD IMMUNITY AND THE 'SECOND WAVE' PROBLEM: MYTH OR TRUTH?

Yes of course it is true. It is as real as the knowledge that there will be new earthquakes, but it is also unpredictable. In order to mention the second wave, it is expected that the first wave will end, and the number of new cases and deaths announced daily will be '0' or close to it for a considerable timeframe. However, in many discussions, it can be seen that everyday hundreds of new cases and dozens of new deaths are recorded as “second wave” discussions. So, it is also a subject of “infodemics” throughout the world. New Zealand is maybe the first country that deserves to claim it has finished the ‘first wave’ in August 2020.

It makes sense to talk about the second wave in flu epidemics. But we cannot simply treat COVID-19 as a flu pandemic. The vulnerable groups, the elderly, those with comorbidities, immunocompromised people should be seriously protected by every appropriate means, because the death rate is above 20% when they are inflicted.

Herd (*i.e.*, "community" for human being) immunity is an accepted method to pursue in the struggle with non-fatal, contagious diseases. It became a method adopted in the 1930s, along with mass vaccination for measles. When the percentage of people who have been immunized in the community (by vaccination or disease) exceed a certain threshold value, the probability of the epidemic to prevail again approaches zero. However, in a disease with a case fatality rate around 5% such as Covid-19, this method becomes controversial. As a matter of fact, England seems to have adopted this method at the beginning of the pandemic, but later on, the cases with a fatality rate of more than 10% announced that they left it amid harsh reaction of healthcare professionals, supported by the public. On March 13, the government's chief health advisor, Sir Patrick Vallance defended the herd immunity policy, reiterating that they would triumph over COVID-19 once nearly 60% of the population became immune. On March 15, epidemiologist Dr. W. Hanage published a report which put forth that a large number of people would die if this method was used. As a result of these discussions, the government reconsidered and initiated closure or 'lock-down' measures on March 23, 2020 (Fig. **3**). (URL: https://www.theguardian.com/commentisfree/2020/mar/15/epidemiologist-britain-herd-immunity-coronavirus-covid-19).

In September 2020, an interesting news has come from Brazil on the immunity status of this developing country. A population-based household survey was performed in the State of Maranhão, in July and August to estimate the seroprevalence of SARSCoV-2 using a serum testing electrochemiluminescence immunoassay (da Silva, 2020). Seroprevalence of total antibodies against SARS-CoV-2 was 40·4% (95%CI 35·6-45·3). The authors concluded that the "herd immunity threshold" (HIT) is not as low as 20%, but at least higher than or equal to around 40%. The infection fatality rate was one of the lowest reported so far, and the proportion of asymptomatic cases was low.

## IS THE 'ORDINARY CITIZEN' ALSO GUILTY? WHICH MISTAKES DID THEY DO IN THE PANDEMIC AND 'NORMALIZATION'?

When the citizens combined incomplete health knowledge and a high motivation to normalize the economy, they tended towards normalization too rapidly. For instance, it has hardly been observed that ordinary citizens react to the crowds in public transport. I do not find it right to make it easy to blame the public as some scientists and politicians do. >We can understand this when we reexamine the "Maslow's order of requirements" scheme, which is still valid today. Under the heading of physiological needs, the motivation to survive, feed, raise offspring and hence, continue their lineage are the top priority instincts for the life. Even the health issue comes next. Therefore, people, regardless of their educational background and what is taught and told to them, prioritize activities related to survival than abstract dangers for health, that is, the risk of being infected with the virus. However, if you do not have problems with physiological needs, that is, if you believe that you have secured your well-being in the future, health issues can be ahead of others. This explains why there are so many different behaviors related to COVID-19 between neighborhoods, and groups with different socioeconomic or cultural backgrounds. In other words, it is natural that those in a region where socioeconomically "comfortable" or those with future security are in the majority do not understand those in the other 'poor' region.

"Maslow's order of requirements" chart helps us understand people's behavior and motivations. Here, priorities move from physiological needs to self-realization, that is, from the bottom to the top.

Turkish people, like many developing countries, have difficulties to comply with masks, physical distance, strict hygiene rules. Mediterranean and Middle Eastern habits, in which the "non-compliance" feature is somehow dominant in cultural codes, can partially explain this. It would be more appropriate for the state to emphasize the issue by using mass media more effectively, not only with sanctions but with effective information including pros and cons of the dangerous disease. Only really educated people can believe in the necessity of the bitter measures and incorporate them in their lives.

What could be the messages for the future?

Even if this epidemic ends after a while, new outbreaks will come. Therefore, long-term evolution of sociocultural codes should be considered. For this, the education of pre-school, school children and women play a key role. Concretizing the virus infection, which is an abstract danger, at a level that will change the lives of people will require serious pedagogical effort and organizational skills. The state should strive to plan and coordinate these in the long run by cooperating with non-governmental organizations.

## HOW DOES THIS DISEASE END?

Community education is very important for the eradication of COVID-19. Increased public awareness is one of the most important factors besides variables such as climatic conditions, vaccination, availability of drugs, and finally, mutation of the virus. Historically, public awareness also played an important role in reducing the tuberculosis, which was very common in most developing countries in the first half of the 1900s.

Another factor is the development of a highly protective vaccine against the disease (discussed in another chapter).

A close scrutiny of the history of vaccine development reveals that even in diseases afflicting populations *en masse*, vaccines were found after many years, and they were never found in many important diseases such as AIDS, Ebolavirus, SARS, and MERS.

**Pearl: Don't panic, get ready. COVID-19 is not a tornado, it is a hurricane. It affects everyone. You will not be harmed if you stand firm.**

## THE SPANISH FLU EXPERIENCES OF 1918: DOES HISTORY LIGHT OUR WAY?

The Spanish flu, which started in Europe between 1918-1920 and travelled to the American continent by ships, turned into a pandemic that affected almost every country and one-third of the world's population at that time, sheds light on the day after 100 years.

Since there are many factors affecting the course of pandemics, one should be very careful in predicting the future. When we look at the state of the disease in its own internal dynamics, we see that there is a disease that is easily contagious, and the specific drug and vaccine have not yet been found. We know similarities of this situation from history. Now, I want to draw attention to the experience in the USA in the 1918 pandemic.

### Why is It Called 'Spanish Flu'?

In fact, although the epidemic affected Europe and the USA very widely, in the chaotic environment of World War I, newspapers in the USA, France, Germany and England were banned from writing the facts about the epidemic, except for the serious illness of the King of Spain and the severe spread of the epidemic in Spain. For this reason, the opinion spread in the world and news has been released that the flu particularly hit Spain. So, it was called a 'Spanish Flu'.

### Is It Different From Other Flu Syndromes?

Yes. Spanish flu emerged with the agent we know from the swine flu epidemic in 2009, coded as H1N1. Young children and the elderly are targets of most influenza outbreaks, although Spanish flu has a higher mortality rate among young adults. Bacterial superinfection has also been shown to be effective in deaths after cytokine storm.

## WHAT HAPPENED IN THE USA?

Philadelphia and St. Louis are two different cities with their own administrative characteristics. It is thought that the epidemic reached the USA with merchant ships coming to Boston in 1918. It was even written that in September 1918, more than 1500 soldiers were infected with the flu in one day after a soldier on a base 35 miles away from Boston was wrongly diagnosed with meningitis.

When the first cases are diagnosed with "Spanish flu", it is remarkable that the two cities follow completely different paths.

Philadelphia welcomes the situation more easily and is slow and reluctant to take action.

With the effect of the underdeveloped medical institutions and civil society, the objections are weak, and an official parade was organized with the participation of thousands of people on September 28, 1918.

Just a few days after this parade, the hospitals in the city are overcrowded with patients presenting with Spanish flu symptoms, fever and respiratory distress, and health institutions are not keeping up with the patient load. After thousands of people have died in this period, the measures are tightened, and the epidemic is brought under control.

### Mass Graves Were Opened in The Usa in September 1918 Due To Massive Death Toll

In St. Louis, on the other hand, an opposite strategy is followed. Immediately after the first case is diagnosed, strict measures are taken, meetings are banned, and almost every field is intervened, from sports matches to political rallies. Mass vaccination has been pursued. The epidemic is thought to be under control, and the practices are suddenly loosened in November 1918, two months after the first measures. Then, there has been a rapid increase in cases from this point on, but it can be taken under control again after months.

As a result, it is easily seen that the number of cases in the two cities follows a different course from each other.

The mistakes made by these two cities at different times and in different ways affected the society in different directions and eventually the increase of cases was reflected in the graphic. In history, these events were called "Philadelphia madness" and "St. Louis complacency".

**SUMMARY:** The Spanish flu pandemic has killed between 20 and 100 million people worldwide. Estimates average 50 million, showing the world's largest pandemic. In just one-year mean life expectancy in America declined by an incredible 12 years, according to the US National Archives.

**CONCLUSION:** The most basic mistake that can be made may be the admission of patients and patients whose general condition deteriorated to the hospital and use hospitals to respond to this, in short, "meeting the tsunami of the pandemic in hospitals". Community education is very important for the eradication of COVID-19. Increased public awareness is one of the most important factors besides variables such as climatic conditions, vaccination, availability of drugs, and finally, mutation of the virus. It will be an effective measure to emphasize the issue by using mass media more effectively, not only with sanctions but with effective information including pros and cons of the dangerous disease.

Although "herd immunity" is an accepted method to pursue in the struggle with non-fatal, contagious diseases, this method appears to be controversial in a disease with a case fatality rate around 4% to 5% such as COVID-19.

Provided with the data of soaring figures of newly diagnosed cases and death toll in many countries worldwide in autumn 2020, governments and public should reevaluate the situation and take efficient measures against the disease. Public mobility, transportation, meetings, and many business activities are known to facilitate the transmission of the disease, which also indicate which sectors should be restricted in order to mitigate the burden.

## REFERENCES

da Silva, AAM, Neto, LGL & de Azevedo, CMPS (2020) https://www.nationalgeographic.com/science/2020/03/uk-backed -off-on-herd-immunity-to-beat-coronavirus-we-need-it/

Huynh, TLD (2020) Does culture matter social distancing under the COVID-19 pandemic? *Saf Sci,* 130104872
[http://dx.doi.org/10.1016/j.ssci.2020.104872] [PMID: 32550745]

IDM Coronavirus InfoHub (2020) https://docs.google.com/document/d/1UZ4eyA qaNnmO4kYKF-Z--IIWA0y0wyR30RRAT-_Wxi9c/preview

Kucharski, AJ, Klepac, P, Conlan, AJK, Kissler, SM, Tang, ML, Fry, H, Gog, JR & Edmunds, WJ (2020) Effectiveness of isolation, testing, contact tracing, and physical distancing on reducing transmission of SARS-CoV-2 in different settings: a mathematical modelling study. *Lancet Infect Dis,* 20, 1151-60.
[http://dx.doi.org/10.1016/S1473-3099(20)30457-6] [PMID: 32559451]

Lauer, SA, Grantz, KH, Bi, Q, Jones, FK, Zheng, Q, Meredith, HR, Azman, AS, Reich, NG & Lessler, J (2020) The incubation period of coronavirus disease 2019 (covid-19) from publicly reported confirmed cases: estimation and application. *Ann Intern Med,* 172, 577-82.
[http://dx.doi.org/10.7326/M20-0504] [PMID: 32150748]

Li, Q, Guan, X, Wu, P, Wang, X, Zhou, L, Tong, Y, Ren, R, Leung, KSM, Lau, EHY, Wong, JY, Xing, X, Xiang, N, Wu, Y, Li, C, Chen, Q, Li, D, Liu, T, Zhao, J, Liu, M, Tu, W, Chen, C, Jin, L, Yang, R, Wang, Q, Zhou, S, Wang, R, Liu, H, Luo, Y, Liu, Y, Shao, G, Li, H, Tao, Z, Yang, Y, Deng, Z, Liu, B, Ma, Z, Zhang,

Y, Shi, G, Lam, TTY, Wu, JT, Gao, GF, Cowling, BJ, Yang, B, Leung, GM & Feng, Z (2020) Early transmission dynamics in Wuhan, China, of novel coronavirus-infected pneumonia. *N Engl J Med,* 382, 1199-207.
[http://dx.doi.org/10.1056/NEJMoa2001316] [PMID: 31995857]

Riou, J & Althaus, CL (2020) Pattern of early human-to-human transmission of Wuhan 2019 novel coronavirus (2019-nCoV), December 2019 to January 2020. *Euro Surveill,* 252000058 [published correction appears in Euro Surveill. 2020 Feb;25(7)].
[http://dx.doi.org/10.2807/1560-7917.ES.2020.25.4.2000058] [PMID: 32019669]

# CHAPTER 3

# Comorbid Diseases and COVID-19: COPD, Smoking, Obesity, Diabetes, Cancer, and Kidney Failure

**Abstract:** COVID-19 can cause disease in almost all ages and all groups. However, those with comorbid diseases are at high risk in terms of the progression of the disease, deterioration such as hospitalization in an intensive care unit (ICU), mechanical ventilation requirement, and the risk of death. Smoking, COPD, coronary artery disease, heart failure, cancer, kidney and liver failure, and obesity have been directly associated with death rates other than advanced age and male gender. Patients with comorbid diseases are older people (mean age 60 y *vs*. 45 y), presented with shortness of breath more commonly , have more severe COVID-19 (30% *vs*. 10%), which directly impacts the clinical course, morbidity, and mortality.

**Keywords:** ACE2 receptors, Cancer, COVID-19, Coronary artery disease, COPD, Heart failure, Kidney failure, Liver failure, Obesity, Pandemic, Smoking.

In an analysis of 1590 patients with COVID-19 in China, at least one comorbidity was found in one-third of critical or severe patients, while only 1/10 of mild patients were found to have the same (Guan, 2020). In accord with this study, we can postulate that having one or more comorbidities and smoking habits directly affected mortality. Now we are sure that patients with comorbid conditions represent a more disadvantaged subpopulation in the universal sample of COVID-19 (Table **1**).

Guan *et al.* reported in their detailed analysis of 1590 COVID-19 cases that having one or more comorbidities negatively affects mortality compared to those with no comorbidities (Guan, 2020).

## THE RELATIONSHIP BETWEEN COVID-19 FATALITY RATE AND COMORBIDITIES

The mortality rate for people who have no co-morbid diseases is 0.9%. Mortality increases with the following diseases (Table **2**).

**Ozgur KARCIOGLU, Selman YENIOCAK and Mandana HOSSEINZADEH**

- Coronary artery disease and heart failure (highest risk)
- Diabetes (DM)
- COPD / asthma
- HT
- Cancer
- Obesity

**Table 1. Characteristics of patients with comorbid diseases compared to others.**

| |
|---|
| • Older people (mean age 60 y *vs.* 45 y), |
| • They have more severe COVID-19 (30% *vs.* 10%), |
| • They are presented with shortness of breath more commonly (41% *vs.* 17%), |
| • Smoke more commonly (11.8% *vs.* 5.4%), |
| • They are presented with nausea / vomiting more commonly (10% *vs.* 4%), |
| • They show a higher rate of abnormalities on the chest radiography (29% *vs.* 15%), |
| • They are admitted into ICU more commonly (13.5% *vs.* 3.8%), |
| • They die more commonly (8.8% *vs.* 1.3%), |

**Table 2. The death rates are given as the odds or rates that people with these chronic conditions will face when infected with COVID-19.**

| Chronic Problems | Mortality Rate (Definite Diagnosis) (%) | Mortality Rate (possible Diagnosis) (%) |
|---|---|---|
| Cardiovascular disease (CVD) | 13.2 | 10.5 |
| Diabetes | 9.2 | 7.3 |
| Chronic respiratory disease | 8.0 | 6.3 |
| Hypertension | 8.4 | 6.0 |
| Cancer | 7.6 | 5.6 |
| None | - | 0.9 |

## Comorbid Diseases and Death In Age Groups

The impact of comorbid diseases on the death rate becomes more prominent with advancing age (Table **3**).

Almost all comorbidities affect both sexes, but some conditions are associated with higher death rates in women or men. Among patients with COVID-19, ischemic heart diseases, COPD, liver diseases and chronic kidney failure are seen more frequently in men. Atrial fibrillation, dementia, heart failure and hypertension are more common in women.

In the largest series published so far, 5,700 patients with a positive PCR test in New York and diagnosed with COVID-19 and hospitalized in 12 hospitals were analyzed (Richardson, 2020). The sample of patients had a median age of 63 and 60% of them are male. It is interesting that 88% of the patients had more than one concomitant disease (Table **4**).

**Table 3. Numbers and rates of the deceased as of May 13 in New York, USA. It is noted that those with comorbid diseases constitute the majority of those who die in all age groups, and this trend is observed more clearly in young people. More than 20% mortality rate over the age of 45 shows that it is a very severe group of COVID-19 patients. (URL: https://www1.nyc.gov/assets/doh/downloads/pdf/imm/covid-19-daily-data-summary-deaths-05132020-1.pdf).**

| Age (years) | # Patients Died | Fatality Rate (%) | Those with Comorbidities (n) | Those with no Comorbidities (n) | Comorbidities Unknown | Percentage of those with no Comorbidities (or Those with no Data) in all Deaths (%) |
|---|---|---|---|---|---|---|
| **0 - 17** | 9 | **0.06** | 6 | 3 | 0 | 0.02 |
| **18 - 44** | 601 | **3.9** | 476 | 17 | 108 | 0.8 |
| **45 - 64** | 3,413 | **22.4** | 2,851 | 72 | 490 | 3.7 |
| **65 - 74** | 3,788 | **24.9** | 2,801 | 5 | 982 | 6.5 |
| **75+** | 7,419 | **48.7** | 5,236 | 2 | 2,181 | 14.3 |
| **TOTAL** | **15,230** | 100 | 11,370 (75%) | 99 (0.7%) | 1,551 (24.7%) | 25.3% |

**Table 4. In the New York series, which includes 5700 patients, it has been reported that cardiovascular and metabolic diseases (obesity and diabetes) have very close association with COVID-19 (Richardson, 2020).**

| **Comorbidities** | **N (%)** |
|---|---|
| Cancer | 320 (6) |
| Hypertension | 3026 (56.6) |
| Coronary artery disease | 595 (11.1) |
| Heart failure | 371 (6.9) |
| COPD | 287 (5.4) |
| Asthma | 479 (9) |
| Obstructive sleep apnea | 154 (2.9) |
| HIV | 43 (0.8) |
| History of organ transplantation | 55 (1) |
| Chronic kidney disease. | 268 (5) |
| End-stage renal disease | 186 (3.5) |
| Diabetes | 1808 (33.8) |

*(Table 4) cont.....*

| | |
|---|---|
| Cirrhosis | 19 (0.4) |
| Chronic Hepatitis B/C | 11 (0.2) |
| Obesity (BMI ≥30)<br>Morbid obesity (BMI ≥35)<br>(among 4170 pts) | 1737 (41.7)<br>791 (19.0) |
| Smokers (among 3567 pts) | 558 (15.6) |

## PULMONARY DISEASES AND COVID-19

The most common chronic respiratory diseases in the community are Asthma, COPD, emphysema and chronic bronchitis. The prevalence of COPD in Turkey is between 19-20%. According to the data of the World Health Organization, COPD is the 4th most common disease in the world. These diseases can often coexist . Asthma inflicts younger patients than the other diseases.

### What is the difference between COPD and COPD-Acute exacerbation (COPD-AA)?

COPD is a structural destruction of the airways as a result of chronic inflammation of the airways, which is seen almost exclusively in smokers, often over the age of 40. The resulting chronic inflammatory response leads to parenchymal tissue damage (emphysema) and impairment in normal tissue repair and defense mechanisms (small airway fibrosis). These changes cause air trapping and progressive airflow restriction. In mild or early-stage COPD, the main symptoms are chronic cough and sputum production. Phlegm is usually white-gray, thick, and sticky. In exacerbations, it often turns green.

### COPD-Acute Exacerbation (COPD-AA)

periods are characterized by fever, flank pain, change in sputum character or amount, odor, and color. According to the definition of the Turkish Thoracic Society, COPD-AA; "... is an acute event characterized by a worsening of the patient's respiratory tract symptoms beyond the normally observed daily change which leads to a change in medication".

Generally, frequent exacerbations are seen in very advanced stages than in the initial stages.

### Could COVID-19 Infection also Cause COPD-AA?

Yes. Causes of COPD-AA can be bacterial, viral, or fungal infections. As can be understood from here, COVID-19 infection is also one of the causes of COPD-AA.

### *Are Patients with COPD or Asthma at High Risk for Contracting COVID-19?*

No, there is no higher risk of getting the disease compared to other people. This has been clearly demonstrated in studies in China and S. Korea (Guan, NEJM, 2020). The Canadian Thoracic Society reported in 2020 publications on both COPD and asthma that neither disease had conveyed an increased risk for COVID-19.

### *Are Patients with COPD at High Risk for Severe COVID-19 and Death?*

Yes, according to the proven data, COVID-19 is severe in those with a previous diagnosis of COPD. In the analysis of 1590 inpatients in China, when age and smoking status are kept under control, COPD, diabetes, hypertension, and obesity predict poor clinical outcomes (Guan, ERJ, 2020). In fact, in this study, COPD stood out as a stronger risk factor than other diseases. In brief, the need for mechanical ventilation and ICU admission is more common in patients with COPD, and death and disability are reported at a significantly higher rate.

### *How are The Follow-up and Treatment of COPD and COPD-AA Cases During The Pandemics?*

There is basically no change in the ongoing treatment of COPD cases and this continuity should be maintained by communicating with the physicians who carry out their follow-up when necessary. Short and long-acting bronchodilators (sympathomimetics) and corticosteroids are the mainstays of treatment.

The main goal is to beware of COVID-19 disease by staying at home, isolation, physical distance, hygiene, and frequent hand washing for at least 20 seconds with cleaners containing at least 60% alcohol. Working from home can be an important solution for most white-collar people. It will be wise for them to have at least one month of treatment with them so that they do not have to leave home.

### *Are Systemic Corticosteroids (CST) Used in COPD-AA During Pandemic?*

Why not? There is no data that inhaled corticosteroids increase the risk of COVID-19. Yes, in COPD-AA cases, it is recommended to take oral prednisone regardless of whether the cause of the exacerbation is COVID-19. In this way, patients can avoid unnecessary ED admissions. Thus, it is thought that they can also be protected from inadvertent contagion of COVID-19.

## Are There Any Changes For Asthma Patients?

The chronic and relapse treatment of asthma exactly should be continued as usual. In summary, keeping asthma under control is the best prevention against a severe COVID-19.

### *How is an Asthma Attack Treated While Infected with COVID-19?*

Corticosteroids and short- or long-acting beta agonists (SABA and LABA) can be used, regardless of a diagnosis of COVID-19. An effective and expedient treatment of asthma is also necessary to alleviate the severity of the respiratory symptoms of COVID-19. Oral prednisone can be used in asthma as well as in COPD, which will reduce hospital admissions.

### *Is the Use of Nebulizers Recommended in The Treatment of Asthma/COPD During The COVID-19 Outbreak?*

Largely no. Instead of a nebulizer, metered dose inhalers should be used. The SARS-CoV-2 virus spread can be reduced in this way.

## Does Smoking and COPD Development Alter Expression of ACE2 Receptors?

Unfortunately, yes. Leung *et al.* reported clear findings on this subject in Canada (Leung, 2020). In this study, it was shown histopathologically that both active smoking and the development of COPD had increased production of ACE2 in the lower respiratory tract. This is a factor in both being inflicted by COVID-19 and having a severe clinical course. In the study, no such clear finding was observed among former smokers, *i.e.*, those who quit. Brake *et al.* reported that ACE2 production increased in smokers, *via* mechanisms mediated by nicotine (Brake, 2020). There is also information published before the pandemic that nicotine reduces ACE2 receptors (Oakes, 2018). Considered to be reduced, there will be an excessive decrease with the ACE2 receptors, which the SARS-CoV-2 virus causes to destroy, increasing the severity of the disease (Usman, 2020). Therefore, smoking cessation and keeping COPD under control is of great importance in the struggle against COVID-19 that will last for more years.

### *Does Smoking Affect Clinical Course?*

Unfortunately, a resounding “yes”. Guan *et al.* reported in their studies, 95% of non-smokers have no comorbidities, while nearly half of smokers have comorbidities such as cardiovascular or lung diseases (Guan, 2020). Again, the majority of COVID-19 cases with COPD and CVD consist of smokers.

In the case series published by Suleyman *et al.* from Detroit, smoking was noted in 22% in discharged patients *vs.* 38.6% in hospitalized patients ($p = 0.002$) (Suleyman, 2020).

One of the variables that statistically significantly affects mortality in the analyzes is smoking ($p = 0.047$).

Smoking increases the risk of contracting COVID-19 and worsens the course of the disease in several ways:

1. By suppressing the ciliary movement in the airways, smoking makes it difficult to remove viruses and bacteria.
2. It increases ACE-2 receptors, which are key to the entry of the virus into the cell.
3. It suppresses the immune system in general, *i.e.*, inhibits antibody production in B lymphocytes by reducing CD4+ 'helper T cells'.
4. Nicotine in the cigarettes also suppresses immunity by increasing catecholamine production.
5. Cardiovascular diseases, pulmonary diseases (COPD, asthma, and chronic bronchitis) progress and worsen with smoking.
6. Nicotine also prevents the production of interleukin-22, which suppresses alveolar inflammation and regenerates damaged cells.

The cilia in the mucous membranes of the airway epithelial cells push harmful particles and microorganisms to the outside (hypopharynx/mouth / nose) with a brush-like motion, thereby protecting the lungs in the long run. Highly active ciliary movement in the top healthy, non-smoker, and bottom most ineffective movements in a person who has been smoking for years.

## *Is Smoking also Effective in Influenza?*

Yes, unfortunately. When the mortality risks of ex-smokers and active smokers are compared with those who have never smoked, the negative effect of smoking is clearly remarkable. Studies show that smokers are inflicted by diseases more commonly due to suppression of immunity (Brake, 2020). Death risk has also been documented to increase with smoking (Han *et al*, 2020).

### *Is COVID-19 More Severe in Smokers?*

Yes, it has been definitively demonstrated that COVID-19 disease progresses more severely in smokers (Guo FR, 2020).

### *What are The Key Findings of Systematic Reviews and Meta-analyzes with High Level of Evidence?*

In the study of Zhao *et al*., who investigated the impact of smoking on COVID-19, the findings of 11 different studies were analyzed together (Zhao *et al*. 2020). While the effect of COPD was 4.38 (Fixed effect model, 95% CI: 2.34-8.20), the effect of smoking alone was found to be 1.98. In other words, being undiagnosed with COPD does not protect smokers from COVID-19.

In a more recent meta-analysis with high level of evidence, the data of 2473 patients with COVID-19 enrolled by 15 studies were analyzed (Alqahtani, 2020). The fatality rate is 7.4%, that is, it is a severe patient group. The percentage of patients known to have COPD is 2% and the rate of smokers is 9%. Cases with COPD have more severe disease, compared to those without COPD (risk of severe disease= 33.4% *vs*. 63%). Current smokers are noted to have a 1.45 times greater risk of severe complications than others (ex- and nonsmokers).

Vardavas *et al*. published a systematic review with findings from the early phase of the pandemic (Vardavas, 2020). In their analysis of 5 studies conducted in China, they reported that smoking increases the probability of a poor clinical course, although the data are limited.

### *What is "Smoker's Paradox" (SP), are There any Justifications?*

Yes, there is. It is known that nicotine suppresses the immune response through its anti-inflammatory effects. It was thought that this might cause a mitigation of the cytokine storm. In 1995, some publications reported that smokers had a better clinical prognosis in coronary artery disease. It is observed that smokers, who constitute a large population especially in developing countries, do not attempt to quit smoking during the pandemic period with this confusion. In fact, in most of the publications, former and active smokers were grouped under the title of "smoker", while a significant decrease was observed in cardiovascular disease and associated mortality rates within a few years with smoking cessation. In more recent studies, the protective effect of smoking has not been demonstrated, on the contrary, a worse clinical course has been observed in smokers (Redfors, 2020).

When the confounding factors are discarded carefully, the protective effect of smoking against COVID-19 cannot be supported by concrete evidence. Putting an emphasis on the protective effect of smoking, especially by physicians, will have a detrimental effect on the public and hamper the efforts to quit smoking.

If we list the potential harms of smoking on COVID-19; (adapted from Usman, 2020).

1. In the use of all tobacco products in the form of cigarettes / hookahs / electronic cigarettes / cigars / pipes; hands are frequently touch face or mouth, which represents the most frequent mechanism in disease transmission.
2. The normal epithelial cover in the respiratory tract is degraded, mucociliary activation decreases, which facilitates infection.
3. Decreased ACE2 receptor production reduces degradation of angiotensin 2, which increases local inflammation, thrombotic events, and vasoconstriction.
4. The increase in ACE2 receptor production prepares the ground for the SARS-CoV-2 virus to attach and enter the cell.
5. The clinical course of COVID-19 worsens as a result of increased coronary and cerebrovascular diseases and COPD in smokers.

In summary, COPD cases should be more careful to avoid the problems associated with COVID-19 and to avoid exacerbations. Risks will be higher with the addition of the effects of seasonal changes. Avoiding smoking is one of the prerequisites for COPD not to worsen. It has been established that smoking increases the risk of severe complications and mortality of COVID-19.

In the fight against COVID-19 that will last for more years, smoking cessation and keeping COPD under control is of great importance. It is of utmost importance that COPD cases do not catch COVID-19 during the pandemic period, because both smoking and COPD will cause a more severe disease. Patients with COPD should not disrupt their ongoing treatment, and medical assistance should be sought, as a new change (change in sputum amount or character, flank pain, fever, increase in shortness of breath) will indicate COPD-AA.

## OBESITY AND COVID-19

Obesity is known to be closely related to immunity. Chronic inflammation is considered to persist in adipose (fatty) tissue in obese individuals.

Obesity increases susceptibility to infections in a large manner. In addition, as a result of chronic adipose tissue inflammation, hypertension, cardiovascular diseases, and dyslipidemias are more common in obese people, each of which boost the risks independently in regard to COVID-19.

## What could be its Mechanism?

It has been observed that ACE2 receptors are also present in adipose tissue. Therefore, ACE2 is more abundant in obese people. Since COVID-19 is the gateway to the cell, it is thought to increase susceptibility to disease.

It is also thought that adipose tissue plays a reservoir role for many microorganisms such as influenza viruses, adenoviruses, HIV, CMV. This phenomenon also suggests that SARS-CoV-2 first settles in the adipose tissue and then spreads throughout the body (Bourgeois, 2019; Kassir, 2020).

## Numerical Data showing the Relationship between Obesity and COVID-19

According to the data announced by CDC in April 2020 regarding patients hospitalized in the USA with the diagnosis of COVID-19, the most common comorbidities detected in patients are hypertension (49%) and obesity (48%) (Garg, 2020).

Among patients with COVID-19, those with critical illness have higher BMI values among the entire patient group (Peng, 2020). Mean BMI value of critical patients is 25.5, *vs.* 22 kg / $m^2$ for the whole group. Perhaps an even more interesting finding is that 88% of the patients who died of COVID-19 have a BMI above 25. The same rate is 19% in survivors ($p < 0.001$).

In France, almost half (47.6%) of patients hospitalized in ICU with COVID-19 have a BMI of> 30 kg / $m^2$, and 28.2% of them> 35 kg / $m^2$ (Simonnet, 2020). This clearly shows that obesity is a risk factor that increases the severity of COVID-19. Likewise, Petrilli *et al* analyzed 5279 patients in New York *via* a retrospective cohort study and reported that obesity is the strongest predictor for critical illness (Petrilli, 2020).

It is also known that obesity increases the coagulation tendency (Movahed, 2019). Thrombosis has been directly associated with deaths in COVID-19 patients.

Finally, obese individuals experience some technical difficulties such as imaging and equipment problems like stretchers, which can impair their management processes (Ryan, 2020, Uppot, 2018).

## Mechanisms of The impact of Obesity on COVID-19

There are numerous different mechanisms *via* which COVID-19 affect the outcome of the patients with the disease (Korakas, 2020) (Fig. **1**).

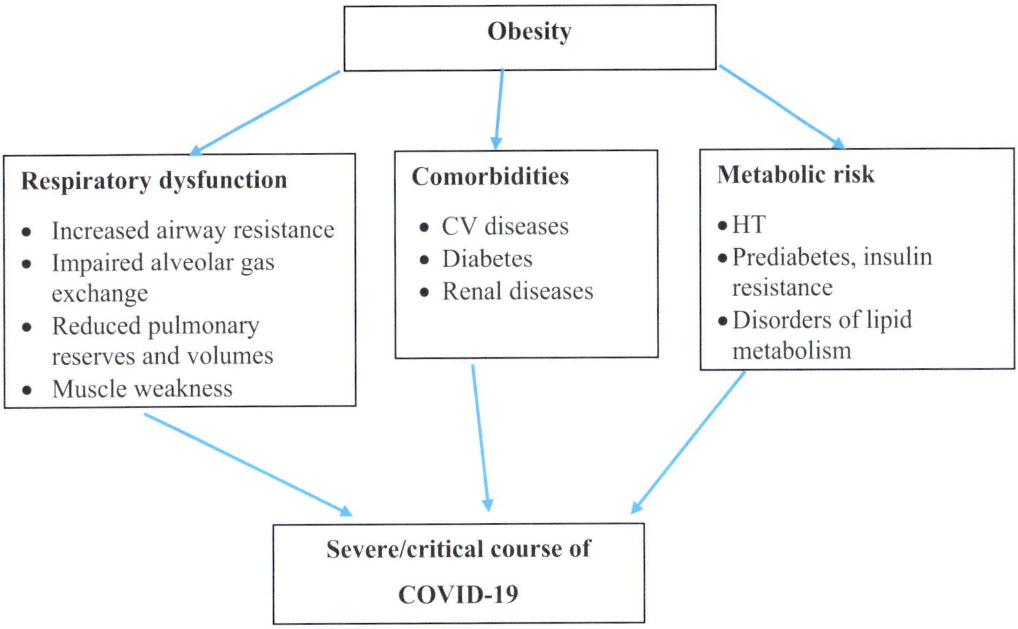


**Fig. (1).** Mechanisms by which obesity causes critical illness.

## The Relationship Between Critical Illness and Obesity:

In the large and consecutive case series Suleyman *et al*. published in Detroit, it has been reported that being over 60 years old, male, HT, DM, CRF, severe obesity (BMI> = 40) and cancer are independent risk factors for admission to ICU (Suleyman, 2020). While the average BMI is 31 for those who were discharged, it is 33.6 for those who were hospitalized ($p = 0.01$).

In a systematic review and meta-analysis, Yang *et al*. reported that severe COVID-19 patients have higher BMI than non-severe ones (WMD=2.67, 95% CI [1.52-3.82]); COVID-19 patients with obesity were more severe and have a worse outcome than those without (OR=2.31, 95% CI [1.3-4.12]) (Yang, 2020).

Respiratory failure developed in 74% of those hospitalized in the ICU and MV was required in 81%. Most of the patients (62.5%) who underwent MV although they were younger than 40 years of age had severe obesity, and this rate was 26% in those who did not. Among the patients with CVD diagnosed with COVID-19, BMI is significantly higher (25.5 kg / $m^2$ and 22 kg / $m^2$) ($p = 0.003$) in the critical group with a severe clinical course (Peng *et al*, 2020). Similarly, BMI was found to be higher in patients who died than those who survived. The percentage of patients with BMI> 25 kg / $m^2$ was 88% in those who died, while 19% in survivors ($p < 0.001$).

So, what shall we do? Metabolic variables should be considered in predicting the course and prognosis of COVID-19 in conjunction with classical markers such as SOFA, d-dimer, and inflammatory markers (Stefan, 2020). These variables are waist and hip circumference, BMI, glucose, and insulin levels.

It has been suggested that obese individuals lose weight and struggle with obesity *via* other methods. This issue should be emphasized for the public as a whole during the pandemic period (Rychter, 2020).

In summary, we recommend that obese individuals be given a special importance and priority in screening for the COVID-19 pandemic. Specialized training should be provided for the treatments to be given to obese individuals in critical care, and equipment preparation (such as obese stretcher, discrete tomography unit) should be arranged. It should be emphasized that the public awareness and struggle against obesity will mitigate the burden from viral and other diseases.

## DIABETES AND COVID-19

The fact that diabetics, whose prevalence is between 8% and 10% in the population under normal conditions, constitute 20% to 34% of the patients hospitalized in intensive care units shows that it is an important problem of public health (Garg 2020, Goyal 2020, Sardu, 2020).

In the SARS epidemic in 2002, it was noted that the mortality and morbidity of patients with diabetes were significantly higher than of nondiabetics (Yang, 2006). In the same study, it has been shown that high levels of blood sugar also pose a risk. Diabetes is second only to hypertension as the most common comorbid disease encountered in individuals with COVID-19.

It has been reported that patients with diabetic patients with COVID-19 are at high risk for severe pneumonia even in the absence of other comorbid diseases. Guo *et al.* reported that both severity of pneumonia and inflammatory markers, IL-6, ferritin, CRP, D-dimer, were also high in diabetics (Guo, 2020). Therefore, it can be postulated that diabetes imposes a high risk for severe disease independent of all other factors.

The risk of ICU admission and morality risk was evaluated in diabetic COVID-19 patients compared to the others (Roncon, 2020). A total of 1382 patients (mean age 51.5 years, 58% males), DM represented the second more frequent comorbidities after arterial HT. Diabetic patients resulted to have a significant increased risk of ICU admission (OR: 2.79, 95% CI 1.85–4.22, $p < 0.0001$, $I2 = 46\%$), and a higher mortality risk (OR 3.21, 95% CI 1.82–5.64, $p < 0.0001$, $I2 = 16\%$)

When 22,254 patients who underwent PCR tests in NYC between March 5 and April 9 were analyzed, DM was recorded in 33%, HT in 37%, CVD in 24%, and CRF in 11% (Kalyanaraman Marcello, 2020). Male gender, advanced age, history of heart disease, presence of DM or CRF are risk factors for both test positivity and death.

Diabetic individuals with COVID have a much higher rate of cardiovascular disease than other patients with COVID (33% *versus* 15%) and give less fever response (59% *versus* 83%) (Guo, 2020). Age and gender distributions and mortality rates have been found similar in this study.

Many laboratory markers such as ALT and LDH were found to be higher in people with diabetes than nondiabetics. Absolute neutrophil count, CRP, D-dimer are also markedly high. Lymphocyte count, erythrocyte and hemoglobin levels were found to be significantly lower in diabetic patients. All these data show that diabetics are at higher risk for excessive and uncontrolled inflammatory response and hypercoagulability.

## In a Diabetic Patient Hospitalized in The COVID-19 Process, There will be 5 Essential Steps of Management

1. Assessment and stabilization in terms of COVID-19.
2. Fluid therapy; monitoring and management of electrolytes such as sodium, potassium, and phosphate.
3. Monitoring and regulation of blood sugar, insulin regimen, prevention of hypoglycemia.
4. Management of complications and additional problems related to diabetes and COVID-19: Kidney failure, pneumonia, ARDS and fever.
5. Managing the impact of COVID-19 itself and hydroxychloroquine and glucocorticoids used in the treatment on blood sugar.

In addition, **metformin**, which is routinely used in the treatment of diabetes, should be discontinued in severe COVID-19 cases with respiratory problems because it can cause acid-base disorders.

It is known that morbidity and mortality decrease in cases of SARS and COVID-19 by performing **on-site blood sugar management** (Sardu, 2020, Yang, 2006).

**Notes on treatment:** It should be known that the usual insulin requirements will increase in the diabetes management of COVID-19 cases and the 'usual' doses will not be sufficient. On the other hand, patients with increased risk of kidney damage due to COVID-19 are at higher risk if they have diabetes as a comorbidity. As CRF will reduce the breakdown of insulin from the kidney, the blood insulin level may rise and paves the way for hypoglycemia.

Due to the disadvantages of insulin administration with continuous infusion, methods of diminishing insulin treatments have been investigated in recent years. For example, "continuous glucose monitoring" (CGM) devices have been developed (Korytkowski, 2020). These will also reduce the close contact between the healthcare worker and the patient during the COVID-19 process.

Although intravenous (IV) insulin administration seems to be standard in critically ill patients against hyperglycemia, some centers may also offer subcutaneous (SC) treatments (Aggarwal, 2020).

In fact, the essence of the matter is to formulate a regimen and strategy fitting best to the individual and the situation, taking into account many variables such as the patient's ability to be fed orally or enterally, the severity of the COVID-19 or other infection, basal metabolic status, and additional diseases.

## CANCER AND COVID-19

It has been suggested that patients with cancer have a higher risk of inflicted by COVID-19 and complications are older and have immunodeficiency more commonly than the others (Liang 2020, Al-Shamsi, 2020). Yu *et al*. reported from Wuhan that cancer patients are at twice the risk of contracting COVID-19 compared to the general population (Yu, 2020).

**What about the other deadly viruses?** In the H1N1 pandemic, it was reported that two-thirds of cancer patients had pneumonia and their 30-day mortality was 18.5% (Dignani, 2014).

### Why are Cancer Patients More Disadvantaged in Terms of COVID-19?

For three reasons:

1. Cancer itself breaks the strength of the immune system and causes predisposition to all infections, including COVID-19.
2. Treatments against cancer, especially chemotherapy, are immunosuppressive. Emergent or mandatory operations also impair the immunity.
3. For the same reasons, these patients experience COVID-19 more severely as they do all infections, and they have a higher risk with regard to intubation, ICU admission and death.

In addition, urgent or emergent hospital visits (such as port insertion, radiotherapy, PET CT, medication renewal, consultations, *etc.*), which are more common for cancer patients than others, also predispose patients to be infected by COVID-19.

**Cancer has been reported to be associated with severe disease.** In a large series, it was reported that the rate of critical illness, mechanical ventilation, and ICU admission was 8% in other patients and 39% in patients with cancer. (Liang, 2020). In a series of 355 patients who died of COVID-19 in Italy, 20% of them were found to be diagnosed with cancer, and since this is a remarkably high rate compared to the society, cancer was thought to pose a high risk for death (Onder, 2020).

*"WHO — China Joint Mission on COVID-19"* reported that among COVID-19 patients in China, the death rate of patients with cancer diagnosed previously was 7.6%, while patients without comorbidities died at a rate of 1.4% *(Report of the WHO – China Joint Mission on Coronavirus Disease 2019 (COVID-19).* Available at https://www.Who.Int/docs/default-source/).

## Are There any More Special Risk Groups among People with Cancer?

Yes. When COVID-19 is diagnosed, those who received chemotherapy or underwent surgery in the previous 1 month have a much higher risk of suffering from severe disease than other cancer cases (3/4 *versus* 6/14) (Liang, 2020). These groups should definitely be given a priority and should be quarantined regardless of their age.

## Can Cancer be Diagnosed During The Pandemic Period, and can Interventions be Performed as Before?

Both yes and no. Since the earlier the cancer diagnosis is made, the higher the survival expectancy, diagnostic interventions should be performed as soon as possible, diagnosis should be established with procedures such as PET CT, biopsy, MRI, and endoscopy, and treatment options should be evaluated. However, on the other hand, the fear of catching COVID-19 can keep patients away from hospitals. While this is understandable to a certain extent, the individual risks of being late must be well balanced with the risks of COVID-19. As a result, although necessary precautions are taken against COVID-19, it is obvious that it would be more correct not to delay attempts for expedient diagnosis.

## Are there Specific Difficulties in Diagnostic Interventions for COVID-19?

Yes. For example, many signs and symptoms such as loss of appetite, muscle-joint pain, and weakness are commonly encountered in cancer patients. Cough, which is a sign of COVID-19, can be easily missed because cough is almost continuous in patients with larynx and lung cancer. There is a similar situation for shortness of breath. Therefore, the physician should evaluate the patient with a more careful history and examination. A decrease in lymphocyte count in blood count (lymphopenia) is an important finding, but lymphopenia can already be seen in cancer patients with the effect of chemotherapy or direct suppression of the production of the blood cells by cancer. As a rule, COVID-19 findings on chest tomography do not masquerade as cancer findings, although there may be some confusing issues.

## Are There Specific Difficulties for Cancer Patients Regarding Care and Treatment?

Unfortunately, yes. Those with cancer constitute one of the most vulnerable groups when resources are limited and certain equipment and resources needed for treatment and care are not sufficient. This has previously been experienced in influenza pandemics (Battershill, 2006). The lack of a particular drug or equipment will be life-threatening in patients receiving certain treatment regimens, especially when alternative agents cannot be preferred, (Alpert, 2019). It is estimated that COVID-19 may also cause difficulties in medical equipment and pharmaceuticals as in past epidemics (Al-Shamsi, 2020). There are 26 cancer drugs on the FDA's drug list published on 21 March 2020 as in a 'shortage' (US Food & Drug Administration; FDA drug shortages. Available at https://www.accessdata.fda.gov/scripts/drugshortages/default.cfm. Accessed March 21, 2020).

## Is there any Difference Regarding the Psychological Conditions of Cancer Patients in this Period?

Yes. Under pandemic conditions, the already fragile social support and psychological conditions of cancer patients will be more handicapped. Getting support from family and caregivers will be difficult due to reasons such as curfew restrictions and anxiety about getting sick. In addition to being older than other people and having comorbidities, they will be more concerned with the awareness that cancer poses a risk in itself.

## THE RISK OF REACTIVE OR MAJOR DEPRESSION WILL BE FURTHER INCREASED

Additional support should be obtained for all these risks. Taking advantage of technology, forming special chat groups *etc.* or other means of counseling other people can also be viable options for a more effective communication.

### What are the General Messages?

- Basically, the criteria used in making decisions such as hospitalization, discharge, intensive care, or operation do not change. For example, in a patient who has obstruction due to bowel cancer, the emergency operation decision does not change due to the pandemic.
- Necessary diagnosis and treatment attempts should not be delayed as much as possible, measures should be taken against COVID-19 and interventions should be performed as warranted.
- In pandemic period, access to environments with a high risk of infection should be minimized, for example, many oncology appointments can be undertaken remotely without going to the hospital.
- Under certain circumstances, some non-vital interventions such as adjuvant chemotherapy may be postponed after the pandemic.
- Decisions such as surgical intervention and hospitalization may result in different directions in pandemic conditions. The physician and the patient should discuss these openly and make a decision.
- Attention should be paid to the social support and psychological conditions of cancer patients and additional support should be obtained.
- Finally, education of cancer cases should be carried out with much more open and close communication in terms of strict adherence to measures such as hand hygiene, physical distance, and masks. For example, it should be stated that the surgical mask may not be enough when it has to go outside, additional protection measures such as a face shield may be required, and the need for them to minimize their time outside. In order to minimize the possibility of malpractice and to protect the patient's health at the highest level, it should be recorded that these points are followed, and the patient's treatment options should be evaluated in accord with this communication.

## RENAL FAILURE (RF), ACUTE KIDNEY INJURY (AKI) AND COVID-19

In the six-week period between 11 March 2020 and 26 April 2020, Montefiore Medical Center (MMC) in Bronx, New York, diagnosed 3345 patients with COVID-19 (Sourial, 2020). 13.1% of the patients were hospitalized in ICU. While renal replacement therapy (RRT) was required at a rate of 0.9% in similar patients in the previous years, RRT was performed in around 5% (n = 164) of COVID-19 cases in this group. For this reason, since routine hemodialysis devices are available, emergency peritoneal dialysis (EPD) option has been introduced. As a result, the authors reported that EPD can be used effectively for patients with RF and AKI for RRT, and that this is an important option in conditions where resources such as the COVID-19 pandemic are suboptimal.

Similarly, RF and AKI have been associated with mortality in COVID-19 patients in some other studies, too. In the study by Zhou *et al.*, who investigated the factors affecting mortality, it was found that high creatinine significantly increased mortality (Zhou S, 2020). While the proportion of patients with creatinine level above 133 micromol / L was 2% in survivors, it was 9% among patients who died (P = 0.045). While the diagnosis of AKI was established in 15% in the whole group, it was reported as 50% in the deaths and 1% in the survivors (p <0.0001). Parallel to this, RRT was performed at a rate of 5% in the whole group, but this rate was found to be 19% in the deceased and "0" in the survivors (p <0.0001). Another remarkable information is that the average time from the onset of the disease to the development of AKI is 15 days

Cornerstones of evolution of signs and symptoms and clinical follow-up from the onset of the disease in two hospitals in Wuhan (Zhou F, 2020, Lancet) revealed that acute kidney injury and cardiac damage are triggered in a similar timeframe (mean 15th day), and the development of secondary infection follows this in around one or two days. Accordingly, death occurs on an average of 19 days.

**Mechanism:** It is thought that AKI occurs during the period called **"cytokine storm"** when overt complaints and symptoms such as fever, muscle aches, respiratory distress, are seen in a fluctuating course and inflammatory markers increased sharply.

## LUNG-KIDNEY AXIS (LKA): A NEW PATHWAY FOR KIDNEY DAMAGE?

Some studies highlighted the relationship between pulmonary, (alveolar) and renal tubular injury, which was termed LKA, especially in patients with ARDS. Before the pandemic period, 357 patients with ARDS (without previous kidney disease) were analyzed in a retrospective study from Cleveland, USA (Panitchote, 2019). The authors pointed out that pneumonia was the cause of ARDS in 83% of patients, and 68% of patients developed AKI. Elderly patients, those with severe disease, DM, and acidosis were more likely to develop AKI in patients with ARDS. Furthermore, severity of AKI was linked with BMI, heart failure, and peak airway pressure. Table **5** summarizes systemic and cytokine-related triggering factors for AKI induced by COVID-19.

**Table 5. Mechanisms and treatment recommendations with special regard to COVID-19.**

| | Mechanism of Action | How Was AKI Induced? | Treatment Recommendations |
|---|---|---|---|
| **Systemic effects** | fluid overload | Renal compartment syndrome | ultrafiltration and diuresis |
| | Endothelial injury, fluid deficits and hypotension | Renal hypoperfusion | Vasoconstrictors, fluid replacement |
| | Rhabdomyolysis | Tubular toxicity | continuous kidney replacement therapy |
| | Endotoxins | Sepsis-induced renal injury | Endotoxin removal using polysterene fibres functionalized with polymyxin-B |
| **Cytokine storm** | Cytokine release syndrome | Direct cytokine injury | Cytokine removal: direct haemoperfusion; plasma adsorption on resin; high-dose continuous kidney replacement therapy |

# CONCLUSION

Comorbid diseases and habits including smoking, COPD, coronary artery disease, heart failure, cancer, kidney and liver failure, and obesity are linked with mortality. Therefore, prevention and management of comorbid diseases should be emphasized both in training of medical community and also the public to improve the clinical course, morbidity and mortality secondary to COVID-19.

# REFERENCES

Aggarwal, A, Rawn, JD, Pendergrass, ML & Garg, RK (2011) Long-acting subcutaneously administered insulin for glycemic control immediately after cardiac surgery. *Endocr Pract,* 17, 558-62. [http://dx.doi.org/10.4158/EP10354.OR] [PMID: 21846617]

Alpert, A & Jacobson, M (2019) Impact of oncology drug shortages on chemotherapy treatment. *Clin Pharmacol Ther,* 106, 415-21. [http://dx.doi.org/10.1002/cpt.1390] [PMID: 30739322]

Alqahtani, JS, Oyelade, T, Aldhahir, AM, Alghamdi, SM, Almehmadi, M, Alqahtani, AS, Quaderi, S, Mandal, S & Hurst, JR (2020) Prevalence, Severity and Mortality associated with COPD and Smoking in patients with COVID-19: A Rapid Systematic Review and Meta-Analysis. *PLoS One,* 15, e0233147. [http://dx.doi.org/10.1371/journal.pone.0233147] [PMID: 32392262]

Al-Shamsi, HO, Alhazzani, W, Alhuraiji, A, Coomes, EA, Chemaly, RF, Almuhanna, M, Wolff, RA, Ibrahim, NK, Chua, MLK, Hotte, SJ, Meyers, BM, Elfiki, T, Curigliano, G, Eng, C, Grothey, A & Xie, C (2020) A Practical Approach to the Management of Cancer Patients During the Novel Coronavirus Disease 2019 (COVID-19) Pandemic: An International Collaborative Group. *Oncologist,* 25, e936-45. [published online ahead of print, 2020 Apr 3]. [http://dx.doi.org/10.1634/theoncologist.2020-0213] [PMID: 32243668]

Battershill, PM (2006) Influenza pandemic planning for cancer patients. *Curr Oncol,* 13, 119-20. [http://dx.doi.org/10.3390/curroncol13040012] [PMID: 17576451]

Bourgeois, C, Gorwood, J, Barrail-Tran, A, Lagathu, C, Capeau, J, Desjardins, D, Le Grand, R, Damouche, A, Béréziat, V & Lambotte, O (2019) Specific biological features of adipose tissue, and their impact on HIV

persistence. *Front Microbiol,* 10, 2837.
[http://dx.doi.org/10.3389/fmicb.2019.02837] [PMID: 31921023]

Brake, SJ, Barnsley, K, Lu, W, McAlinden, KD, Eapen, MS & Sohal, SS (2020) Smoking upregulates angiotensin-converting enzyme-2 receptor: a potential adhesion site for novel coronavirus SARS-CoV-2 (COVID-19). *J Clin Med,* 9, E841.
[http://dx.doi.org/10.3390/jcm9030841] [PMID: 32244852]

*Coronavirus Disease 2019 (COVID-19) Daily Data Summary (NYC).* https://www1.nyc.gov/assets/doh/downloads/pdf/imm/covid-19-daily-data-summary-deaths-05132020-1.pdf

Dignani, MC, Costantini, P, Salgueira, C, Jordán, R, Guerrini, G, Valledor, A, Herrera, F, Nenna, A, Mora, C, Roccia-Rossi, I, Stecher, D, Carbone, E, Laborde, A, Efron, E, Altclas, J, Calmaggi, A & Cozzi, J (2014) Pandemic 2009 Influenza A (H1N1) virus infection in cancer and hematopoietic stem cell transplant recipients; a multicenter observational study. *F1000 Res,* 3, 221.
[http://dx.doi.org/10.12688/f1000research.5251.1] [PMID: 25469231]

Garg, S, Kim, L & Whitaker, M (2020) Hospitalization rates and characteristics of patients hospitalized with laboratory-confirmed coronavirus disease 2019—COVID-NET. *14 states,* 69, 458-64. MMWR Morb Mortal Wkly Rep

Garg, S, Kim, L, Whitaker, M, O'Halloran, A, Cummings, C, Holstein, R, Prill, M, Chai, SJ, Kirley, PD, Alden, NB, Kawasaki, B, Yousey-Hindes, K, Niccolai, L, Anderson, EJ, Openo, KP, Weigel, A, Monroe, ML, Ryan, P, Henderson, J, Kim, S, Como-Sabetti, K, Lynfield, R, Sosin, D, Torres, S, Muse, A, Bennett, NM, Billing, L, Sutton, M, West, N, Schaffner, W, Talbot, HK, Aquino, C, George, A, Budd, A, Brammer, L, Langley, G, Hall, AJ & Fry, A (2020) Hospitalization Rates and Characteristics of Patients Hospitalized with Laboratory-Confirmed Coronavirus Disease 2019 - COVID-NET, 14 States, March 1-30, 2020. *MMWR Morb Mortal Wkly Rep,* 69, 458-64.
[http://dx.doi.org/10.15585/mmwr.mm6915e3] [PMID: 32298251]

Goyal, P, Choi, JJ, Pinheiro, LC, Schenck, EJ, Chen, R, Jabri, A, Satlin, MJ, Campion, TR, Jr, Nahid, M, Ringel, JB, Hoffman, KL, Alshak, MN, Li, HA, Wehmeyer, GT, Rajan, M, Reshetnyak, E, Hupert, N, Horn, EM, Martinez, FJ, Gulick, RM & Safford, MM (2020) Clinical Characteristics of COVID-19 in New York City. *N Engl J Med,* 382, 2372-4.
[http://dx.doi.org/10.1056/NEJMc2010419] [PMID: 32302078]

Guan, WJ, Ni, ZY, Hu, Y, Liang, WH, Ou, CQ, He, JX, Liu, L, Shan, H, Lei, CL, Hui, DSC, Du, B, Li, LJ, Zeng, G, Yuen, KY, Chen, RC, Tang, CL, Wang, T, Chen, PY, Xiang, J, Li, SY, Wang, JL, Liang, ZJ, Peng, YX, Wei, L, Liu, Y, Hu, YH, Peng, P, Wang, JM, Liu, JY, Chen, Z, Li, G, Zheng, ZJ, Qiu, SQ, Luo, J, Ye, CJ, Zhu, SY & Zhong, NS China Medical Treatment Expert Group for COVID-19 (2020) Clinical characteristics of coronavirus disease 2019 in China. *N Engl J Med,* 382, 1708-20.
[http://dx.doi.org/10.1056/NEJMoa2002032] [PMID: 32109013]

Guan, WJ, Liang, WH, Zhao, Y, Liang, HR, Chen, ZS, Li, YM, Liu, XQ, Chen, RC, Tang, CL, Wang, T, Ou, CQ, Li, L, Chen, PY, Sang, L, Wang, W, Li, JF, Li, CC, Ou, LM, Cheng, B, Xiong, S, Ni, ZY, Xiang, J, Hu, Y, Liu, L, Shan, H, Lei, CL, Peng, YX, Wei, L, Liu, Y, Hu, YH, Peng, P, Wang, JM, Liu, JY, Chen, Z, Li, G, Zheng, ZJ, Qiu, SQ, Luo, J, Ye, CJ, Zhu, SY, Cheng, LL, Ye, F, Li, SY, Zheng, JP, Zhang, NF, Zhong, NS & He, JX China Medical Treatment Expert Group for COVID-19 (2020) Comorbidity and its impact on 1590 patients with COVID-19 in China: a nationwide analysis. *Eur Respir J,* 55, 2000547.
[http://dx.doi.org/10.1183/13993003.00547-2020] [PMID: 32217650]

Guan, WJ, Liang, WH, Zhao, Y, Liang, HR, Chen, ZS, Li, YM, Liu, XQ, Chen, RC, Tang, CL, Wang, T, Ou, CQ, Li, L, Chen, PY, Sang, L, Wang, W, Li, JF, Li, CC, Ou, LM, Cheng, B, Xiong, S, Ni, ZY, Xiang, J, Hu, Y, Liu, L, Shan, H, Lei, CL, Peng, YX, Wei, L, Liu, Y, Hu, YH, Peng, P, Wang, JM, Liu, JY, Chen, Z, Li, G, Zheng, ZJ, Qiu, SQ, Luo, J, Ye, CJ, Zhu, SY, Cheng, LL, Ye, F, Li, SY, Zheng, JP, Zhang, NF, Zhong, NS & He, JX China Medical Treatment Expert Group for COVID-19 (2020) Comorbidity and its impact on 1590 patients with COVID-19 in China: a nationwide analysis. *Eur Respir J,* 55, 2000547.
[http://dx.doi.org/10.1183/13993003.00547-2020] [PMID: 32217650]

Guo, FR (2020) Smoking links to the severity of COVID-19: An update of a meta-analysis. *J Med Virol,* 92,

2304-5. [published online ahead of print, 2020 May 5].
[http://dx.doi.org/10.1002/jmv.25967] [PMID: 32369203]

Guo, W, Li, M, Dong, Y, Zhou, H, Zhang, Z, Tian, C, Qin, R, Wang, H, Shen, Y, Du, K, Zhao, L, Fan, H, Luo, S & Hu, D (2020) Diabetes is a risk factor for the progression and prognosis of COVID-19. *Diabetes Metab Res Rev,* e3319, e3319. [published online ahead of print, 2020 Mar 31].
[http://dx.doi.org/10.1002/dmrr.3319] [PMID: 32233013]

Han, L, Ran, J, Mak, YW, Suen, LK, Lee, PH, Peiris, JSM & Yang, L (2019) Smoking and Influenza-associated Morbidity and Mortality: A Systematic Review and Meta-analysis. *Epidemiology,* 30, 405-17.
[http://dx.doi.org/10.1097/EDE.0000000000000984] [PMID: 30789425]

Kalyanaraman Marcello, R, Dolle, J & Grami, S (2020) Characteristics and Outcomes of COVID-19 Patients in New York City's Public Hospital System. *Preprint medRxiv.*

Kassir, R (2020) Risk of COVID-19 for patients with obesity. *Obes Rev,* 21, e13034.
[http://dx.doi.org/10.1111/obr.13034] [PMID: 32281287]

Korakas, E, Ikonomidis, I, Kousathana, F, Balampanis, K, Kountouri, A, Raptis, A, Palaiodimou, L, Kokkinos, A & Lambadiari, V (2020) Obesity and COVID-19: immune and metabolic derangement as a possible link to adverse clinical outcomes. *Am J Physiol Endocrinol Metab,* 319, E105-9.
[http://dx.doi.org/10.1152/ajpendo.00198.2020] [PMID: 32459524]

Korytkowski, M, Antinori-Lent, K & Drincic, A (2020) A Pragmatic Approach to Inpatient Diabetes Management during the COVID-19 Pandemic. *J Clin Endocrinol Metab,* 105, dgaa342.

Leung, JM, Yang, CX, Tam, A, Shaipanich, T, Hackett, TL, Singhera, GK, Dorscheid, DR & Sin, DD (2020) ACE-2 expression in the small airway epithelia of smokers and COPD patients: implications for COVID-19. *Eur Respir J,* 55, 2000688.
[http://dx.doi.org/10.1183/13993003.00688-2020] [PMID: 32269089]

Liang, W, Guan, W, Chen, R, Wang, W, Li, J, Xu, K, Li, C, Ai, Q, Lu, W, Liang, H, Li, S & He, J (2020) Cancer patients in SARS-CoV-2 infection: a nationwide analysis in China. *Lancet Oncol,* 21, 335-7.
[http://dx.doi.org/10.1016/S1470-2045(20)30096-6] [PMID: 32066541]

Movahed, MR, Khoubyari, R, Hashemzadeh, M & Hashemzadeh, M (2019) Obesity is strongly and independently associated with a higher prevalence of pulmonary embolism. *Respir Investig,* 57, 376-9.
[http://dx.doi.org/10.1016/j.resinv.2019.01.003] [PMID: 30770232]

Oakes, JM, Fuchs, RM, Gardner, JD, Lazartigues, E & Yue, X (2018) Nicotine and the renin-angiotensin system. *Am J Physiol Regul Integr Comp Physiol,* 315, R895-906.
[http://dx.doi.org/10.1152/ajpregu.00099.2018] [PMID: 30088946]

Onder, G, Rezza, G & Brusaferro, S (2020) Case-Fatality Rate and Characteristics of Patients Dying in Relation to COVID-19 in Italy. *JAMA,* 323, 1775-6. [published online ahead of print, 2020 Mar 23].
[http://dx.doi.org/10.1001/jama.2020.4683] [PMID: 32203977]

Panitchote, A, Mehkri, O, Hastings, A, Hanane, T, Demirjian, S, Torbic, H, Mireles-Cabodevila, E, Krishnan, S & Duggal, A (2019) Factors associated with acute kidney injury in acute respiratory distress syndrome. *Ann Intensive Care,* 9, 74.
[http://dx.doi.org/10.1186/s13613-019-0552-5] [PMID: 31264042]

Peng, YD, Meng, K, Guan, HQ, Leng, L, Zhu, RR, Wang, BY, He, MA, Cheng, LX, Huang, K & Zeng, QT (2020) [Clinical characteristics and outcomes of 112 cardiovascular disease patients infected by 2019-nCoV]. *Zhonghua Xin Xue Guan Bing Za Zhi,* 48, 450-5.
[http://dx.doi.org/10.3760/cma.j.cn112148-20200220-00105] [PMID: 32120458]

Petrilli, CM, Jones, SA, Yang, J, Rajagopalan, H, O'Donnell, L, Chernyak, Y, Tobin, KA, Cerfolio, RJ, Francois, F & Horwitz, LI (2020) Factors associated with hospital admission and critical illness among 5279 people with coronavirus disease 2019 in New York City: prospective cohort study. *BMJ,* 369, m1966.
[http://dx.doi.org/10.1136/bmj.m1966] [PMID: 32444366]

Redfors, B, Furer, A, Selker, HP, Thiele, H, Patel, MR, Chen, S, Udelson, JE, Ohman, EM, Eitel, I, Granger,

CB, Maehara, A, Kirtane, AJ, Généreux, P, Jenkins, PL, Ben-Yehuda, O & Stone, GW (2020) Effect of smoking on outcomes of primary PCI in patients with STEMI. *J Am Coll Cardiol,* 75, 1743-54. [http://dx.doi.org/10.1016/j.jacc.2020.02.045] [PMID: 32299585]

*Report of the WHO–China Joint Mission on Coronavirus Disease 2019 (COVID-19).* https://www.Who.Int/docs/default-source/

Richardson, S, Hirsch, JS, Narasimhan, M, Crawford, JM, McGinn, T, Davidson, KW, Barnaby, DP, Becker, LB, Chelico, JD, Cohen, SL, Cookingham, J, Coppa, K, Diefenbach, MA, Dominello, AJ, Duer-Hefele, J, Falzon, L, Gitlin, J, Hajizadeh, N, Harvin, TG, Hirschwerk, DA, Kim, EJ, Kozel, ZM, Marrast, LM, Mogavero, JN, Osorio, GA, Qiu, M & Zanos, TP the Northwell COVID-19 Research Consortium (2020) Presenting Characteristics, Comorbidities, and Outcomes Among 5700 Patients Hospitalized With COVID-19 in the New York City Area. *JAMA,* 323, 2052-9. [http://dx.doi.org/10.1001/jama.2020.6775] [PMID: 32320003]

Roncon, L, Zuin, M, Rigatelli, G & Zuliani, G (2020) Diabetic patients with COVID-19 infection are at higher risk of ICU admission and poor short-term outcome. *J Clin Virol,* 127, 104354. [http://dx.doi.org/10.1016/j.jcv.2020.104354] [PMID: 32305882]

Ryan, DH, Ravussin, E & Heymsfield, S (2020) COVID 19 and the patient with obesity—the Editors speak out. *Obesity (Silver Spring),* 28, 847. [http://dx.doi.org/10.1002/oby.22808] [PMID: 32237212]

Rychter, AM, Zawada, A, Ratajczak, AE, Dobrowolska, A & Krela-Kaźmierczak, I (2020) Should patients with obesity be more afraid of COVID-19? *Obes Rev,* 21, e13083. [http://dx.doi.org/10.1111/obr.13083] [PMID: 32583537]

Sardu, C, D'Onofrio, N, Balestrieri, ML, Barbieri, M, Rizzo, MR, Messina, V, Maggi, P, Coppola, N, Paolisso, G & Marfella, R (2020) Outcomes in Patients With Hyperglycemia Affected by COVID-19: Can We Do More on Glycemic Control? *Diabetes Care,* 43, 1408-15. [http://dx.doi.org/10.2337/dc20-0723] [PMID: 32430456]

Simonnet, A, Chetboun, M, Poissy, J, Raverdy, V, Noulette, J, Duhamel, A, Labreuche, J, Mathieu, D, Pattou, F & Jourdain, M LICORN and the Lille COVID-19 and Obesity study group (2020) High prevalence of obesity in severe acute respiratory syndrome coronavirus-2 (SARS-CoV-2) requiring invasive mechanical ventilation. *Obesity (Silver Spring),* 28, 1195-9. [http://dx.doi.org/10.1002/oby.22831] [PMID: 32271993]

Sourial, MY, Sourial, MH, Dalsan, R, Graham, J, Ross, M, Chen, W & Golestaneh, L (2020) Urgent Peritoneal Dialysis in Patients With COVID-19 and Acute Kidney Injury: A Single-Center Experience in a Time of Crisis in the United States. *Am J Kidney Dis,* 76, 401-6. [http://dx.doi.org/10.1053/j.ajkd.2020.06.001] [PMID: 32534129]

Stefan, N, Birkenfeld, AL, Schulze, MB & Ludwig, DS (2020) Obesity and impaired metabolic health in patients with COVID-19. *Nat Rev Endocrinol,* 16, 341-2. [http://dx.doi.org/10.1038/s41574-020-0364-6] [PMID: 32327737]

Suleyman, G, Fadel, RA, Malette, KM, Hammond, C, Abdulla, H, Entz, A, Demertzis, Z, Hanna, Z, Failla, A, Dagher, C, Chaudhry, Z, Vahia, A, Abreu Lanfranco, O, Ramesh, M, Zervos, MJ, Alangaden, G, Miller, J & Brar, I (2020) Clinical Characteristics and Morbidity Associated With Coronavirus Disease 2019 in a Series of Patients in Metropolitan Detroit. *JAMA Netw Open,* 3, e2012270. [http://dx.doi.org/10.1001/jamanetworkopen.2020.12270] [PMID: 32543702]

Suleyman, G, Fadel, RA, Malette, KM, Hammond, C, Abdulla, H, Entz, A, Demertzis, Z, Hanna, Z, Failla, A, Dagher, C, Chaudhry, Z, Vahia, A, Abreu Lanfranco, O, Ramesh, M, Zervos, MJ, Alangaden, G, Miller, J & Brar, I (2020) Clinical Characteristics and Morbidity Associated With Coronavirus Disease 2019 in a Series of Patients in Metropolitan Detroit. *JAMA Netw Open,* 3, e2012270. [http://dx.doi.org/10.1001/jamanetworkopen.2020.12270] [PMID: 32543702]

U.S. Food & Drug Administration. *FDA drug shortages.* https://www.accessdata.fda.gov/scripts/drugshortages/default.cfm

Uppot, RN (2018) Technical challenges of imaging & image-guided interventions in obese patients. *Br J Radiol,* 91, 20170931.
[http://dx.doi.org/10.1259/bjr.20170931] [PMID: 29869898]

Usman, MS, Siddiqi, TJ & Khan, MS (2020) Is there a smoker's paradox in COVID-19? *BMJ Evid Based Med.* [published online ahead of print, 2020 Aug 11]. bmjebm-2020-111492.

Vardavas, CI & Nikitara, K (2020) COVID-19 and smoking: A systematic review of the evidence. *Tob Induc Dis,* 18, 20.
[http://dx.doi.org/10.18332/tid/119324] [PMID: 32206052]

Yang, J, Hu, J & Zhu, C (2020) Obesity aggravates COVID-19: a systematic review and meta-analysis. *J Med Virol* [published online ahead of print, 2020 Jun 30].
[http://dx.doi.org/10.1002/jmv.26677] [PMID: 32603481]

Yang, JK, Feng, Y, Yuan, MY, Yuan, SY, Fu, HJ, Wu, BY, Sun, GZ, Yang, GR, Zhang, XL, Wang, L, Xu, X, Xu, XP & Chan, JC (2006) Plasma glucose levels and diabetes are independent predictors for mortality and morbidity in patients with SARS. *Diabet Med,* 23, 623-8.
[http://dx.doi.org/10.1111/j.1464-5491.2006.01861.x] [PMID: 16759303]

Yu, J, Ouyang, W, Chua, MLK & Xie, C (2020) SARS-CoV-2 Transmission in Patients With Cancer at a Tertiary Care Hospital in Wuhan, China. *JAMA Oncol,* 6, 1108-10. [published online ahead of print, 2020 Mar 25].
[http://dx.doi.org/10.1001/jamaoncol.2020.0980] [PMID: 32211820]

Zhao, Q, Meng, M, Kumar, R, Wu, Y, Huang, J, Lian, N, Deng, Y & Lin, S (2020) The impact of COPD and smoking history on the severity of COVID-19: A systemic review and meta-analysis. *J Med Virol,* 92, 1915-21. Epub ahead of print
[http://dx.doi.org/10.1002/jmv.25889] [PMID: 32293753]

Zhou, F, Yu, T, Du, R, Fan, G, Liu, Y, Liu, Z, Xiang, J, Wang, Y, Song, B, Gu, X, Guan, L, Wei, Y, Li, H, Wu, X, Xu, J, Tu, S, Zhang, Y, Chen, H & Cao, B (2020) Clinical course and risk factors for mortality of adult inpatients with COVID-19 in Wuhan, China: a retrospective cohort study. *Lancet,* 395, 1054-62.
[http://dx.doi.org/10.1016/S0140-6736(20)30566-3] [PMID: 32171076]

Zhou, S, Yang, Y, Zhang, X, Li, Z, Liu, X, Hu, C, Chen, C, Wang, D & Peng, Z (2020) Clinical Course of 195 Critically Ill COVID-19 Patients: A Retrospective Multicenter Study. *Shock,* 54, 644-51. [published online ahead of print, 2020 Aug 20].
[http://dx.doi.org/10.1097/SHK.0000000000001629] [PMID: 32826818]

# CHAPTER 4

# Risks and Losses of Healthcare Workers in the Pandemic Era

**Abstract:** The rapid spread of the disease has strained the health system and increased the risk of infection on healthcare workers (HCW). HCW is the group with the highest risk of transmission among all professions. Within COVID-19 deaths, HCW is overrepresented when compared to all other groups. The prevalence of the disease in the general population maintains a certain correlation with the prevalence in HCW. Resuscitative interventions and airway procedures that trigger aerosolization pose the greatest risk for disease transmission to HCW. Therefore, the use of PPE is vital. Proper training and education of HCW are invaluable in this pandemic era. Since the viral load taken in these procedures is higher than the contamination outdoors, it can be thought that the disease progresses more severe ly in the HCW than the others. In case of all viral outbreaks, hospitals should prepare and follow strict guidelines regarding ventilation of the workplaces and contact precautions.

**Keywords:** Aerosolization, COVID-19, Healthcare professionals, Healthcare workers, Nosocomial spread, Outbreak, Pandemic, Transmission.

COVID-19 disease caused by SARS-COV-2 has a clinical course with severe Acute Respiratory Distress Syndrome (ARDS) in a group of patients, which is a global health problem we face since December 2019 . As of September, there are more than 28 million patients documented in the world, more than 900,000 deaths, and almost a 4% fatality rate. The rapid spread of the disease has strained the health system and increased the risk of infection on healthcare workers (HCW) (Wei *et al.*, 2020).

**Pearl: HCW is the group with the highest risk of transmission among all professions. Within COVID-19 deaths, HCW is overrepresented when compared to all other groups.**

It has been reported that 3.5% to 20% of HCW is infected, with a mortality rate of 0.53% to 1.94% (Jennifer, 2020). In line with the data collected from all over the

Ozgur KARCIOGLU, Selman YENIOCAK and Mandana HOSSEINZADEH

world, the number of HCW that died due to COVID-19 as of July 1 has reached 1800 people from 64 countries. In Turkey, the number of physicians who died of COVID-19 until August 2020 reached 27, while 53 HCW died in total.

The prevalence of the disease in the general population maintains a certain correlation with the prevalence in HCW. Dates are based on the symptom onset day.

COVID-19 is generally transmitted by direct contact or droplets. With actions such as coughing, sneezing, intubation, tracheostomy, cardiopulmonary resuscitation (CPR), aerosols may be spread into the air and cause contamination.

## PHENOMENA PROVEN TO INCREASE THE RISK OF COVID-19 TRANSMISSION IN HCW

- Working under extreme workload and stress.
- Inadequate free time for rest, impairment of sleep quality.
- Working in high-risk units such as ED, ICU, and wards, including patients with infections.
- Lack of adaptation to working conditions.
- Inability to apply flexible working hours.
- Being unable to get paid sick leave.
- Lack of reserve employees.
- Work and environmental factors (ambient temperature, low air quality, noise *etc.*)

Based on these risks, strict protective measures should be pursued for HCW, especially ICU and ED, during all kinds of contacts with the patient, especially procedures such as CPR. Intubation boxes could be used during medical procedures concerning aerosol release. PPE (gloves, apron, protective glasses, face shields, surgical mask, FFP3 mask) should be used in contact with the patient. Hand and respiratory hygiene should be provided. Staff should be trained on PPE selection and use. HCW should act assuming all patients are infected by COVID-19, especially in endemic regions for the disease. In case of a viral outbreak, hospitals should prepare and follow strict guidelines regarding ventilation of the workplaces and contact precautions.

### Is COVID-19 Risky for HCW?

The COVID-19 pandemic increases the risk of physical illness, mental trauma, and death for all HCWs. It should be ensured that HCW operates in safe environments. Protecting HCWs should be the priority of the public authority.

The group defined as HCW is physicians, nurses and those who work in ancillary services (such as document recording, archive, human resources, cleaning) in the hospital. The riskier groups among HCW are those working in intensive care, ED, infection, and internal medicine clinics, who are in close contact with the patient, family physicians in primary care, and the nurses in these units.

In a case series of 138 patients hospitalized for COVID-19 pneumonia in Wuhan, China, hospital-acquired (nosocomial) infections were found responsible for 41.3% of all COVID-19 transmissions. In the same study, 29% (n: 40) of the patients hospitalized due to COVID-19 pneumonia are HCW (Wang *et al*, 2020).

SARS-COV2 can travel long distances as aerosol droplets smaller than 5 μm. Depending on the ambient conditions, they can fly in the air for 2-4 hours. Human coronavirus can survive up to 5 days at 22-25 ° C, while the humidity is 40-50% in inanimate objects.

It has been reported that SARS COV2 can stay alive for up to 9 days on certain surfaces at room temperature. In an experimental study, it was observed that SARS COV2 has a viability of 72 hours on plastic surfaces, 48 hours on stainless steel and 8 hours on copper (COVID-19: Guidance for infection prevention and control in healthcare settings. Version 1.0).

## How much Risk COVID-19 Impose on HCW?

The data on the number and distribution of infected HCW are very limited in the world. In line with the data obtained from 30 countries, it is stated that an average of 6% (between 0 to 18%) of all confirmed COVID-19 cases are HCW. When calculated over 3.5 million cases, International Council of Nurses calculated that 210 thousand HCWs are infected, in the first period of the pandemic (ICN 2020-International Council of Nurses). When we extrapolate this hypothesis to August 2020, there should be almost a million HCW among 23 million inflicted cases. For example, 20% of HCWs have been infected in Italy (Godderis *et al*, 2020).

## HEADLINES FROM VARIOUS COUNTRIES

- On February 11, 2020, 1716 HCWs were diagnosed with COVID 19 according to the records of the Chinese disease control and prevention center (Wei *et al*, 2020).
- 19% of the patients with occupational records in the USA are HCW. Only 8 to 10% of these cases were hospitalized (CDC - MMWR, 2020).
- According to data from the Brazilian Ministry of Health, as of 6 August 2020, at

least 232,992 HCW were diagnosed with COVID-19, 196 of which died (https://www.voanews.com/covid-19-pandemic/icrc-essential-workers-brazil-face-high-risk-coronavirus-fight).

- As of July 2020, 7.985 HCW have been diagnosed with COVID-19 in Ukraine (https://qha.com.tr/haberler/ukrayna-da-koronavirus-durumu-yaklasik-8-bin-saglik-calisani-kovid-19-a-caught/226251/).
- Since February, 138 **HCW** have 'officially' died in Iran due to COVID-19 (https://www.haber7.com/dunya/haber/2997333-koronaviruste-son-dak-ka-development-brazya-meksika-ve-ndistanda-olu-sayisi-artista/?detail=2).
- In accord with the data collected by Medscape from 64 countries, the number of HCW who lost their lives due to COVID-19 reached 1800 people as of July 1 (https://www.medscape.com/viewarticle/927976).

**As of September 2020, Americas, India, Russia, South Africa and some parts of Europe and Asia had substantial rates of HCW killed or injured by the COVID-19.**

In a study conducted to analyze the personnel and environmental protection status of an advanced medical center in Wuhan, Zhang *et al.* reported that No SARS-CoV-2 RNA was detected in 48 air and environmental samples after regular disinfection and cleaning (Zhang *et al*, 2020).

Before the COVID-19 outbreak, 82.64% of the HCWs had already known the proper procedure of wearing masks and other personal protective equipment (PPE). Of note, 99.8% of 634 participants entering the inpatient areas have undergone occupational protection trainings. 7.8% experienced different types of occupational exposure, which mainly caused by the damage of PPE. In conclusion, a 'bundle approach' including intensive training, strengthened personal protection, strict environmental disinfection and timely remedial measures for occupational exposure had ensured the safety of the HCW (Zhang *et al*, 2020).

## THE SITUATION IN TURKEY

The Turkish Medical Association (TMA) has accessed and evaluated the information of 902 HCW with COVID-19 *via* online forms. Of those, 77.8% had been employed in hospitals, 18.2% in primary care institutions (mainly Family Health Centers), 2.4% in administrative units and 1.4% in cleaning works. 13.4% of those diagnosed with COVID-19 are employees of internal medicine and its sub-branches, 9.3% ED, 7.0% were working in chest diseases, 5.0% in operating rooms and ICU and 1.9% of them in laboratories.

Turkish Minister of Health, Dr. Fahrettin Koca announced that on April 29, 2020, COVID-19 infection was identified in 7428 HCW. On June 1, the TMA's Monitoring Board for COVID-19 shared with Human Rights Watch (HRW) that up to 11,000 HCWs were also infected by COVID-19 (https://www.hrw.org/tr/news/2020/06/09/375368).

In Turkey, the number of physicians died of COVID-19 till September 2020 reached to 28, while HCWs were 55 (https://www.ttb.org.tr/kollar/covıd19/haber_goster.php?guid=80783f90- d651-11ea-9c50-7fbe39e4ca48) .

## SITUATIONS INCREASING THE RISK OF INFECTION TO HCW

Analyzing 118 COVID-19-infected HCWs in Wuhan, China, Bai *et al.* reported that a large proportion of cases were on night shifts (75% *vs.* 40% in non-infected HCWs) stated that they had been working too much and under pressure (67% *vs.* 32% in non-infected HCWs) (Bai, 2020).

Furthermore, the researchers applied the Pittsburgh Sleep Quality Index (PSQI) and The Nurse Stress Index (NSI) and found that higher scores on both scales increased the likelihood of being infected with COVID-19. In brief, poor sleep quality and working under stress boosted the risk of COVID-19. Mean shift time during which personal protective equipment (PPE) is used without breaks is calculated as 4 hours for both doctors and nurses. Adverse effects (80%) were reported as temperature (51%), thirst (47%), pressure areas (44%), headache 28%), inability to use a bath (27%) and burnout (20%). All of these effects have been associated with the shift times in which PPE had to be used (Tabah *et al*, 2020).

Close and protracted contact with a patient with COVID-19 includes these procedures:

- Taking a sample from the respiratory tract (throat swab)
- Intubation
- Aspiration of airway secretions
- Non-invasive ventilation
- High-flow oxygen therapy
- CPR
- Nebulizer use
- Endoscopic procedures
- Bronchoscopy
- Videolaryngoscopy

- Dental procedures
- Oral ENT and ophthalmological examination
- Insertion of central catheters

Resuscitative interventions pose the greatest risk for disease transmission to HCW. Therefore, the use of PPE is vital. Since the viral load taken in these procedures is higher than the contamination outdoors, it can be thought that the disease progresses more severe in the HCW than the others.

## Findings

14 HCW who contacted two patients hospitalized in Neurosurgery Clinic in Wuhan without knowing that they had COVID-19 were analyzed and published. Mean age of these cases was 36, and 10 (28%) of them were women. The most common complaints were muscle pain, weakness/fatigue, fever, and cough (between 100% and 71%). The frequency of diarrhea was 64% at the beginning and gradually decreased. In the initial workup, 79% had leukopenia and 43% lymphopenia, and bilateral ground glass opacities were noted in 86% in chest CT (Wei, 2020).

## Precautions and Measures

Based on the risks, HCW should take the highest possible precautions in all contacts with the patient, especially procedures such as CPR. Being informed on the degree of environmental contamination of SARS-CoV-2 is important in improving safety practices for HCW.

In the study conducted by Guo *et al*. In Wuhan, China, it was found that the virus was widely distributed on floors, computer mice, trash cans and hospital bed railings, and it was found in the air around 4 m away from the patients. The highest positivity rates are in order, computer mice, garbage cans, hospital bed handrails, doorknobs. According to the results of the study, it was determined that there was more contamination in ICU compared to wards. Therefore, more stringent protective measures should be taken by the HCW staffed in the ICU.

Half of the samples taken from shoe soles of HCW in ICU were tested positive. Therefore, medical personnel shoe soles can act as carriers. Before leaving units containing COVID-19 patients, it is important for people to disinfect their shoe soles.

The efficiency of plastic box barriers to protect HCWs during medical procedures related to aerosol dispersion have been investigated. It has been noted that these barriers are more effective in preventing the spread than conventional approaches. Intubation boxes, which surround the patient's head and have two holes used by the intubating person to put in arms, are one of the methods to prevent aerosolization (Figs. **1 A & B**). In cough and droplet simulation studies with fluorescent dyes, it was observed that the laryngoscopist reduced the spread to the gloves and arms (Jazuli *et al*, 2020).

A B

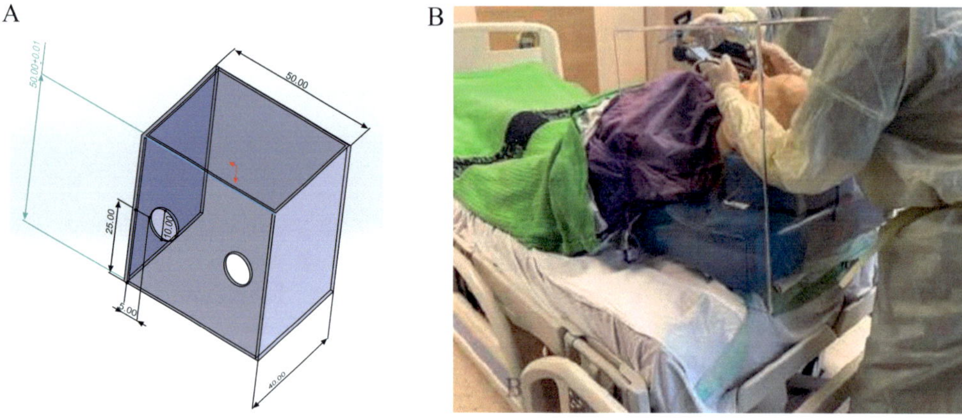


**Fig. (1A & 1B).** Intubation boxes, which surround the patient's head and have two holes used by the intubating person to put in arms, are methods to prevent aerosolization (https://litfl.com/should-we-use-an-aerosol-box-for-intubation/).

Sporadic positive results were obtained from the gloves and sleeves of the medical personnel. This shows that HCW should apply hand hygiene immediately after any contact with the patients.

Staff should be trained on PPE selection and use. In case of a viral outbreak, hospitals should prepare and follow strict guidelines regarding ventilation of the workplaces and contact precautions.

## Personal Protective Equipment

1. Gloves and aprons
2. **Eye protection:** Birshoff *et al*. were the first to report the intraocular spread of influenza virus. This trend has also been found for the current COVID 19 pandemics. Despite all the protective clothing and N95 mask, one of the experts was found to be infected. The initial finding was unilateral conjunctivitis. For this reason, protective glasses and face shields are recommended.
3. **Masks and respirators:** Surgical masks are liquid resistant. They filter particles, droplets, and bacteria. Since they are not designed with a tight sealing

feature, they allow unfiltered air to enter from the edges. They do not have the ability to filter very small particles. They do not provide respiratory protection. They only prevent large droplets or infectious body fluids from passing directly through the mucosal membrane of the mouth and nose. When worn by patients, they reduce the amount and concentration of large infectious particles during coughing, sneezing, and talking, reducing the risk of contamination to other people. The failure rate of surgical masks has been reported to be 10% to 90%.

4. **Gas masks:** N95 masks and "*Powered Air Purifying Respirators*" (PAPR)

**N95 masks:** SARS-COV2 is recommended for HCW to work at a distance of less than 2 meters to suspected patient. Birschoff *et al.* studied with influenza contact models and reported that people who wear N95 and protective goggles experienced 90% effective protection. Studies on the long-term effectiveness of N95 masks are limited and most of them are laboratory studies.

It has been established that in the H1N1 pandemic, most of the HCW can only tolerate the use of N95 for 8 to 12 hours. Furthermore, many HCWs are reluctant to wear N95, use it in breaks and wear it continuously for a maximum of 4 hours. N95 masks should be discarded when contaminated, damaged, or made it difficult to breathe.

In highly suspected SARS-CoV-2 cases, N95 masks used should be disposable. It has been reported that N95 masks render communication difficult, cause excessive heat, pain and pressure on the face, headache, itching and burning in the eyes, cause nausea, dizziness, concentration difficulty, and impair practice of procedures.

**PAPR (*Powered Air Purifying Respirators*):** An engine powered by a battery filters the air and distributes it through the box with positive pressure from the hood or face piece. Thanks to this positive pressure, contaminated air outside cannot enter. The most commonly used masks are filter face masks and PAPRs. Respirators provide more effective protection than masks in aerosol dispersion. If available, PAPRs should be used in high-risk procedures.

Compared to N95, PAPRs have a higher protection factor (APF 25). They filter 99.97% of the 0.3 m particles and are resistant to oil. Long term use is more comfortable than other devices, with no adaptation problem. It covers the entire face and head. However, its cost is high.

The protective equipment recommendations in the SARS-CoV epidemic in 2003 and the recommendations for COVID-19 are slightly different. For SARS-COV in 2003, it was advocated that both masks and surgical masks had similar protection, and the infection reduction rate was 80%. However, while N95 masks are not promoted for COVID-19 in the USA, FFP3 (BS EN 149.200 compliant) masks are recommended.

After the processes that emit aerosol, the rooms must be ventilated mechanically or naturally. Natural ventilation should be at least 6 air changes per hour, negative ventilation should be 12 air changes per hour *(COVID-19: Guidance for infection prevention and control in healthcare settings. Version 1.0).*

## Sequence of Control Measures

- Early evaluation and triage of cases
- Report the patients
- Fulfilling control measures
- Reserve a separate place for suspected or confirmed COVID-19 patients
- Training of staff, patient, and visitor in regard to standard infection control and transmission-based measures
- Expediting measures to limit contamination
- Restricting visitor access
- Restrict symptomatic staff from working until they are fully recovered
- Development of planning and implementation strategies for overflow capacity

## Infection Protection and Control Measures

1) Standard infection control measures

2) Contagion-based measures

### 1. Standard Precautions

a. **Patient evaluation and triage:** COVID-19 patients should be evaluated and isolated/separated from others immediately.
b. **Hand hygiene:** Before and after contact with the patient, after removing the PPE, hand hygiene must be provided. If there is visible dirt and contamination on the hands, hand washing with soapy water, if not, hand hygiene should be provided with an alcohol-based hand disinfectant. Hand washing should take at least 40-60 seconds to inactivate the virus. Alcohol-based hand sanitizer should be easily accessible to all personnel.
c. **Respiratory and cough hygiene:** Patients should use wipes during coughing and sneezing and wear a liquid-resistant surgical face mask in closed areas.
d. **PPE (Disposable gowns/clothes/gloves, goggles/face shields):** All personnel should be trained about which PPE to use and where to get them.
e. **Management of used clothes:** All dirty clothes should be left in the patient

room or in the designated collection area, and the containers for clothes should be in the easiest place to reach.

f. **Personnel Uniforms and Clothes:** These must be protected by wearing PPE. There should be a separate designated dressing room for HCW. Specialized laundry services should be used for staff uniforms. If this cannot be achieved, it should be carried home in disposable plastic bags. It should be separated from other laundry at home.
g. **Management of bloodstain and bloody fluid splashes:** Management varies according to the contaminated material. If PPE is contaminated with blood, urine, vomit, faeces, or if it comes into contact with an infected patient, wipe it with a disposable cloth / paper towel or detergent, rinse and dry. Chlorinated disinfectant solution is applied and dried.
h. **Medical and non-medical waste management:** These should be managed in accordance with the procedures.

### Contamination-Based Precautions

Droplet precautions should be known to all HCW besides standard precautions.

**Duration of Precautions:** Patients should be kept in isolation until the patient's fever and respiratory symptoms have resolved. If the symptoms of the patients regressed and are clinically improved, they may be recommended to be discharged home and continue isolation at home.

### Separating Inpatients

a. **Negative pressure isolation rooms:** Negative pressure rooms are not always required to prevent COVID 19 transmission, but early stage and high risk COVID-19 patients can be isolated in these rooms.
b. **Separate room (Single room):** Patients should be isolated in separate rooms if possible. However, in periods when the epidemic increases, single isolation rooms may be insufficient.
c. **Separate areas in the room:** If a single room cannot be provided, patients should be hospitalized in separate areas from other COVID 19 patients. The distance between patients should be guaranteed to be at least 1 meter. Curtains can be used between patients. The area where the patient entrances are reserved should be accessed from another door. Other patients, healthcare professionals and visitors should not use these doors.
d. **Separation of personnel:** If the number of personnel is sufficient, those who care for COVID-19 patients and those who care for other patients should be separated.
e. **Separation of Visitors:** Patient visitors should be restricted, only the main

caregiver of nursing patients and parents of children should be accepted. Visitors should also wear PPE and be informed about hand hygiene.

## Patient Transfer and Transport

a. **In-hospital transfer:** Patients should not be transferred to another area unless necessary, and if they have to, they should definitely use a surgical mask. Patients should not be kept in public areas.
b. **Patient transfer from primary care units to other facilities:** Ambulance team should be warned. The transferred center should be informed that the patient has COVID-19.
c. **Transfer between hospitals:** Patients should not be transferred unless medically mandated (dialysis, cardiac angioplasty, *etc*.).
d. **PPE**
    a. Fluid resistant surgical face masks:
        - All nose and mouth should be covered
        - Masks should not hang around the neck.
        - Should not be touched after wearing
        - It must be replaced when it is damaged or wetted.
        - It should be taken off after leaving the patient room.
        - Must be worn once and thrown into medical waste bin.
    b. FFP3 masks:
        - It should be used in ICU and similar units during procedures that emit aerosol.
        - Must be disposable and liquid resistant.
        - All personnel should be trained in proper fitting.
        - It should be compatible with other protective equipment (such as eye protection).
        - It should not be used if proper facial adaptation is not provided and breathing becomes difficult.
        - FFP3 must be used with the face shields if it is not liquid resistant.
e. **Aerosol-related interventions:** The following aerosol-related interventions should be performed in a separate area only in the presence of the necessary personnel, with disposable gowns, gloves, eye protection and FFP3 mask.
    - Intubation, extubation
    - Tracheotomy, tracheostomy
    - Manual ventilation
    - Open aspiration
    - Bronchoscopy
    - Noninvasive ventilation (NIV) • BiPAP, CPAP
    - Surgical and postmortem interventions

- High frequency oscillating ventilation (HFOV)
- High flow nasal oxygen (HFNO)
- Some dental procedures

f. **Equipment Management and Environmental maintenance**

a. Equipment:

- Patient care equipment should be for single use, if possible.
- Reusable equipment should be placed away from the patient care area.
- Equipment should be cleaned at regular intervals between each patient or after use, after contamination with blood or bloody fluids.
- Ventilators must be protected with high efficiency filters (HEPA filter).
- Closed system aspirators should be used.

b. Environmental care:

- Patient isolation / examination rooms should be decontaminated at least once a day.
- Examination rooms should be decontaminated after every suspected / diagnosed COVID-19 patient.

g. **Measures for healthcare personnel to work during the epidemic period:**

- HCW with symptoms should not come to work.
- Where possible, staff dealing with suspected patients should not care for other patients.
- Risky or pregnant HCW should not work in services with patients with COVID-19.
- A multifaceted and global strategy to protect HCW from high-risk infection should be developed.

**Pearl: In regions where the disease is endemic, HCW should be protected by acting with a presumption that all patients have COVID-19.**

## Psychosocial Problems in HCW During The Pandemics

In addition to all these, the mental health of HCW is also of utmost importance. In a study comparing medical (n = 927) and non-medical HCW (n = 1255) with special regard to psychosocial problems experienced during the COVID-19 pandemic, insomnia (38.4% *vs*. 30.5%, $p < 0.01$), anxiety (13% *vs*. 8.5%, $p < 0.01$), depression (12.2% *vs*. 9.5%; $p < 0.04$), somatization (1.6% *vs*. 0.4%; $p < 0.01$), and obsessive-compulsive symptoms (5.3% *vs*. 2.2%; $p < 0.01$) were significantly more common in medical HCW. Having an organic disease, living in the countryside, female sex, assuming the risk of contact with a COVID-19 patient are the most common risk factors for insomnia, anxiety, obsessive-compulsive symptoms, and depression (Zhang WR *et al*, 2020).

In a study conducted in terms of mental health on a total of 1521 healthcare workers in China, 147 of whom had a community health /ED experience during the pandemic era, 1374 of whom had no experience, those who had worked in an ED performed worse (Cai *et al*, 2020). Again, in a study conducted in China, it was observed that healthcare personnel who had direct contact with the patient were more exposed to anxiety symptoms (Liu CY *et al*, 2020).

According to the findings of a multicenter study conducted with 1563 HCW in Guangzhou, the rate of depression was 51%, anxiety 45%, insomnia 36% and distress symptoms 73% in HCWs (Liu *et al*, 2020).

In a recent systematic review and meta-analysis, Pappa *et al.* highlighted very high prevalence rates of depression, anxiety, and insomnia among healthcare workers during the COVID-19 pandemic: 22.8%, 23.2% and 34%, respectively (Pappa *et al*, 2020). The authors emphasized on the need to institute solutions to alleviate mental health risks and adjust interventions for HCW worldwide.

Salazar *et al.* searched for the mental disturbances from which HCW suffered most (Salazar *et al*, 2020). They have compared the complaints and symptoms HCW reported in COVID-19 pandemics with those recorded in SARS and MERS outbreaks. Results indicated that COVID-19 lead to insomnia more frequently than the other disease outbreaks, while SARS was associated in insomnia more commonly than the others did (Fig. **2**) .

Many HCWs working during the pandemic stayed in different places from their families in order not to infect their families with the virus. The fear of infecting the family of those who do not have the opportunity to stay away from the family can also lead to psychosocial problems.

For all these reasons, more psychological and social support should be given to HCW in the front line during the pandemic period. Suspected HCW should be given effective mental health measurements and offered special support.

## What kind of Interventions can be Pursued to Support The Resilience and Mental Health of Frontline HCW During The Pandemic?

It is a harder question to address sufficiently. Pollock *et al.* very recently searched for these vital answers (Pollock *et al*, 2020). The authors are "moderately confident that the following two factors were barriers to intervention implementation: frontline workers, or the organizations in which they worked, not being fully aware of what they needed to support their mental well-being; and a lack of equipment, staff time or skills needed for an intervention". They also pointed out that the following three factors were facilitators of intervention implementation: interventions that could be adapted for local needs; having effective communication, both formally and socially; and having positive, safe, and supportive learning environments for frontline workers. Also, the knowledge or beliefs, or both, that people have about an intervention can act as either barriers or facilitators to implementation of the intervention. These issues should be subjected to further population-based research which can enlighten the possible measures for these impairments for HCW.

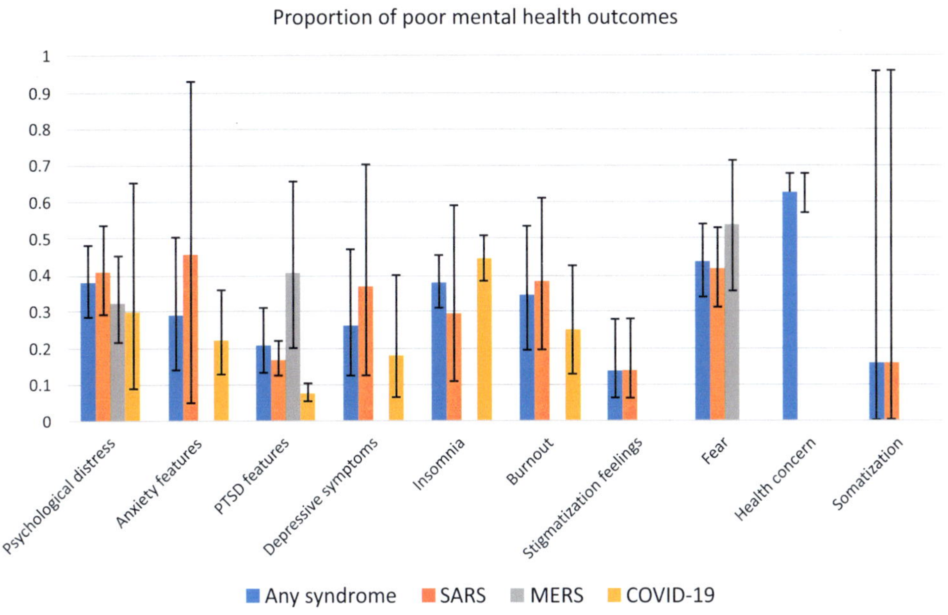


**Fig. (2).** Distribution of the complaints and symptoms HCW reported in COVID-19 pandemics in comparison to those recorded in SARS and MERS outbreaks. (Adapted from Salazar *et al.* 2020).

## IS THERE ANY GOOD NEWS TO CONVEY?

Yes. A recently published systematic review and meta-analysis pointed out that although HCW carry the highest risk for contracting the disease, they have a less severe clinical course and a significantly lower mortality risk when compared to the general population (Sahu *et al*, 2020). The overall proportion of HCW (varies with the regions and countries) who had the disease among all COVID-19 patients was 10%. The incidence of severe or critical disease in HCW (10%) was significantly lower ($p < 0.001$) than the incidence of severe or critical disease in all COVID-19 positive patients (29%). Likewise, the death toll among HCW (0.3%) is remarkably lower ($p < 0.001$) when compared to the whole population (2.3%). This can be attributed to easier access to healthcare, testing and treatment measures by the HCW as compared to the lay people worldwide, especially in underdeveloped regions.

HCWs on all the world need the support and appreciation of the public and governments not to remain heroes, just to get credit that they deserve.

**Pearl: Protecting HCWs should be the priority of the public authority or 'state'. In other words, it is out of question to protect a society where HCW cannot be protected.**

**Summary: How Should Healthcare Professionals Work in the Hospital During the Pandemic Period?**

- A uniform should be worn at the hospital
- Uniforms worn in the hospital should be washed with normal detergent at least 60 degrees each time, and if possible, they should not be worn inside the house.
- Separate shoes, or slippers should be reserved at the hospital, they should be removed before entering the house, or left at the hospital
- Hands should be washed up to the elbows before leaving the hospital.
- Cell phone should be wiped with disinfectant when leaving the hospital
- Stethoscopes should not be hung around the neck.
- No nail polish should be used
- Long hair should be tied
- Nails should be kept short
- Jewellery that prevents washing such as watches, rings, and the like should not be worn in the hospital.

## CONCLUSION

Findings show that most countries have failed to protect their HCW. The COVID-19 pandemic increases the risk of physical illness, mental trauma, and death for all HCWs. These entities should be examined separately, and it should be ensured that the HCW works in safe environments.

If it is necessary to make concrete suggestions, medical needs, storage, and distribution programs including PPE should be developed during pandemic periods. A rational system for equipment distribution, allocation and utilization should be formed with the participation of professional associations, chambers, and trade unions. Only in this way is the damage to both HCW and society minimized and preparation for the next pandemic can be implemented as required.

# REFERENCES

Bai, Y, Wang, X & Huang, Q (2020) SARS-CoV-2 infection in health care workers: a retrospective analysis and model study. *Preprint from medRxiv.* [http://dx.doi.org/10.1101/2020.03.29.20047159]

Cai, W, Lian, B, Song, X, Hou, T, Deng, G & Li, H (2020) A cross-sectional study on mental health among health care workers during the outbreak of Corona Virus Disease 2019. *Asian J Psychiatr,* 51102111 [http://dx.doi.org/10.1016/j.ajp.2020.102111] [PMID: 32361388]

CDC COVID-19 Response Team (2020) Characteristics of Health Care Personnel with COVID-19 - United States, February 12–April 9, 2020. Weekly / April 17, 69, 477-81.

COVID-19: Guidance for infection prevention and control in healthcare settings. Version 1.0. (2020) COVID-19: a new work-related disease threatening healthcare workers. *Occup Med (Lond),* 70, 315-6.

Godderis, L, Boone, A & Bakusic, J (2020) COVID-19: a new work-related disease threatening healthcare workers. *Occup Med (Lond),* 70, 315-6. [http://dx.doi.org/10.1093/occmed/kqaa056] [PMID: 32359148]

Jazuli, F, Bilic, M, Hanel, E, Ha, M, Hassall, K & Trotter, BG (2020) Endotracheal intubation with barrier protection. *Emerg Med J,* 37, 398-9. [http://dx.doi.org/10.1136/emermed-2020-209785] [PMID: 32482759]

Ha, JF (2020) The COVID-19 pandemic, personal protective equipment and respirator: A narrative review. *Int J Clin Pract,* 74e13578 [http://dx.doi.org/10.1111/ijcp.13578] [PMID: 32511834]

Liu, CY, Yang, YZ, Zhang, XM, Xu, X, Dou, QL, Zhang, WW & Cheng, ASK (2020) The prevalence and influencing factors in anxiety in medical workers fighting COVID-19 in China: a cross-sectional survey. *Epidemiol Infect,* 148e98 [http://dx.doi.org/10.1017/S0950268820001107] [PMID: 32430088]

Liu, S, Yang, L, Zhang, C, Xiang, YT, Liu, Z, Hu, S & Zhang, B (2020) Online mental health services in China during the COVID-19 outbreak. *Lancet Psychiatry,* 7, e17-8. [http://dx.doi.org/10.1016/S2215-0366(20)30077-8] [PMID: 32085841]

Pappa, S, Ntella, V, Giannakas, T, Giannakoulis, VG, Papoutsi, E & Katsaounou, P (2020) Prevalence of depression, anxiety, and insomnia among healthcare workers during the COVID-19 pandemic: A systematic review and meta-analysis. *Brain Behav Immun,* 88, 901-7. [http://dx.doi.org/10.1016/j.bbi.2020.05.026] [PMID: 32437915]

Pollock, A, Campbell, P, Cheyne, J, Cowie, J, Davis, B, McCallum, J, McGill, K, Elders, A, Hagen, S, McClurg, D, Torrens, C & Maxwell, M (2020) Interventions to support the resilience and mental health of frontline health and social care professionals during and after a disease outbreak, epidemic or pandemic: a mixed methods systematic review. *Cochrane Database Syst Rev,* 11CD013779 [PMID: 33150970]

Sahu, AK, Amrithanand, VT, Mathew, R, Aggarwal, P, Nayer, J & Bhoi, S (2020) COVID-19 in health care workers - A systematic review and meta-analysis. *Am J Emerg Med,* 38, 1727-31. [http://dx.doi.org/10.1016/j.ajem.2020.05.113] [PMID: 32738467]

Salazar de Pablo, G, Vaquerizo-Serrano, J, Catalan, A, Arango, C, Moreno, C, Ferre, F, Shin, JI, Sullivan, S, Brondino, N, Solmi, M & Fusar-Poli, P (2020) Impact of coronavirus syndromes on physical and mental health of health care workers: Systematic review and meta-analysis. *J Affect Disord,* 275, 48-57. [http://dx.doi.org/10.1016/j.jad.2020.06.022] [PMID: 32658823]

Tabah, A, Ramanan, M, Laupland, KB, Buetti, N, Cortegiani, A, Mellinghoff, J, Conway Morris, A, Camporota, L, Zappella, N, Elhadi, M, Povoa, P, Amrein, K, Vidal, G, Derde, L, Bassetti, M, Francois, G, Ssi Yan Kai, N & De Waele, JJ (2020) Personal protective equipment and intensive care unit healthcare worker safety in the COVID-19 era (PPE-SAFE): An international survey. *J Crit Care,* 59, 70-5. [http://dx.doi.org/10.1016/j.jcrc.2020.06.005] [PMID: 32570052]

Wang, D, Hu, B, Hu, C, Zhu, F, Liu, X, Zhang, J, Wang, B, Xiang, H, Cheng, Z, Xiong, Y, Zhao, Y, Li, Y, Wang, X & Peng, Z (2020) Clinical Characteristics of 138 Hospitalized Patients With 2019 Novel Coronavirus-Infected Pneumonia in Wuhan, China. *JAMA,* 323, 1061-9. [http://dx.doi.org/10.1001/jama.2020.1585] [PMID: 32031570]

Wei, XS, Wang, XR & Zhang, JC A cluster of health care workers with COVID-19 pneumonia caused by SARS-CoV-2. *J Microbiol Immunol Infect,* S1684-1182, 30107-9.

Zhang, M, Wang, L, Yu, S, Sun, G, Lei, H & Wu, W (2020) Status of occupational protection in the COVID-19 *Fangcang* Shelter Hospital in Wuhan, China. *Emerg Microbes Infect,* 9, 1835-42. [http://dx.doi.org/10.1080/22221751.2020.1803145] [PMID: 32726187]

Zhang, WR, Wang, K, Yin, L, Zhao, WF, Xue, Q, Peng, M, Min, BQ, Tian, Q, Leng, HX, Du, JL, Chang, H, Yang, Y, Li, W, Shangguan, FF, Yan, TY, Dong, HQ, Han, Y, Wang, YP, Cosci, F & Wang, HX (2020) Mental Health and Psychosocial Problems of Medical Health Workers during the COVID-19 Epidemic in China. *Psychother Psychosom,* 89, 242-50. [http://dx.doi.org/10.1159/000507639] [PMID: 32272480]

# CHAPTER 5

# What Kind of Disease is this? Signs and Symptoms, Predictors of Clinical Course and Management

**Abstract:** COVID-19 affects almost every organ and system in the body, depending on the severity of the disease, viral load, and host factors. In definition, the complex (ACE2) receptors – protein S of the virus leads to the involvement of various tissues and organs. ACE2 receptors are present on most cells, inducing cardiovascular symptoms, kidney disease, and neurological involvement. Complaints and findings such as fever, dry cough, and weakness are predominant in many large series . However, shortness of breath almost invariably predicts a more severe disease course in most patients. More rarely, neurological, gastrointestinal, or dermatological complaints and findings are also noted, mostly in conjunction with other signs. Laboratory and radiological adjuncts are mostly the keys for an expedient diagnosis and management, especially in institutions with a high number of admissions in a time unit. The clinician should be alert on how to interpret hallmarks of the disease, which can predict a grave outcome and severe course in any given patient.

**Keywords:** Clinical course, COVID-19, Outbreak, Pandemic, Signs and symptoms.

In a myriad of case reports, complaints and findings such as fever, dry cough, and weakness are predominant. There is fever in 35% to 98% of the reported cases, fatigue / weakness in 65% to 70%, dry cough in 60%, shortness of breath in 30% to 60%, and muscle pain in 50% to 70%. These percentages can vary substantially, depending on the geographical and temporal variation, as well as sampling characteristics, *etc*. (Table **1**).

As a rule, vital signs (pulse rate, blood pressure, consciousness, temperature) may be normal on presentation to the hospital. Likewise, asymptomatic cases have been reported in the literature with a wide range between 17 and 87%.

**Ozgur KARCIOGLU, Selman YENIOCAK and Mandana HOSSEINZADEH**

## DO PATIENTS WHO ARE DIAGNOSED NECESSARILY HAVE SYMPTOMS?

A total of 2824 cases were included in a study conducted during the rise of the epidemic in Italy (Poletti, 2020). It was reported that only 31% of the patients who were diagnosed serologically or with RT-PCR developed symptoms at the time of diagnosis.

**Table 1. Common symptoms of COVID-19 in the first months of the pandemic. Data source: CCDC 2020 (data as of February 11, 2020).**

| Symptoms | Percentage (%) |
| --- | --- |
| Diarrhea | 3 |
| Hemoptysis | 5 |
| Headache | 8 |
| Sputum production | 28 |
| Myalgia | 44 |
| Cough | 76 |
| Fever | 98 |

Patients without fever / respiratory symptoms

- 4% under 60

Symptomatic patients in the range of 18%-65%

- 18% under 20
- 65% over the age of 80

Critical patients

- under 60 years old 0.54%
- 6.6% over the age of 60

The risk of turning into a critical patient is higher in men.

- Among those with RT PCR +, those who were symptomatic and those without symptoms were found to have similar viral loads (Oran, 2020).
- The presence / absence of symptoms on presentation was not associated with gender

**The rate of critical cases in men between the ages of 60-80 is significantly higher than that of women. Women are more likely to be symptomatic then men between the ages of 20-40.**

## ASYMPTOMATIC AND SYMPTOMATIC... IS THERE A 3RD WAY?

Yes. A group of cases were called **'presymptomatic'** because they were first asymptomatic and then symptomatic (Oran, 2020). Since this can be seen in a group between 10% and 89%, there are large variations according to geography and population. For example, asymptomatic cases have been reported up to 96% in 4 different prisons in the USA, which suggests that patients and/or officials have difficulty reporting and recording their symptoms (So, 2020). This can occur because the recommended 6 feet of separation for social distancing necessitates an approximate 28 sq. foot area for each detainee, which exceeds the minimum 25 sq. foot standard published by the American Correctional Association (Irvine, 2020).

Publishing a systematic review of more than 24,000 adult diagnosed cases, Grant *et al.* reported the total death rate as 7% and listed the complaints on presentation as follows: (Grant, 2020):

Fever 78%

Cough 57%

Fatigue 31%

NIV was performed in 19% of hospitalized patients (44 studies)

17% of them prompted admission to ICU (33 studies)

ETI + MV was performed in 9% (45 studies)

ECMO was applied in 2% (12 studies)

In conclusion, the authors reported that fever and cough were the most common complaints, but a diagnosis could not be made solely on the basis of symptoms in a significant proportion of patients (Grant, 2020)

The rate of fever and cough in confirmed cases is reported differently in different countries. Fever is noted in an average of 78% of cases and a dry or productive cough is observed in 57% (Grant, 2020).

Fever is not present in the patient every time in the clinical course, it waxes and wanes or follows a fluctuating curve. Therefore, the absence of fever in a patient at a given time point does not prove that the patient did not have fever, but that we could not find it at that time. If the patient says that he has a fever while at home or workplace, he/she should be believed in.

Sputum production has been reported at a rate of or 1/3. Gastrointestinal complaints (diarrhea-vomiting, abdominal pain) can be found around 10% to 40%. While tachypnea is found in 1 of 3 cases, it is mostly recorded in cases admitted to ICU.

The most important point is that no patient can be exactly like another, and the 'classical' pattern of findings and complaints should not be sought fully in a given patient.

Fever and cough were more common in children than in adults. Shortness of breath and muscle-joint pain are seen mostly in adults and the elderly.

**Less Common Findings (Chen, 2020)**

Headache in 8% of cases.

Hemoptysis (bleeding with coughing) in 5% of cases.

Diarrhea has been reported in up to 2% of cases in Chen's series. However, the frequency of diarrhea is much higher in cases in many countries. Whether this is due to the mutation of the virus or unique characteristics of these populations is open to research.

**Periods in the Course of the Disease**

While a significant improvement is observed within 3-5 days in other flu syndromes, COVID-19 cases gradually worsen within 7-8 days.

In most series 80% to 90% of the cases are mild. Especially when we go to younger ages, this rate is very close to 100%.

- Mild cases: improve within 2 weeks.
- Severe-critical cases result in (death or recovery) 3 to 6 weeks.
- Time from onset of illness (first symptom) to development of severe / critical condition: 1 week.
- The process varies between 2 to 8 weeks in fatal cases.

## How Long Does It Take To Progress/Deteriorate?

- After the first symptom until the development of dyspnea (shortness of breath): An average of 5 days,
- From the first symptom to hospitalization: An average of 7 days,
- After the first symptom until the development of ARDS (respiratory distress syndrome): An average of 8 days.

Within the one-year period of pandemics, the medical community has accumulated extensive experience on real cases, albeit we should keep in mind that each new case has his/her unique characteristics (Table **2**).

**Table 2. A few examples of real cases are shown below.**

| Age, Gender | First Finding, (Day 1) | New Findings and Fever | Course and Outcome |
|---|---|---|---|
| **40, F** | Low-grade fever, hyposmia | 2nd day 38C fever | 6th day, treatment at home |
| **61, M** | Shaking, flu-like cold | 6th day 39C fever | 8th day, apparent pneumonia, admission to hospital |
| **72, F** | 38C fever lasting for minutes, anosmia | 5th day presents to hospital after a bus trip for two days | 6th day, signs of pneumonia, admission to hospital |
| **43, M** | Shaking chills, weakness | 4th day muscle pain and persistent cough | 6th day, treatment at home |
| **45, M** | Muscle pain and weakness | Not recorded | 7th day, signs of pneumonia, and diarrhea, admission to hospital |
| **44, M** | fever, weakness, cough and sore throat, admission to hospital. | Severe pneumonia and dyspnea on exertion at 4th and 5th day. | 7th day ARDS, died at 8th day. |

**A Brief Look at the Stages of the Disease in Special Regard to Severity:** First of all, one can view management principles of COVID-19 infection in accord with symptom severity. The patients can be examined in an array of severity subgroups, from noncomplicated disease to septic shock or irreversible respiratory compromise (Tables **3** and **4**).

## Can A Mild-looking Patient Worsen Quickly?

Yes. Below are the tomographic images of a case from Istanbul. A 20-year-old male patient has dramatic progression in CT scans taken in consecutive days. The case, who presented with mild shortness of breath and swelling in the jaw at the first visit, was discharged after CT. The next day, when he presented with increased dyspnea and worsening in his general status, images compatible with

COVID-19 pneumonia were marked on CT. He was monitored in intermediate ICU without need for intubation.

## WHICH MARKERS CAN WE USE TO PREDICT CLINICAL WORSENING?

The most important variable predicting the severity of the cases is respiratory failure and low blood oxygen levels resistant to treatment. Apart from that, patients who get worse develop ARDS, sepsis and septic shock (Table **5**).

**Table 3. World Health Organization- WHO examined COVID-19 infection at the following stages in the guide published at the end of January 2020.**

| | |
|---|---|
| **Noncomplicated** disease | **Signs of viral URI; may include fever, cough, sore throat, weakness, nasal congestion, headache, and muscle aches. The elderly and immunocompromised may present with atypical symptoms.** |
| **Mild pneumonia** | Patients with pneumonia without evidence of severe disease. Cough and shortness of breath may be marked.<br>Respiratory rates: <2 months, 60 bpm; 2–11 months, ≥50 bpm; 1--5 years old, ≥40 bpm |
| **Severe pneumonia** | **Adolescent or adult:** fever or suspected respiratory infection, plus one of the following: RR> 30 bpm, severe respiratory distress, or $SpO_2$ <90% (at room air).<br>**Child:** Cough or shortness of breath, plus one of the following: central cyanosis or $SpO_2$ <90%; severe breathing difficulties (*e.g.,* wheezing, retractions in chest muscles); red flags in pneumonia: difficulty breastfeeding or drinking liquids, drowsiness / unconsciousness, or seizures. Other signs of pneumonia: chest retractions, tachypnea: Respiratory rates: <2 months≥60 bpm; 2–11 months, ≥50 bpm; 1–5 years, ≥40 bpm. Diagnosis is clinical, chest x-ray can only rule out certain complications. |
| **Acute Respiratory Distress Syndrome (ARDS)** | **Onset:** De novo or worsening respiratory signs and symptoms within one week after the triggering event<br>**Imaging:** Bilateral opacities not limited to effusion, lobar or pulmonary collapse, nodules.<br>**Pulmonary edema:** Respiratory failure not explained by HF or fluid overload. It should be evaluated with Echo/POCUS.<br>**Oxygenation (adult):**<br>Mild ARDS: 200 mmHg $<PaO_2 / FiO_2 \leq 300$ mmHg (PEEP or CPAP ≥5 cmH2O, or non-ventilated)<br>Moderate ARDS: 100 mmHg $<PaO_2 / FiO_2 \leq 200$ mmHg (PEEP ≥5 cmH2O, or non-ventilated)<br>Severe ARDS: $PaO_2 / FiO_2 \leq 100$ mmHg (PEEP ≥5 cmH2O, or non-ventilated)<br>If $PaO_2$ cannot be checked, $SpO_2 / FiO_2 \leq 315$ suggests ARDS |

*(Table 3) cont.....*

| | |
|---|---|
| **Noncomplicated disease** | **Signs of viral URI; may include fever, cough, sore throat, weakness, nasal congestion, headache, and muscle aches. The elderly and immunocompromised may present with atypical symptoms.** |
| **Sepsis** | **Adult:** Life-threatening organ dysfunction due to dysregulated host response accompanying infection (altered mental status, tachypnea / respiratory distress, low $O_2$ saturation, decreased urine output, tachycardia, hypotension, cold extremities, coagulopathy findings in laboratory work up, *i.e.,* thrombocytopenia, acidosis, high lactate, or hyperbilirubinemia<br>**Child:** Suspected or proven infection and presence of ≥2 SIRS criteria |
| **Septic shock** | Resistant hypotension despite fluid resuscitation, MAP>= 65 mmHg only with vasopressors and lactate> 2 mmol / L |

**Table 4. A brief overlook at the management principles in accordance with symptom severity.**

| **Management principles are driven primarily by the severity of signs and symptoms of the disease** |
|---|
| • Asymptomatic patients can be followed in outpatient basis to assess the emergence of signs and complaints.<br>• If only mild symptoms (esp. lasting longer than 7 days) are present, and pneumonia is not detected, the patient can be kept in quarantine at home.<br>• More severe patients with the following criteria should be admitted to a hospital for close monitoring. |
| o evidence of pulmonary involvement,<br>o over 60 years of age,<br>o presence of comorbidities (COPD/CHF/ severe persistent HT<br>o severe extrapulmonary manifestations (fever, GI signs, headache, *etc.* |

**Table 5. Markers predicting clinical deterioration.**

| **Age (significant increase in risk with every 10-year increase).** |
|---|
| Tachypnea (every one-unit increase in bpm) |
| Abnormal blood gases ($PaO_2$ (≥60 *vs.* <60 mm Hg) |
| $PaCO_2$ (every 1 mmHg increment) |
| $PaO_2$ to $FiO_2$ (every 10-units' increment) |
| Imaging findings; (consolidation) |
| Coronary heart disease. |
| Hemoglobin (every 1 g / dL increase) |
| leukocytosis; (> $10x10^9$) |
| lymphocytopenia; (> $1x10^9$) |
| procalcitonin; (each 1 ng / mL increase) or (≥0.5 *vs.* <0.5 ng / mL) |
| IL-6 (interleukin-6); (≥100 *vs.* <100 pg / mL) |
| serum ferritin; (per 100 ng / mL increase) or (≥336.2 *vs.* <336.2 ng / mL) |
| CRP (C-reactive protein); (each 1 mg / dL increment) or (≥5 *vs.* <5 mg / dL) |
| aspartate aminotransferase (AST); (every 10 U / L increment) or (≥ 50 *vs.* <50 U / L) |

*(Table 5) cont.....*

| |
|---|
| **Age (significant increase in risk with every 10-year increase).** |
| Direct bilirubin (≥0.3 *vs.* <0.3 mg / dL) |
| LDH-lactate dehydrogenase; (every 100 U / L increment) or (≥250 *vs.* <250 U / L) |
| creatinine; (each 1 mg / dL increment) or (≥ 1.10 *vs.* <1.10 mg / dL) |
| fibrinogen; (every 100 mg / dL increment) |
| troponin I; (every 1000 ng / L increment) or (≥20 *vs.* <20 ng / L) |
| D-dimer: (each 1 μg / L increment) or (≥ 0.35 *vs.* <0.35 μg / L) |

Factors predicting clinical deterioration in COVID-19 patients hospitalized in Italy were tried to be highlighted (Cecconi, 2020). 29% of the group with an average age of 69 got worse, 41 people were hospitalized in ICU and 36 of them died.

In this study, a prognostic index was established using respiratory rate, $PaO_2$ / $FiO_2$ ratio, coronary heart disease history, CRP, and creatinine level. This score has been found to have high predictive accuracy (Cecconi, 2020).

## RADIOLOGICAL CRITERIA

Many researchers have tried to identify patients who will deteriorate with COVID-19 using radiological criteria. 65 adult patients (42 males, 65%) with PCR-confirmed COVID-19 diagnosis in the Munich cohort were analyzed retrospectively. Patients showed mild or severe symptoms. The lesions found in patients were scored between “incompatible with COVID” (Grade 0) and “confluent lesions (Grade 5), which included more than 50% of the lung parenchyma. The mean CT severity score was 4.0 in intensive care patients, while it was 2.9 in other patients with confirmed diagnosis (Burian, 2020) (Fig. **1**).

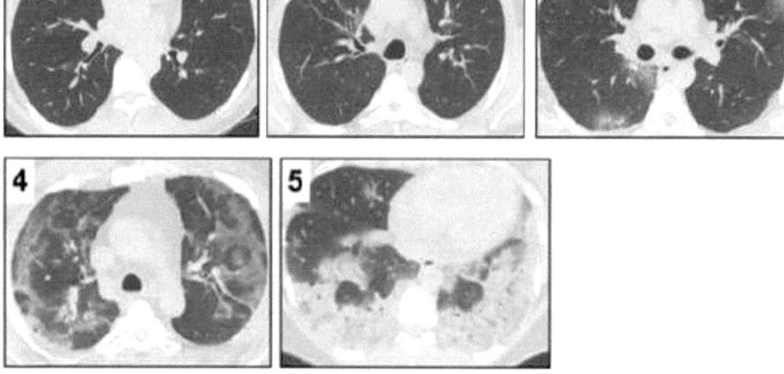


**Fig. (1).** CT images illustrating 5 different stages that predict the risk of ICU admission on tomography (Burian, 2020). It was also found that CRP, leukocyte elevation, and lymphocyte depletion were significantly associated with worsening in patients.

- Grade 1: No typical signs suggestive of COVID
- Grade 2: Solitary GGO in a single lobe
- Grade 3: bilateral, multiple GGO
- Grade 4: Confluent (merging) GGO and consolidations
- Grade 5: Confluent lesions involving more than 50% of the lung parenchyma

Although scoring systems such as Wells' criteria, 'Pulmonary Embolism Rule out Criteria' (PERC) and Geneva scoring system are used to exclude pulmonary embolism, Karimzadeh *et al*. stated that these would be insufficient to exclude PE occurring concurrent with COVID-19 (Karimzadeh, 2020). Basically, these scoring systems calculate the risk in patients who are not hospitalized, but rather in patients who have been admitted to the ED.

**Factors affecting admission to ICU** are variables that predict deterioration in general and death (Table **6**).

**Table 6. Criteria to estimate need for admission to ICU and death.**

| **• Respiratory failure: Low oxygen in the blood despite oxygen administration** |
|---|
| • Hypotension: low blood pressure despite adequate fluid administration. |
| • De novo organ failures: Failure in organs and systems such as kidney, heart, liver, and coagulation functions. |
| • Pre-existing organ failure: Heart, kidney, liver failure, chronic lung disease, coronary artery disease. |
| • People with high viral load, such as healthcare workers or family members who are in close contact with the COVID-19 patients. |
| • Advanced age and male gender. |

## TYPICAL CASE

A 54-year-old taxi driver admitted to the ED with weakness, fever, and occasional cough for 4 to 5 days. There is no known history of any disease. On arrival, the body temperature was 37.7C, no other vital sign abnormality was noted. Lymphopenia and eosinopenia were detected ın the work up. Non-contrast chest CT showed patchy GGO in both lung areas (Fig. **2**). The patient was hospitalized into ward, hydrated, and closely followed up.

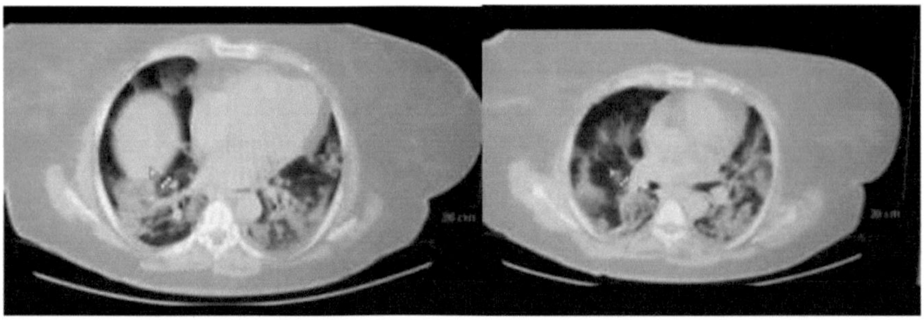

**Fig. (2).** Criteria that should be used to distinguish cold, flu and COVID-19 from each other. With such visual aids in public education, the frequency of ED admissions and EMS calls will be reduced, and necessary cases will be cared for.

**Differential diagnosis:** Patients with shortness of breath and findings suggestive of pneumonia on CT should be evaluated in regard to a myriad of diseases (Tables **7** and **8**).

**Table 7. Some diseases involving the lungs that should be considered in the differential diagnosis of COVID-19.**

| |
|---|
| **• Pulmonary embolism** |
| • Bacterial pneumonia: such as streptococci, staphylococci, Hemophilus, Klebsiella, Moraxella |
| • Other viral pneumonia: Respiratory viruses that trigger influenza A and B, such as H1N1, H5N1, H2N2, H2N3 |
| • Occupational diseases such as asbestosis, pneumoconiosis |
| • Lung cancer |
| • Lung-affecting diseases such as atelectasis and bronchiectasis |
| • Infectious exacerbations in those with COPD and chronic bronchitis |

**Table 8. Features that can be used to distinguish symptoms of COVID-19 from upper respiratory tract infections caused by other viruses.**

| | **COVID-19** | **Common Cold-Rhinitis** | **Flu** | **Allergy/ Asthma** |
|---|---|---|---|---|
| **Fever / shaking chills** | common | Rare | common | Not expected |
| **Weakness/ fatigue** | common | +/- | common | +/- |
| **Shortness of breath** | Can be severe | Not expected | Not expected | +/- |
| **Anosmia** | Common, +/- | +/- | +/- | Not expected |
| **Cough (mostly dry and persistent)** | common | Not expected | +/- | +/- |
| **Pain (mostly muscle)** | Common, +/- | Rare | common | Not expected |
| **Sneeze** | Not expected | Common | +/- | common |

*(Table 8) cont.....*

| | COVID-19 | Common Cold-Rhinitis | Flu | Allergy/ Asthma |
|---|---|---|---|---|
| **Runny nose** | +/- | Common | +/- | common |
| **Epiphora- injection in the eyes** | Not expected | - | +/- | common |
| **Sore throat** | Common, +/- | Common | +/- | Not expected |
| **Diarrhea** | +/- | - | rare | +/- |

## HOW ARE COVID AND COUGH RELATED?

It is known that cytokine storm, which is a hyperactive inflammatory response, triggers COVID-19 symptoms (such as fever, muscle pain, sore throat, respiratory tract irritation). These characteristics have also been shown to be related to the severity of the disease.

The high level of CRP, IL-6 and other inflammatory markers in severe patients indicates that the pro-inflammatory response plays an important role in COVID-19 infection (Martinez-Urbistondo, 2020).

### Cough In Terms of Contagiousness

There is contagiousness from 2-3 days before the symptom onset. Asymptomatic / presymptomatic people can infect the disease. It has been reported that transmission from presymptomatic patients is 48% to 62% (Ganyani 2020) (Fig. **3**, Table **9**).

**Table 9. What has changed in the patient who presented with cough in COVID-19?**

| |
|---|
| • **During the pandemic period, it was necessary to exclude COVID-19 in the majority of patients in the EDs and primary care facilities.** |
| • Focal point of medicine has shifted: «*primum est covid-19?*» instead of «*primum nihil nocere*» was instituted. |
| • Since COVID-19 could not be ruled out immediately, the physicians had to assume that every patient had COVID-19. |
| • Tests for exclusion had to be performed in the patient who presented with a COVID-unrelated complaint, |
| • Time and costs spent for patient care boosted. |

In the Cochrane analysis published in July 2020, 16 studies were included, and more than 7700 patients were evaluated (Struyf, 2020). When the symptoms were examined in terms of sensitivity leading to the diagnosis of COVID-19, only 6 complaints were found to have a sensitivity more than 50%.

Cough, sore throat, fever, myalgia / arthralgia, fatigue, and headache are symptoms with a sensitivity of at least 50% in the diagnosis of COVID-19.

### Pharmacological Methods To Relieve Cough

- NSAIDs: prostaglandin synthesis inhibition (useful in ACEI-related cough)
- Corticosteroids: effective in asthma cough
- Sodium cromoglycate shows its effects only after 36-48 hours
- Expectorant and mucolytic agents: help to eliminate sputum by reducing its viscosity
- Antihistamines and sedatives: The antitussive effect of first-generation antihistamines such as diphenhydramine is due to their central and peripheral anticholinergic activities.
- Butamirate citrate: It is a non-opioid antitussive with a central effect on receptors in the brain stem. It has also been reported that it reduces bronchospasm with peripheral effect and has anti-inflammatory and anticholinergic effects. Therefore, it is thought to be effective in cough with both acute and chronic etiology.
- Opioids: Morphine and codeine reduce cough by inhibition of the cough center in the brain. It is not used in USYE.
- Dextromethorphan: Opioid derivative, centrally effective non-narcotic antitussive. It is included in many over the counter cough relievers.
- Placebo can also be effective in selected cases.

## GASTROINTESTINAL COMPLAINTS AND FINDINGS IN THE COURSE OF COVID-19

Although GI symptoms are not among the main complaints (fever, shortness of breath, dry cough) that are sought primarily in COVID-19 cases, they can be encountered frequently. Abdominal pain, diarrhea, nausea, vomiting, loss of appetite and sense of taste (ageusia) are the most frequently noted GI complaints. Although GI complaints are generally considered as atypical complaints in these cases, they can be an important complement to the main findings and can help in the diagnosis of the disease. Although rarely, GI complaints may occur as the main complaint or finding at the time of admission to the hospital. Atypical or infrequent findings may also cause patients to be difficult to identify and stay in the hospital for a longer period of time.

When 1141 cases were examined in the initial period of the epidemic in China, it was reported that 183 (16%) presented with GI complaints (Luo, 2020). Among these, the most commonly reported were loss of appetite, nausea and vomiting, diarrhea, and abdominal pain. As a rule, this patient group had leukopenia, lymphopenia, increased CRP, and mild liver enzyme elevation, while renal functions were normal (Table **10**). In 96% of the cases, there was findings on CT of the chest, so it was a severe group of patients.

**Table 10. In order of frequency, GI complaints in patients with confirmed COVID-19 and laboratory findings (Luo, 2020).**

| Complaints | Laboratory Findings |
|---|---|
| loss of appetite | leukopenia (mean 2.7x $10^9$/L) |
| nausea | Lymphopenia (mean 0.53x $10^9$ / L) |
| vomiting | increased CRP |
| diarrhea | liver enzyme elevation |
| abdominal pain | normal kidney function |

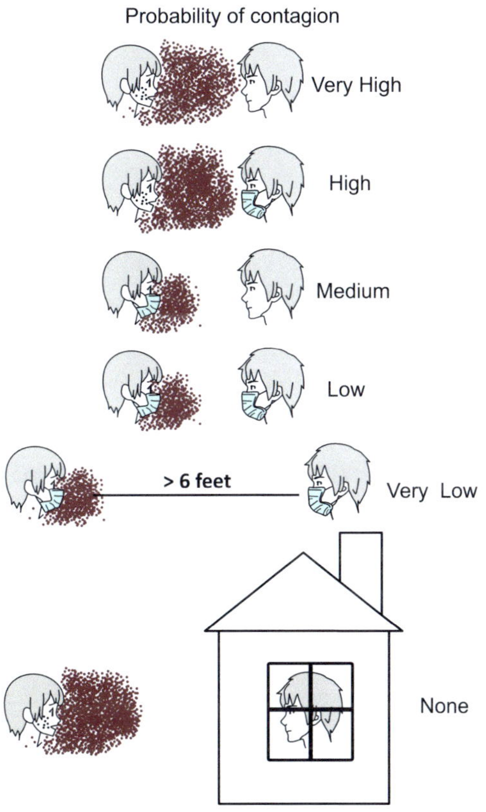


**Fig. (3).** The risk of contamination, which increases significantly with coughing, can be reduced with the use of a mask, but cannot be reset. This reveals that cough should also be treated separately.

Cheung *et al*. published a systematic review and found that GI symptoms were present at a rate of 17.6% in the entire pool analyzed (Cheung, 2020). There are studies reporting that the clinical course of patients with GI complaints is worse than others.

**The Importance of GIS in the Pathophysiology of the Virus:** The virus is excreted with faeces during acute illness. Even when nasopharyngeal swabs become negative, viral RNA can remain positive in the episode. Fecal-oral transmission is present in 10.5% to 53% of patients. It has been also noted that fecal RNA excretion is more prominent in severe patients and may accompany liver enzyme elevation.

Three adult cases (40, 44, and 53 years) who presented with abdominal findings mimicking acute abdomen syndrome and were diagnosed with COVID-19 have been published (Ahmed, 2020). The cases did not require surgical intervention. Although all three cases had COVID-19 pneumonia, epiploic appendagitis was found as a cause of abdominal pain in one, lower lobe pneumonia in one, and nonspecific abdominal pain in the other.

In Italy, COVID-19 pneumonia was diagnosed concurrent with ruptured diaphragm with gastric perforation in a young woman with fever and dry cough for 5 days (Poggiali, 2020).

In the analysis of 182 pediatric cases with a median age of 6 in China (Du, 2020), fever and cough were the two most common complaints with 43% and 44%. About 11% of cases had GI symptoms, most of which were diarrhea, abdominal discomfort and vomiting. It was recovered in 97.8% with a mild course. The presence of intussusception and sepsis in the only child who died actually reveals the importance of GI symptomatology.

De Souza *et al.* published a systematic review of 38 studies reported that diarrhea was seen in 8.1% patients and nausea and vomiting in 7.1% patients (de Souza, 2020).

## CORONA FACTS: WHICH IS CORRECT?

Misunderstandings and misconceptions are the phenomena which pose greatest threat to the measures and precautions taken against a disease. These can sometimes pave the way to economic crises, and, sometimes, to vital consequences for the individual. There is a continuous flow of information, but "getting informed" is not so easy in this turmoil and quagmire, which is also called an "Infodemics" somewhere. Here, we tried to indicate some truths instead of some false beliefs propagated in the society.

Our world will never be the same again. Our generation has gone through SARS in 2002, bird flu outbreaks between 2003 and 2006, swine flu in 2009, MERS in 2012, but –probably the worst one among all- we were shaken by a pandemic in 2020 that we had not experienced before. As the attention of our citizens, like the rest of the world, is focused on this issue, there is a continuous flow of information, but "getting informed" is not so easy in this turmoil and quagmire. Some authors have ironically called this an "Infodemics". Sometimes we get stuck in the search for the truth. Here, we aimed to present some false (F) beliefs and truths (T) regarding them.

F: I wear gloves and finish the job. I wish it would not burst from here and there if I wear them all day.

T: The glove you wear for more than 30 to 60 minutes and touch the environment (handrail, handle, inside the subway or bus) is not different from your bare hands. It is infectious.

F: When I go shopping, I go to the most expensive market where high-class people hang out, no problem.

T: Did you write your will? Much has been said that COVID-19 spread from poor Chinese fishermen eating bats. Indeed, it was spread from the wealthy Chinese such as those who went to Milan's fashion week who ate fancy & expensive 'exotic' things. The virus does not distinguish between people, class, *etc*. After all, if you should protect yourself from COVID-19 everywhere, if you want to caress your grandchildren.

F: Thermal cameras will do the job, we can rely on them.

T: Yes, people with high fever can be caught with the thermal cameras, but you can see the COVID by inspection, electron microscope or other tests in afebrile people. "The ill patient" is not something detectable just by fever. People study for six years for this.

F: I wear a mask with a fancy pattern, and I will feel comfortable.

T: The mask is primarily to prevent the sick person from spreading drops around. It is correct to wear a mask when entering crowded places and in high-risk environments (such as bazaars and shops in big cities) in an environment where the epidemic is rising. Simple (surgical) masks are sufficient for this. Do not waste your money.

F: Some masks are thin; I blow it out. I would not wear it.

T: Put a wet wipe into the mask and make sure that it does not slip away. Just be practical.

F: I feel bored, take off the mask, put it in my pocket, then walk and wear it if necessary, in any dangerous place.

T: Not like that. You should wear it constantly, as it will not be clear who you will meet at any dangerous situation outside. The mask is not enough, stay away from people who are coughing, clogging, ill- looking.

F: It lives in animate milieu and does not live in inanimate surfaces.

T: You think so. 9 hours in plastic, up to 6 days in steel, 6 hours on wood… Even 3 hours in the air. As the hours pass, especially in high temperature and dry environment, the number of viruses decreases, although they can decrease to the numbers that will not cause disease. You can still go safely to places that smell of bleach (in terms of loving grandchildren).

Q: The virus is transmitted by air, is it correct?

Both yes and no. The presence of the virus in the air hours later does not necessarily indicate that they are at a level that can be really contagious. It is clear that you won't be loaded by the virus as much as a doctor intubating the patient. The gossip with your friend for over 10 minutes at a distance of <=1 m is risky. Say hello and be a little antisocial.

F: I have lots of money, can get one of these most expensive masks, you know, those with funny filters.

T: Nope. N95 (FFP2) is 95% protective, you remove the virus from the air you get from outside, but you give out the viruses directly. So, you become more infectious than any other ways. Do not come to your physician for examination by attaching this, we will break.

F: Only if someone cough on us, we can get ill.

T: No, it is also transmitted through food, breath, by not adherence to toilet hygiene (we call it the bad name, fecal-oral route).

F: Let us wash all edible things with vinegar.

T: We do not have that sort of water shortage yet. Vinegar is no different from other liquids we use for washing (we call them $H_2O$). If we have really run out of water, we can use vinegar. Let us cook the cookable meals, enough.

F: If we pour alcohol or chlorinated disinfectants on us?

T: your clothes cn change colours, or you can get burned. Killing the virus is very easy, indeed. They easily die with liquid containing 0.1% sodium hypochlorite (bleach), 62-71% ethanol, or 0.5% hydrogen peroxide. If we put this into practice; Mixing 5 tablespoons (1/3 of the glass) of bleach in 3.5-4 L water will cause fear to the enemy. Pour it on you? You can get poisoned or burn to kill 3 to 5 viruses.

F: A great leader said inject them?

T: Do not do it before writing your will. It is not what can be injected into the body. We are very lucky. it's still science deciding upon serious situations.

F: We are protected by being vaccinated.

T: Pneumonia, influenza, *etc*. vaccines that have been used so far are inefficient against COVID-19. However, the pneumonia vaccine which is useful for risk groups for COVID-19, as it will protect against agents that can cause co-infection.

F: I suck and defeat the virus by sniffing and blowing salt water into our nose.

T: It has never been recorded that the virus of those who did it died. Do it as a hobby, anyway?

F: We kill the virus by drinking 60-70 degrees hot water, tea, *etc*.

T: Beware, you burn your throat.

F: Young people do not need to be afraid since they kill only the elderly.

T: The elderly, our mothers, our fathers die with viruses brought by young people. Be concerned and take action.

Anyone at any age can become sick (infected) with coronavirus. The only difference between the elderly and those with comorbid/concomitant diseases is that they have a more severe disease. Do not be so comfortable just because you are young.

F: These viruses do not survive in the cold.

T: Weather conditions cannot kill coronaviruses. The virus is actually bear-like and likes cold and wet-humid places. Since our climate is in a transition zone between bear and zebra, there will be partial relief with the warming of the weather, but do not rely too much on.

F: These viruses do not survive in the heat and sun.

T: Weather conditions cannot kill coronaviruses. Brazil and Mexico have high numbers of suffering people. By the way, the disease is not transmitted with mosquito bites.

F: it passes to as *via* animals.

T: There is no transition from animals such as pets and dogs.

F: It is transmitted from us to the animals.

T: There is no transition from people to animals such as domestic cats and dogs.

F: bath kills the virus

T: Bath and illness have nothing to do with. Let us justify it, it can help lower your fever. It is good to take a shower, especially in hot weather, we can prevent the transmission of the virus left in our body through face-to-eye exposure. So again, the key point is not to take your hands to the face.

F: What if we eat garlic, sumac, or something?

T: Good for your health, of course, but the virus does not die with it. Maybe the smell would keep people away from you.

T: I think Anatolian local tradesmen selling garlic would be pleased by such an action. Garlic both regulates your blood pressure and keeps people away from you. Will they go further than the critical limit of 1.5 m, it depends on how much garlic you will eat.

F: Hand dryers kill the virus

T: It does not kill. There is no information on this subject except for the absurdity of one US high bureaucrat. The opposite is purely scientific.

F: We kill with ultraviolet (UV) light.

T: UV light devices should not be used for virus killing / sterilization purposes in living places. Causes skin irritation. I should add that research are going on, like Martians on earth.

F: Let us ingest antibiotics.

T: Antibiotics may be effective on bacterial superinfection, which is rarely seen in

COVID infection. You should still see a doctor.

F: I fear of the shoes I traveled outside so I throw them into the machine every day in order to get off the virus.

T: Not that much. If there is a child/toddler crawling at home, lift it out of reach, it is enough. Keep it in a sachet that did not happen either. The shoe-borne disease report is not even included in 10 million patients.

F: I always wear the mask, even when doing sports.

T: It is not suitable to use in active sports. It is enough not to do sports in cramped, stuffy environments and in closed areas with a team or crowd.

F: Using the mask for a long time caused carbon dioxide ($CO_2$) poisoning.

T: It does not cause any poisoning. You cannot breathe while talking, or swallow. Have you ever noticed? With the mask, you can easily breathe.

F: 5 G mobile networks help spread the coronavirus.

T: Viruses do not spread over radio networks or mobile networks. It is spread by the infected person's coughs, sneezes, *etc*., or through contaminated surfaces. In countries that have never met 5 G, coronavirus infection is spreading rapidly.

## CONCLUSION

COVID-19 affects almost every organ and system in the body, depending on the severity of the disease, viral load, and host factors. Complaints and findings such as fever, dry cough and weakness are predominant in many large series. However, shortness of breath almost invariably predicts a more severe disease course in most patients. More rarely, neurological, gastrointestinal, or dermatological complaints and findings are also noted, mostly in conjunction with other signs. Laboratory and radiological adjuncts are mostly the key for an expedient diagnosis and management, especially in institutions with a high number of admissions in a time unit. The clinician should be alert on how to interpret hallmarks of the disease which can predict a grave outcome and severe course in any given patient.

## REFERENCES

Ahmed, AOE, Badawi, M, Ahmed, K & Mohamed, MFH (2020) Case Report: COVID-19 Masquerading as an Acute Surgical Abdomen. *Am J Trop Med Hyg,* 103, 841-3. [published online ahead of print, 2020 Jun 9]. [http://dx.doi.org/10.4269/ajtmh.20-0559] [PMID: 32524962]

Burian, E, Jungmann, F, Kaissis, GA, Lohöfer, FK, Spinner, CD, Lahmer, T, Treiber, M, Dommasch, M, Schneider, G, Geisler, F, Huber, W, Protzer, U, Schmid, RM, Schwaiger, M, Makowski, MR & Braren, RF

(2020) Intensive Care Risk Estimation in COVID-19 Pneumonia Based on Clinical and Imaging Parameters: Experiences from the Munich Cohort. *J Clin Med,* 9, E1514.
[http://dx.doi.org/10.3390/jcm9051514] [PMID: 32443442]

Cecconi, M, Piovani, D, Brunetta, E, Aghemo, A, Greco, M, Ciccarelli, M, Angelini, C, Voza, A, Omodei, P, Vespa, E, Pugliese, N, Parigi, TL, Folci, M, Danese, S & Bonovas, S (2020) Early Predictors of Clinical Deterioration in a Cohort of 239 Patients Hospitalized for Covid-19 Infection in Lombardy, Italy. *J Clin Med,* 9, E1548.
[http://dx.doi.org/10.3390/jcm9051548] [PMID: 32443899]

Chen, N, Zhou, M, Dong, X, Qu, J, Gong, F, Han, Y, Qiu, Y, Wang, J, Liu, Y, Wei, Y, Xia, J, Yu, T, Zhang, X & Zhang, L (2020) Epidemiological and clinical characteristics of 99 cases of 2019 novel coronavirus pneumonia in Wuhan, China: a descriptive study. *Lancet,* 395, 507-13.
[http://dx.doi.org/10.1016/S0140-6736(20)30211-7] [PMID: 32007143]

Cheung, KS, Hung, IFN, Chan, PPY, Lung, KC, Tso, E, Liu, R, Ng, YY, Chu, MY, Chung, TWH, Tam, AR, Yip, CCY, Leung, KH, Fung, AY, Zhang, RR, Lin, Y, Cheng, HM, Zhang, AJX, To, KKW, Chan, KH, Yuen, KY & Leung, WK (2020) Gastrointestinal Manifestations of SARS-CoV-2 Infection and Virus Load in Fecal Samples From a Hong Kong Cohort: Systematic Review and Meta-analysis. *Gastroenterology,* 159, 81-95.
[http://dx.doi.org/10.1053/j.gastro.2020.03.065] [PMID: 32251668]

*Chinese Center for Disease Control and Prevention (CCDC) (2020a) General questions COVID-19 Prevention and Control.* http://www.chinacdc.cn/en/COVID19/202002/P02020030635 8351973919.pdf a

de Souza, TH, Nadal, JA, Nogueira, RJN, Pereira, RM & Brandão, MB (2020) Clinical manifestations of children with COVID-19: A systematic review. *Pediatr Pulmonol,* 55, 1892-9. [published online ahead of print, 2020 Jun 3].
[http://dx.doi.org/10.1002/ppul.24885] [PMID: 32492251]

Du, H, Dong, X & Zhang, JJ (2020) Clinical Characteristics of 182 Pediatric COVID-19 Patients With Different Severities and Allergic Status. *Allergy.*
[http://dx.doi.org/10.1111/all.14452] [PMID: 32524611]

Ganyani, T, Kremer, C, Chen, D, Torneri, A, Faes, C, Wallinga, J & Hens, N (2020) Estimating the generation interval for coronavirus disease (COVID-19) based on symptom onset data, March 2020. *Euro Surveill,* 25
[http://dx.doi.org/10.2807/1560-7917.ES.2020.25.17.2000257] [PMID: 32372755]

Grant, MC, Geoghegan, L, Arbyn, M, Mohammed, Z, McGuinness, L, Clarke, EL & Wade, RG (2020) The prevalence of symptoms in 24,410 adults infected by the novel coronavirus (SARS-CoV-2; COVID-19): A systematic review and meta-analysis of 148 studies from 9 countries. *PLoS One,* 15, e0234765.
[http://dx.doi.org/10.1371/journal.pone.0234765] [PMID: 32574165]

Irvine, M, Coombs, D, Skarha, J, Del Pozo, B, Rich, J, Taxman, F & Green, TC (2020) Modeling COVID-19 and Its Impacts on U.S. Immigration and Customs Enforcement (ICE) Detention Facilities, 2020. *J Urban Health,* 97, 439-47.
[http://dx.doi.org/10.1007/s11524-020-00441-x] [PMID: 32415422]

Karimzadeh, S, Raut, A & Nguyen Tien, H (2020) COVID-19 and pulmonary embolism: diagnostic imaging trends. *J Nucl Med.* [published online ahead of print, 2020 May 22]

Luo, S, Zhang, X & Xu, H (2020) Don't Overlook Digestive Symptoms in Patients With 2019 Novel Coronavirus Disease (COVID-19). *Clin Gastroenterol Hepatol,* 18, 1636-7.
[http://dx.doi.org/10.1016/j.cgh.2020.03.043] [PMID: 32205220]

Macera, M, De Angelis, G, Sagnelli, C, Coppola, N & Vanvitelli Covid-Group, (2020) Clinical Presentation of COVID-19: Case Series and Review of the Literature. *Int J Environ Res Public Health,* 17, 5062.
[http://dx.doi.org/10.3390/ijerph17145062] [PMID: 32674450]

Martinez-Urbistondo, M, Mora-Vargas, A, Expósito-Palomo, E, Castejón, R, Citores, MJ, Rosado, S, de Mendoza, C, Baños, I, Fernández-Cruz, A, Daimiel, L, San-Cristóbal, R, Vargas, JA & Martinez, JA (2020)

Inflammatory-Related Clinical and Metabolic Outcomes in COVID-19 Patients. *Mediators Inflamm,* 2020, 2914275.
[http://dx.doi.org/10.1155/2020/2914275] [PMID: 33273888]

Oran, DP & Topol, EJ (2020) Prevalence of Asymptomatic SARS-CoV-2 Infection : A Narrative Review. *Ann Intern Med,* 173, 362-7.
[http://dx.doi.org/10.7326/M20-3012] [PMID: 32491919]

Poggiali, E, Vercelli, A, Demichele, E, Ioannilli, E & Magnacavallo, A (2020) Diaphragmatic Rupture and Gastric Perforation in a Patient with COVID-19 Pneumonia. *Eur J Case Rep Intern Med,* 7, 001738.
[http://dx.doi.org/10.12890/2020_001738] [PMID: 32523933]

Poletti, P, Tirani, M, Cereda, D, Trentini, F, Guzzetta, G, Marziano, V, Buoro, S, Riboli, S, Crottogini, L, Piccarreta, R, Piatti, A, Grasselli, G, Melegaro, A, Gramegna, M, Ajelli, M & Merler, S (2020) Age-specific SARS-CoV-2 infection fatality ratio and associated risk factors, Italy, February to April 2020. *Euro Surveill,* 25
[http://dx.doi.org/10.2807/1560-7917.ES.2020.25.31.2001383] [PMID: 32762797]

So, L & Smith, G (2020) *In four US state prisons, nearly 3,300 inmates test positive for coronavirus — 96% without symptoms*www.reuters.com/article/us-health-coronavirus Reuters. 25 April 2020. Accessed at www.reuters.com/article/us-health-coronavirus -prisons-testing-in-idUSKCN2270RX on

Struyf, T, Deeks, JJ, Dinnes, J, Takwoingi, Y, Davenport, C, Leeflang, MM, Spijker, R, Hooft, L, Emperador, D, Dittrich, S, Domen, J, Horn, SRA & Van den Bruel, A Cochrane COVID-19 Diagnostic Test Accuracy Group (2020) Signs and symptoms to determine if a patient presenting in primary care or hospital outpatient settings has COVID-19 disease. *Cochrane Database Syst Rev,* 7, CD013665.
[http://dx.doi.org/10.1002/14651858.CD013665] [PMID: 32633856]

# CHAPTER 6

# Diagnosis of COVID-19: Which Tests To Do? Laboratory and Radiological Adjuncts To Recognition

**Abstract:** As the organism is afflicted by COVID-19 as a whole, recognition of the disease can sometimes pose difficulties for healthcare workers. Laboratory and radiological workup are necessary for expedient diagnosis in most cases. Although considered as a gold standard, the need for certified laboratories, expensive equipment, and trained staff are drawbacks of RT-PCR tests to be applied to large numbers of people as screening tests . Chest radiography is recommended as an initial test for any patient with suspicion of the disease, while chest tomography is more sensitive to demonstrate specific lesions and the extent of the disease inflicting lungs.

**Keywords:** CD4/CD8 ratio, Complete blood count, COVID-19, CRP, Neutrophil/lymphocyte ratio, Outbreak, Pandemic, RT-PCR.

## DIAGNOSTIC PROTOCOL FOR CORONAVIRUS DISEASE (COVID-19)

Amplification of viral RNA by RT-PCR for the detection of SARS-CoV-2 virus, which has caused the pandemic, functions as the gold standard for confirmation of infection but has a long processing time and shows false-negative rates of 15% to 40%. In addition, the need for certified laboratories, expensive equipment, and trained staff drives many countries to limit RT-PCR tests to only individuals with prominent respiratory symptoms. Therefore, there is a need for alternative, cheaper, and more accessible tests for expedient diagnosis. Combining the appropriate cut-off values for some hematological parameters can help identify false positive / negative RT-PCR tests. Blood test analyses can be used as an alternative to RT-PCR to identify COVID-19 positive patients in countries with great shortages of RT-PCR reagents and / or specialist laboratories. In addition, the identification of biomarkers that can predict the severity and prognosis of the disease is also necessary to guide clinical care (Fig. **1**).

**Ozgur KARCIOGLU, Selman YENIOCAK and Mandana HOSSEINZADEH**

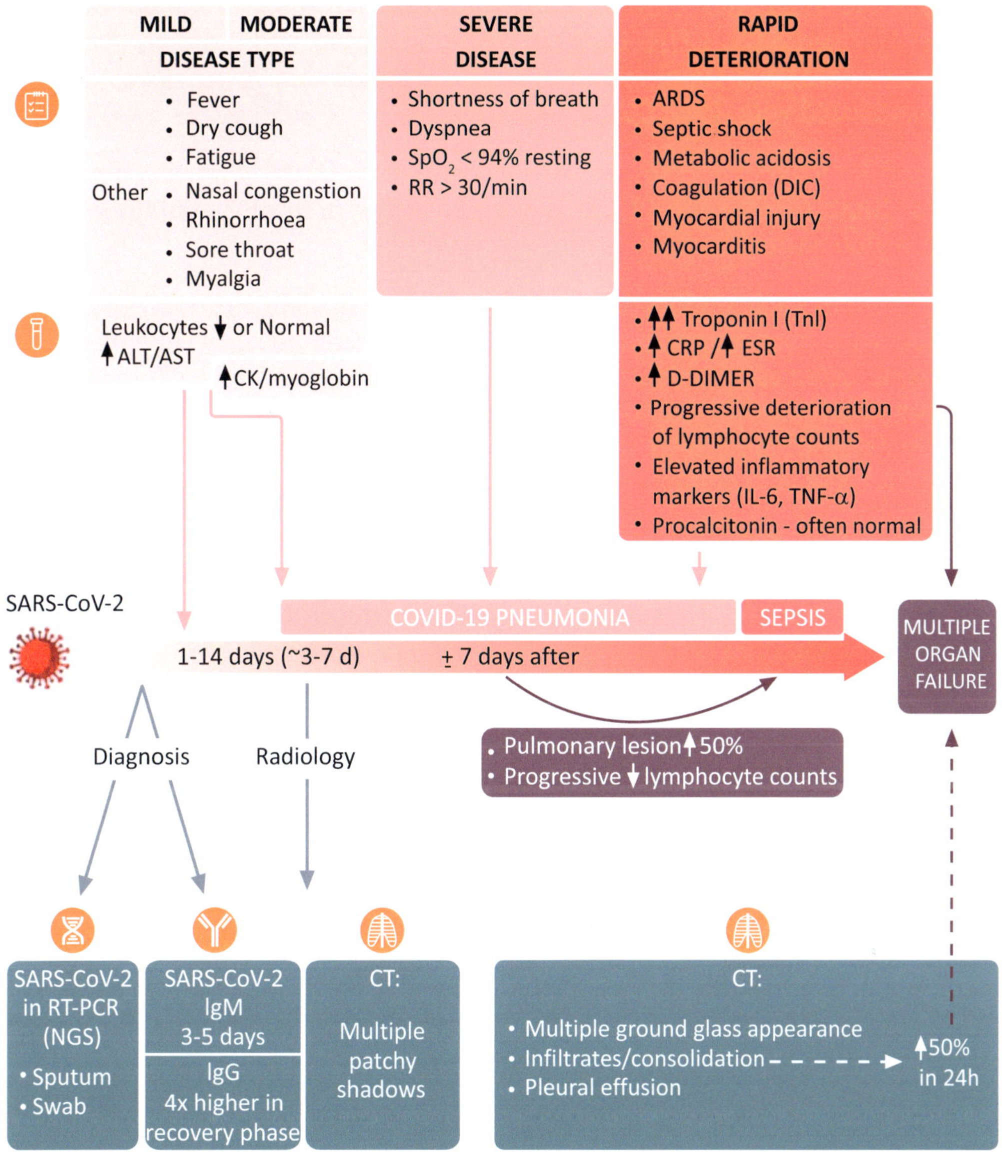


**Fig. (1).** Clinical findings and laboratory indicators of mild, moderate, severe, and critical forms of COVID-19 disease.

## LABORATORY TESTS

**Complete blood count (CBC):** Important clues can be found. Lymphocyte count decreases in 4/5 of the cases (lymphopenia). Half of the cases have eosinopenia. Wang *et al*. found the median lymphocyte count as 800 x 106 / L in patients with COVID-19 pneumonia (Wang, 2020). There is no difference between patients admitted into the ICU and others. In a retrospective study, lymphopenia, leukocytosis, elevated ALT, LDH, Hs-cTnI, creatine kinase, and d-dimer, serum ferritin, IL-6, prothrombin time, creatinine, and procalcitonin levels were also found to be associated with death (Zhou *et al.*, 2020).

The median of the leukocyte count in patients with COVID-19 is mostly found within normal limits (4500 x106 / L). It is slightly higher in those hospitalized in ICU but still within normal limits.

It has been shown in adult studies that increased leukocyte and neutrophil counts are associated with poor prognosis. However, radiological changes suggesting pneumonia were detected in only one of three cases with abnormal leukocyte or neutrophil counts among 10 symptomatic children. Lymphopenia was reported in only two infants in all studies. It was thought that the reason for not detecting significant lymphopenia in children might be the low incidence of severe cases.

It was reported that 80% of critical patients and 25% of mild cases had lymphopenia, and it was suggested that it might be related to the course of the disease in adult studies. As a result, a consistent laboratory change has not yet been determined in children with COVID 2019. Lymphocyte count and CRP can be monitored as signs of severe infection and PCT possible bacterial co-infection. (Henry BM, 2020).

Lastly, it has been established that there may be changes in laboratory parameters according to the stages of the disease. For example, in the early stages of the disease, the peripheral WBC count is normal or low, and the lymphocyte count is reduced. Some patients have elevated liver enzymes, lactate dehydrogenase (LDH), muscle enzymes, and myoglobin. High troponin is seen in some critically ill patients. Most patients have markedly elevated C-reactive protein and erythrocyte sedimentation rate along with a normal procalcitonin. In severe cases, D-dimer increases, and peripheral blood lymphocytes gradually decrease. Severe and critically ill patients often have high inflammatory factors (Table **1**).

Various biomarkers have been identified that could potentially be helpful in risk stratification models for predicting critical and mortal COVID-19 patients. Variables that can be used as a marker for potential progression to critical diseases in patients hospitalized with respiratory distress are:

- WBC count
- Lymphocyte count
- Platelet count
- IL-6 level

- Serum ferritin level

When the parameters of fatal patients compared to the survivors are examined some variables are marked to discern the dead from survivors:

- Increased in the dead survivors:

- WBC number
- Total bilirubin
- Creatine kinase
- Serum ferritin
- IL-6

**Table 1. Summary of laboratory changes in patients with critical or fatal COVID-19.**

| Biochemical Markers | Inflammatory Biomarkers | Hematological + Coagulation Markers |
|---|---|---|
| ↑Albumin | ↑ Erythrocyte sedimentation rate | ↑ WBC count |
| ↑Alanine aminotransferase | ↑ CRP | ↑ Neutrophil count |
| ↑ Aspartate aminotransferase | ↑ Serum ferritin | ↓ Lymphocyte count |
| ↑Total bilirubin | ↑ Procalcitonin | ↓ Platelet count |
| ↑ Blood urea nitrogen | ↑ IL-2R | ↓ Eosinophil count |
| ↑ Creatinine | ↑ IL-6 | ↓ Hemoglobin |
| ↑ Creatine kinase | ↑ IL-8 | ↑ Prothrombin time |
| ↑Lactate dehydrogenase | ↑ IL-10 | ↑ D-dimer |
| ↑ Myoglobin | | |
| ↑ Cardiac troponin I | | |

- Declined in the dead more than survivors:

- Lymphocyte count
- Platelet count

In a meta-analysis of Diagnostic and prognostic value of hematological and immunological markers in COVID 19 infection, Elshazli *et al.* disclosed that ICU admission was associated with higher levels of WBCs (OR = 5.21), neutrophils (OR = 6.25), D-dimer (OR = 4.19), and prolonged PT (OR = 2.18) (Elshazli *et al.* 2020). They also reported that patients with high IL-6 (OR = 13.87), CRP (OR = 7.09), D-dimer (OR = 6.36), and neutrophils (OR = 6.25) had the highest likelihood of mortality (Table **2**).

**Table 2. Receiver operating characteristics results for severity of COVID-19 ( Elshazli *et al.* 2020 ) (Bold values indicate significance at *P* < 0.05).**

| Lab test | AUC | Threshold | Sensitivity | Specificity | P-value |
|---|---|---|---|---|---|
| WBC | 0.801 ± 0.09 | 5.47 | 85.7 | 85.7 | **0.007** |
| Neutrophil | 0.831 ± 0.09 | 3.74 | 78.5 | 100 | **0.003** |
| Lymphocyte | 0.867 ± 0.06 | 0.98 | 81.2 | 87.5 | **<0.001** |
| Platelets | 0.836 ± 0.11 | 177.6 | 71.4 | 71.4 | **0.035** |
| PT | 0.583 ± 0.17 | 12.9 | 50.0 | 83.3 | 0.63 |
| Procalcitonin | 0.845 ± 0.09 | 0.06 | 80.0 | 90.0 | **0.007** |
| D-dimer | 0.876 ± 0.08 | 0.48 | 88.9 | 77.8 | **0.007** |
| CRP | 0.875 ± 0.08 | 38.2 | 84.6 | 92.3 | **0.001** |
| IL-6 | 0.632 ± 1.6 | 22.9 | 71.4 | 71.4 | 0.40 |

## Cytokines and Related Findings

Significantly elevated blood cytokine and chemokine levels in patients with COVID-19 infection, including IL1-β, IL1RA, IL7, IL8, IL9, IL10, FGF2, GCSF, GMCSF, IFNy, IP10, MCP1, Mip1a, Mip1ß, PDGFB, TNFa and VEGFA has been recorded. In some of the severe cases admitted to the ICU, high levels of pro-inflammatory cytokines, including IL2, IL7, IL10, GCSF, IP10, MCP1, Mip1a and TNFa, have been cited as the distinguishing factor for increased disease severity.

A workup of IL-6 should be noted as a potential prognostic indicator in severe COVID 2019 in children.

## Laboratory Values Can Also Highlight The Stages of The Disease

Stage 1: Lymphopenia and neutrophilia are prominent in CBC.

Stage 2: Lymphopenia, transaminases and systemic inflammatory markers are elevated. Meanwhile, serum PCT values are expected to be normal.

Stage 3: A small subset of COVID-19 patients progress to stage 3, where systemic hyperinflammatory state ensues.

Studies have shown increased levels of IL-2, IL-6, IL-7, G-CSF, macrophage stimulating factor 1α (MSP 1α), TNF-α, CRP, ferritin, D-dimer, troponin and NT-proBNP in patients with severe outcome (Siddiqi, 2020).

**D-dimer:** Advanced age at the time of admission, high SOFA score and d-dimer> 1 µg / mL were found to be associated with death during hospitalization. Therefore, advanced age, high SOFA score and d-dimer over 1 µg / mL defined as potential risk factors are parameters that can be evaluated in early identification of patients who will have a poor prognosis.

Laboratory and radiology examinations can be planned in accord with the COVID-19 stages (Siddiqi, 2020).

**Stage 1:** Lymphopenia and neutrophilia are prominent in complete blood count.

**Stage 2:** Lymphopenia, transaminases and systemic inflammatory markers are elevated. An increase in serum procalcitonin values is not expected.

**Stage 3:** A small proportion of COVID-19 patients progress to stage 3 where systemic hyper-inflammation ensues. Studies have shown an increase in IL-2, IL-6, IL-7, GCSF, macrophage stimulating factor 1α (MSP 1α), TNF-α, CRP, ferritin, D-dimer, troponin and NT-proBNP levels in patients with severe prognosis.

## CD4/CD8 Ratio: A Promising Marker?

Maybe. CD4/CD8 ratio assessed on presentation (in the ED or primary care facilities) can be viewed a risk factor for severe disease and/or deterioration in the course. It can be used for early prediction of progression towards ICU in patients with COVID-19.

Total counts of T cells, CD4 cells, and CD8 cells were reported to be significantly decreased in critically ill patients with COVID-19 (Liu *et al.* 2020, and Wan *et al.* 2020). In another study, Wang *et al.* put forth that, in the context of lymphopenia, low CD8 cell count and increased CD4/CD8 ratio were associated with the inflammatory status of COVID-19 patients (Wang *et al.* 2020). In the study by Pallotto *et al.*, low CD4 and CD8 count were noted in both the critically ill and the non-critically ill group and the CD4/CD8 ratio were significantly higher in those with critical COVID-19 (Pallotto *et al*, 2020).

## *Can The Neutrophil-lymphocyte Ratio Be Used For Diagnostic Purposes?*

Yes. It has been reported that if the NLR rate is above 4.94 in the first day in COVID-19 cases in Louisiana, its power to predict intubation is very high (Tatum, 2020). The mortality rate of the cohort is 18.4%. In the same study, it was shown that NLR values above the cut-off values on the $2^{nd}$ and $5^{th}$ days can predict mortality.

Liu *et al.* reported that the accuracy of NLR being> 3.13 is high in predicting critical disease in China (Liu, 2020). Even though they are over 50 years of age, critical disease is only 9% in those with NLR <3.13, while in the same group, patients with NLR> 3.13 progress to 50% critical disease . As a result, they reported that patients over the age of 50 and with a NLR of> 3.13 are prone to emergent hospitalization in ICU .

## PATHOLOGICAL FINDINGS

Detection of COVID-19 in the laboratory can be performed in two ways: Visualization of the virus (SARS-CoV-2) itself (*e.g.*, under the microscope), or identification of its surrogates such as the adaptive immune response against the virus. The decision on which method is safe and correct depends mainly on the stage of the infection.

The preferred method to be used in the diagnosis of COVID-19 virus (SARS-CoV-2) is nucleic acid determination. The nucleic acid can be detected in nasopharyngeal swabs, sputum, lower respiratory tract secretions, blood, feces, and other samples using PCR. "Real-time PCR (RT-PCR)", which is used to confirm the diagnosis and accepted as the gold standard in the world, can be performed in advanced laboratories. These tests may be ordered by the physician to guide the treatment by distinguishing it from bacterial and other infections in patients who meet the "probable case" definition.

Mostly, three specific genes have been identified for this: Open Reading Frame 1a / b (ORF1a / b), Nucleocapsid protein (N) and Envelope Protein (E) genes. It is more accurate to obtain samples from the lower respiratory tract (sputum or airway extraction). However, as much as possible, use in combination with other samples provides more accurate results. Samples should be treated and examined as soon as possible after collection.

Nasal swab detects 2/3 of cases, while pharyngeal swab can detect only around 1/3 of cases. Nasal swabs may be preferred in unidentified patients. It should be kept in mind that bronchoalveolar lavage fluids has the most accurate identification rates among all.

Samples should be taken correctly as soon as possible in suspected patients for RT-PCR testing. Swabs should be taken from the nose and throat, and also from the trachea for those with breathing difficulties or those have already been intubated.

In a systematic review, accuracies of identification of SARS-CoC-2 in different samples from airway, that is, sputum, nasopharyngeal and oropharyngeal swabs and demonstrated that sensitivity of sputum was the highest (73%) and oropharyngeal swab was the lowest (43%) (Table **3** ) (Mohammadi *et al*, 2020).

**Table 3. PCR test positivity rates (Adapted from Wang *et al.* 2020).**

| S. No. | Sample Type | % Positivity |
|---|---|---|
| 1 | Bronchoalveolar lavage fluid | 93% |
| 2 | Fibrobronchoscope biopsy | 46% |
| 3 | Sputum | 72% |
| 4 | Nasal swab | 63% |
| 5 | Pharyngeal swab | 32% |
| 6 | Stool | 29% |
| 7 | Blood | 1% |
| 8 | Urine | 0 |

Half of those patients with a positive RT-PCR test are asymptomatic. It was also reported that lesions were seen in CT in more than half of asymptomatic patients . COVID-19 should be suspected if the patient becomes symptomatic even if the test is negative.

On February 20, 2020, PCR test was performed on almost everyone on the Japanese cruise ship and 17% positivity (n = 619) was found (Japanese National Institute of Infectious Diseases).

## ANTIBODY TEST OR SEROLOGICAL FINDINGS

The average incubation period of COVID-19 lasts for 5.1 days. Specific IgM antibodies can be detected within 3-5 days after symptom onset. Therefore, the rapid test should be used at least 3-5 days after the onset of symptoms.

IgG, known as permanent antibody, reaches at least 4-fold titration during recovery compared to the acute phase. Antibody testing may be more effective and cost-effective instead of antigen testing in areas where coronavirus is common. It is important to check IgM and IgG in cases where antigen test cannot be performed widely in the early period and adequate isolation cannot be provided, especially after the first positive case (Fig. **2**).

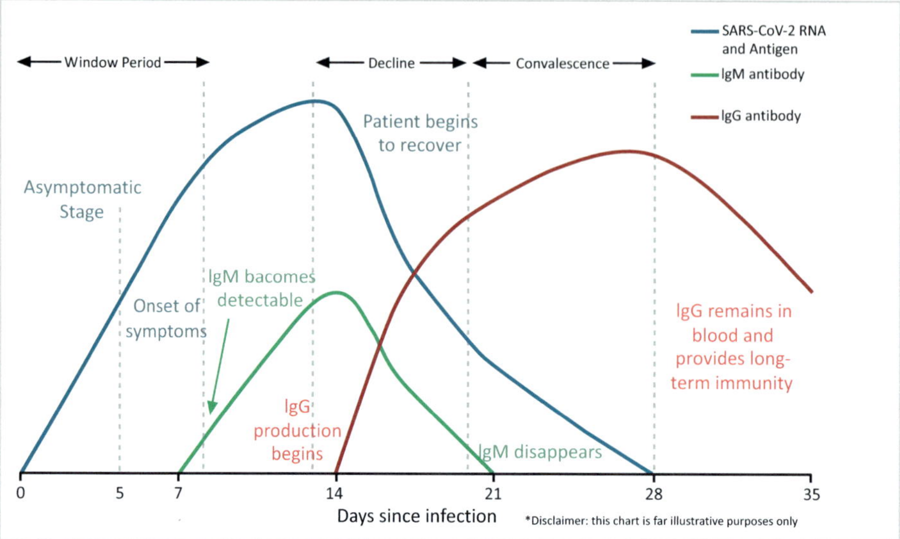


| Test results | | | Clinical Significance |
|---|---|---|---|
| PCR | IgM | IgG | |
| + | - | - | Patient may be in the window period of infection. |
| + | + | - | Patient may be in the early stage of infection. |
| + | + | + | Patient is in the active phase of infection. |
| + | - | + | Patient may be in the late or recurrent stage of infection. |
| - | + | - | Patient may be in the early stage of infection. PCR result may be false-negative. |
| - | - | + | Patient may have had a past infection, and has recovered. |
| - | + | + | Patient may be in the recovery stage of an infection, or the PCR result may be false-negative. |

**Fig. (2). A.** Interpretation of PCR. **B.** Antibody tests (IgM and IgG) positive and negative results.

## Do Antibody Tests Give Accurate Results In The Early Period After Infection?

Both yes and no. In a Cochrane review that performed a meta-analysis of 57 publications over 54 study cohorts, Deeks *et al*. reported that antibody tests in the first week yielded results with very low sensitivity (Deeks, 2020). Therefore, it cannot play a diagnostic role. However, it may have a value in patients with negative RT-PCR tests and late presentation.

## How Accurate Results Do Igg, M, and a Give?

Antibody tests have a very low sensitivity (30%) in detecting COVID-19 in the first week after symptom onset. In the second week, this value increases, and we see peak levels in the third week.

In addition,

- Antibody tests may be useful in revealing a past SARS-CoV-2 infection when performed 15 days or longer after the onset of symptoms.
- Its use in public health studies is controversial due to the high risk of 'bias', its reliability is low, in accord with some small studies in the literature.
- Its accuracy has been mostly evaluated in hospitalized patients, therefore its performance at low antibody titers in mild or asymptomatic cases in the community is unknown.

Tests should be ordered with respect to the patient and the severity of the signs and symptoms. Countries (South Korea, New Zealand, and China), which performed many tests and identified the cases at an early stage, managed to control the disease in the most expedient and effective way. Especially New Zealand has come close to ending the process with very low mortality in this way.

## CHEST IMAGING - RADIOLOGICAL EXAMINATIONS

Highly suspicious cases should be screened by radiography (CXR) and tomography (chest CT), apart from serological / microbiological examinations.

Radiological findings are the most important adjuncts of the clinical findings and sometimes it can be a more important indicator than tests. In studies comparing CT and PCR tests, it has been noted that tomography can recognize the disease with very high accuracy, and furthermore, it demonstrates severity and extent of involvement. When used with a rational strategy and avoiding unnecessary radiation, CT helps us to detect patients in early stages.

## Which Should We Choose? X-ray, CT, USG, or MR?

CT has a priority in diagnosis. It is recommended not to be used in every patient as a screening test (Acr.org.2020). Although these two sentences seem to contradict each other, it means that CT should be taken diagnostically in cases with certain clinical findings and not for 'everyone'. CT scans should be performed to exclude lung involvement or to understand its prevalence, if the clinical status of any given patient indicates strong suspicions of COVID-19.

Although it is not a contraindication in children and pregnant women, it should be used with restrictions, but should be obtained if it would cause significant changes in treatment modalities.

The reason why CT is prominent in many regions of the world is its high sensitivity, as well as the ability to make additional diagnoses such as PE and bacterial pneumonia, or alternative diagnoses that can change the treatment, such as pneumothoraces or abscesses (Scialpi, 2020). In critically ill COVID-19 patients with pneumonia, PE needs to be ruled out.

It has also been recommended to repeat CT when there is an important clinical change in recovering patients.

The advantages of USG over CT are that it does not give radiation, is noninvasive, cheap, and reproducible (Peng 2020, Buonsense, 2020). However, its drawbacks are that it is operator-dependent, has low sensitivity, and fails to visualize deep-seated and intrapulmonary lesions (Sofia 2020, Huang 2020).

The most common early-stage findings noted with USG in COVID-19 patients are B-lines, patch-like consolidations, and irregular pleural lines (Huang, 2020). Since these findings are also found in other viral pneumonias, USG is thought to be not a good screening test (Tsai, 2014). It is known that the most common CT finding in COVID-19 patients is ground glass opacities (GGO) (Lei, 2020). The fact that GGO is most common in the posterobasal region explains the difficulty of reaching and diagnosing with USG at the bedside.

USG is still useful in patients with or suspected COVID-19, because the risk of pulmonary embolism is increased in these patients, USG can be used to rule out massive PE and DVT (Rouhezamin, 2020). As a result, USG can be used in the diagnosis and management of COVID-19, being aware of its limitations (Khalili, 2020).

CT identifies patients with COVID-19, but it cannot distinguish from other viral infections (H1N1, SARS-CoV and MERS-CoV). Therefore, we can postulate that the use of CT as a screening test will be a wrong choice. CT should not be used as a first test but should be used with certain criteria for symptomatic patients who will be hospitalized (Acr.org. (2020).

CXR may detect findings in the lungs. In the early stage, imaging shows multiple small irregular shadows and interstitial changes that are more prominent in the peripheral region of the lungs. As the disease progresses, imaging shows multiple GGO and infiltrates in both lungs. In severe cases, pulmonary consolidation may occur. However, pleural effusion is rare.

### *Tomography (CT):*

Weaknesses of the RT-PCR test with obtaining and performing it are debated widely. It has been suggested in some publications that chest CT can be used as a screening test instead of PCR, and positive results have been reported. As in diagnosis, thorax CT is used to highlight the progression of the disease, to monitor the effectiveness of the treatment and to decide on discharge. However, it should be kept in mind that CT cannot rule out some diseases definitely, and the isolation and quarantine measures of suspicious cases should not be ignored because they are only CT negative.

### *Artificial Intelligence (AI) for Covid-19 Diagnosis from Chest CT:*

In a multinational study on CT images to detect GGOs Warman *et al.* employed an AI-driven object detection model in search of COVID-19 (Warman, 2020). The model predicted COVID-19 with an accuracy of 96.8%, AUC-ROC of 0.966, sensitivity of 98.3%, precision of 95.9%, and specificity of 94.9%. The authors claimed that the model can discern COVID-19 GGOs from alternative diagnoses, which suggested that GGOs can be disease-specific.

### *Radiological Features:*

Although CXR is not adequately sensitive to detect GGOs and demonstrate normal findings in early stages of the disease, it can be employed with its low radiation, low cost, and easy application, even at the bedside. The sensitivity and accuracy of the CXR studies increase with the severity of the disease.

Some 'typical' imaging findings are visualized in CT images of most patients with COVID-19. Therefore, CT can also be used as a diagnostic tool such as RT-PCR (Zhao *et al*, 2020). However, in a radiological analysis study in which 101 patients were enrolled, it was reported that no CT findings were detected in 8% of the cases. It is recommended to use PCR test along with radiological screening for expedient diagnosis (Zu ZY *et al.*).

Characteristics of the radiological findings of COVID-19 are listed below, and percentages are given in Table **4**.

- Radiological findings are evident from the beginning.
- While GGO are frequent in the first days or weeks, consolidation and reticular densities are more frequent as the disease progresses.

CT findings are basically nonspecific and may be confused with other viral pneumonias.

- Subpleural / peripheral localization is prominent in the distribution of lesions.
- Often multiple lesions (at least 3 or more) involving multiple segments are noted.
- The most common lobe involved is the right lower lobe.
- Usually patchy lesions are seen, there may also be larger lesions or nodules.
- GGO and consolidation are the most common lesions among all.
- Interlobular septal thickening can be added to GGO (cobblestone view).
- There may be bronchial wall thickening.
- Air bronchograms and cavitations can be seen rarely.
- Pleural fluid and lymphadenopathy are rare, may lead to other diagnoses.
- Radiological progression is an indicator of poor clinical outcome.

**Table 4. Radiological findings and their percentages in patients.**

| | |
|---|---|
| **87%** | **Peripheral distribution** |
| **86%** | **GGO** |
| **82%** | **Bilateral involvement (100% in emergency admissions)** |
| **78%** | **Diffuse (24% in non-emergency group)** |
| **71%** | **Vascular enlargements** |
| **64%** | **Consolidation + GGO** |
| **54%** | **Lower lobe predominant** |
| **54%** | **Multifocal** |
| **52.5%** | **Bronchiectasis** |
| **48%** | **Reticulation** |
| **43%** | **Consolidation** |
| **29%** | **Bronchial wall thickening** |

## *CT Scoring Systems for Severity:*

Lieveld *et al.* aimed to validate the "COVID-19 Reporting and Data System (CO-RADS)" at the ED in order to compare COVID-19 CT data across different settings and countries, and whether the corresponding CT severity score (CTSS) was associated with prognosis (Lieveld, 2020). CO-RADS employs a scoring system from 0 to 5 to classify pulmonary involvement from very unlikely to very likely, respectively. The system had an area under the curve (AUC) compared to SARS-CoV-2 PCR of 0.91 (CI 0.89-0.94). The optimal CO-RADS cut-off was 4, with a sensitivity of 89.4% and specificity of 87.2%. After correcting for confounders, the CTSS was significantly positively associated with hospital and ICU admission, and mortality.

In another scoring system, Li *et al.* employed a modified semi-quantitative CT scoring system, in which the lung was divided into six zones by the level of tracheal carina and the level of inferior pulmonary vein bilaterally on CT (Li, 2020). GGOs, consolidation, crazy-paving pattern and overall lung involvement were rated by Likert scale of 0-4 or binary as 0 or 1. Global severity score for each targeted pattern was calculated as total score of six zones. Overall lung involvement score in the second week demonstrated predictive value for severity with a sensitivity of 81.0% and specificity of 69.2%

The sensitivity of thoracic CT in the diagnosis of COVID-19 is quite high, especially when evaluated together with serial CT images, and it provides a chance to detect 93% of previously RT-PCR negative patients. Contact history, clinical findings and imaging data should be considered more sensitive in the diagnosis of COVID-19 in those with a negative RT-PCR test.

Xia *et al.* Investigated the changes in thoracic CT findings due to COVID-19 pneumonia in the study they conducted on 21 pediatric cases from the onset of the disease to the recovery period (Xia *et al.*, 2020). Semi-quantitative method was used for CT scoring. Accordingly, the scoring system was used as follows: The 5 lobes of the lung are evaluated separately, and the total score for each patient ranged between 0 (no involvement) and 25 (maximum involvement):

0 = no involvement,
1 = <5% involvement,
2 = <25% involvement,
3 = 26% - 49% involvement,
4 = 50% -75% involvement,
5 => 75% involvement.

Another interesting point is that the thoracic CT findings in patients who are to be discharged after the PCR tests become negative are also quite colorful. Analysis of 125 COVID-19 cases revealed bilaterally distributed GGO in the lungs of 79.2% and fibrosis in 44.8% (Du, 2020). The right lower lobe was the most commonly involved area, and the lesions were usually between –570 to –470 HU. In the follow-up performed within 2-13 days, GGO decreased in both size and density. In quantitative analysis, it was observed that lung lesion volumes were also decreased (Fig. **3**).

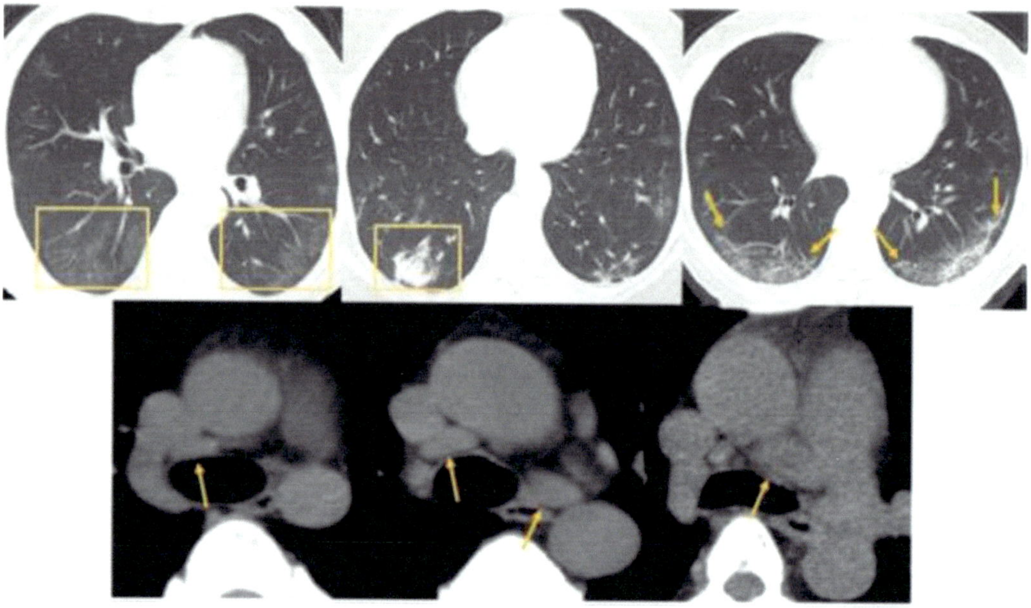

**Fig. (3).** Regression in thoracic CT findings in patients preparing for discharge.

(A) Multiple homogenous GGOs with very low density (box); (B) small consolidation with air bronchograms (box) in the right lung; (C) fibrosis with reticulation (arrow) in the subpleural regions of both lungs; (D,E,F) mediastinal lymph nodes with the short-axis diameter <10 mm (D), 10–15 mm (E) and >15 mm (F) (arrow).

## CLINICAL CLASSIFICATION

Approximately 81% of the patients exhibit mild symptoms, while 14% show severe symptoms requiring hospitalization, and 5% are critical patients requiring ICU follow-up.

**Mild Cases:** Clinical symptoms are mild and there is no sign of pneumonia on imaging.

**Moderate Cases:** Radiological findings of pneumonia and fever and respiratory symptoms, without marked respiratory distress.

## Severe Cases

### *Adult Cases who Meet Any of the Following Criteria:*

- Respiratory distress (30 bpm).
- Oxygen saturation ≤ 93%.
- Arterial partial pressure of oxygen ($PaO_2$) / fraction of inspired oxygen ($FiO_2$) 300 mmHg (1 mmHg = 0.133 kPa).
- Cases with chest imaging with significant progression of lesions for longer than 24 to 48 hours should be managed as severe cases.

### *Pediatric Cases That Meet Any Of the Following Criteria:*

- Tachypnea (Respiratory rate 60 bpm for babies under 2 months; 50 bpm for 2-to-12 month infants; 40 bpm for 1-5 years old and 30 bpm for 5 years and older children) regardless of fever and restlessness;
- Oxygen saturation ≤92% by finger pulse oximeter obtained at rest.
- Difficulty breathing (moaning, nasal breathing and infrasternal, supraclavicular and intercostal retractions), cyanosis and intermittent apnea.
- Drowsiness and convulsions.
- Feeding difficulties and signs of dehydration.

Critical Cases

Cases that meet any of the following criteria:

- Respiratory failure which prompts mechanical ventilation;
- Shock;
- Other organ failures necessitating ICU care.

Patients can present very differently from each other (Table **5**). Encephalopathy, diabetic ketoacidosis, renal failure, myocarditis, pericarditis, new onset congestive heart failure and *de novo* atrial fibrillation may be encountered.

## CASE EXAMPLES

Case scenarios and corresponding radiological views are provided (Figs. **4** - **8**) .

## CASE EXAMPLE AND TIME COURSE OF THE DISEASE

54-year-old Korean male patient, weighing 96 kg and having a BMI of 25.5, developed symptoms (fever and dry cough) in 5 to 7 days. Lymphopenia and eosinopenia were most prominent on the 6th day in his work up. Ceftriaxone was started on the 4th day of the disease, azithromycin on the 7th day, and lopinavir 200 mg / ritonavir 50 mg on the 10th day. On the 9th day, findings of pneumonia were marked on chest CT. The day after lopinavir + ritonavir treatment has been commenced, a decrease in viral load was detectable. What he had read about isolation and his illness from the mass media triggered depression and suicidal thoughts in the patient. Staying in a negative pressure room was also thought to contribute to changes in the patient's psychology. After the 15th day, the patient was discharged with radiological and clinical improvement.

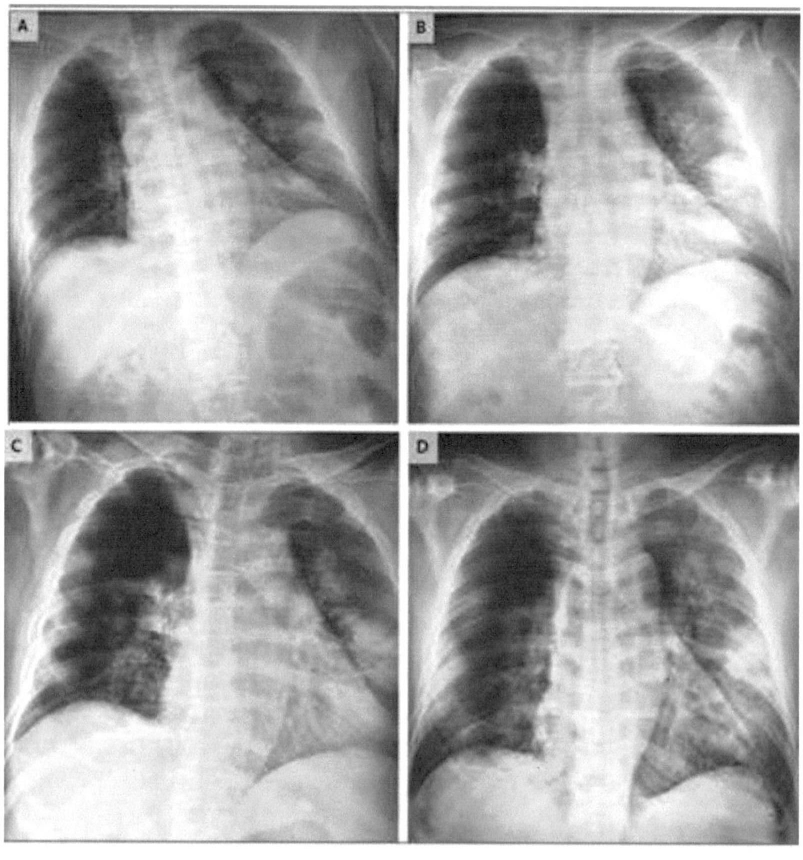


**Fig. (4).** Radiographic changes within 6 days of hospitalization in a 65-year-old male patient with a history of hypertension, diabetes, coronary artery disease, and lung cancer. (Day 0-A), (Day 3-B), (Day 5-C), (Day 6-D). The patient received oxygenation and supportive therapy for his shortness of breath, and he improved significantly within 1 week after treatment with antivirals and broad-spectrum antibiotics (Phan *et al*, 2020).

**Table 5. Clinical early warning indicators of serious and critical patients**

| Adults | Children |
|---|---|
| Lymphocytes gradually decrease | Altered mental status |
| Inflammatory factors in peripheral blood such as IL-6 and C-reactive proteins are progressively elevated; | Increased respiratory rate |
| Lactate is elevated gradually; | Lactate is elevated gradually |
| Lung lesions progress rapidly in a short time. | The visualization of infiltrations in both lungs or more than one lobe, pleural effusion, or rapid progression of lesions in a short time; |
| | Underlying diseases (congenital heart disease, chest deformity, abnormal hemoglobins and severe malnutrition *etc.*) or infants with immune deficiency or long-term use of immunosuppressant medication. |

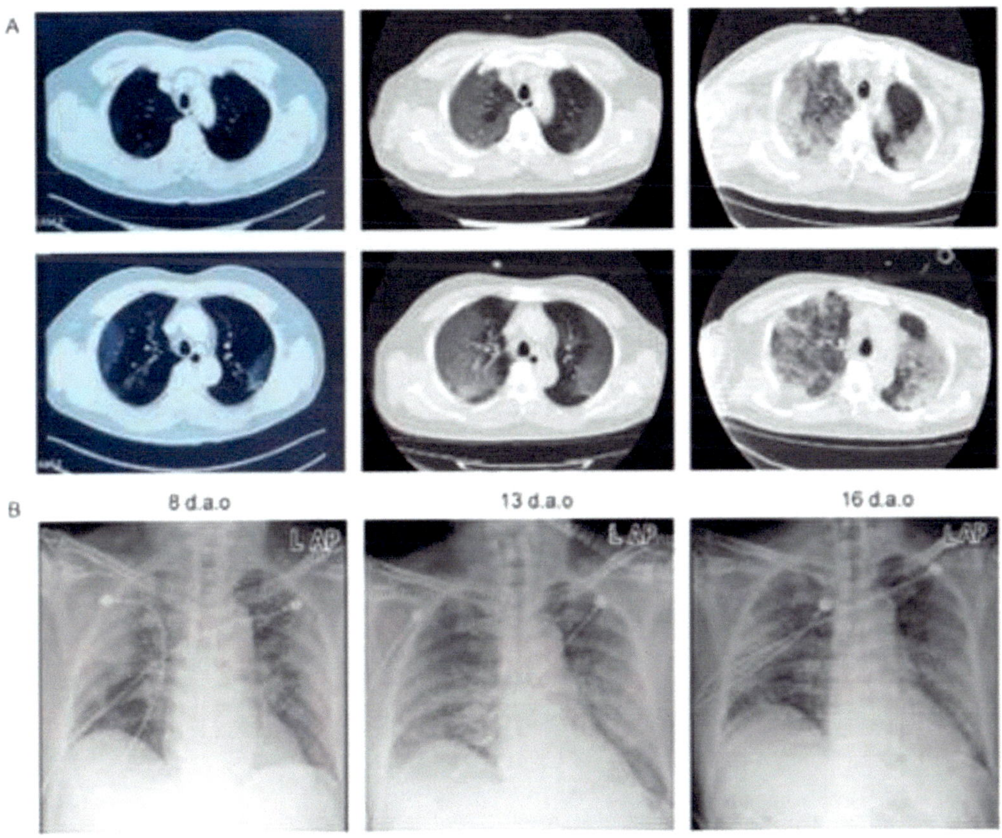


**Fig. (5).** 66-year-old Chinese male patient. Findings on CT and simultaneous CXR at 8, 13 and 16 days after the onset of the complaints.

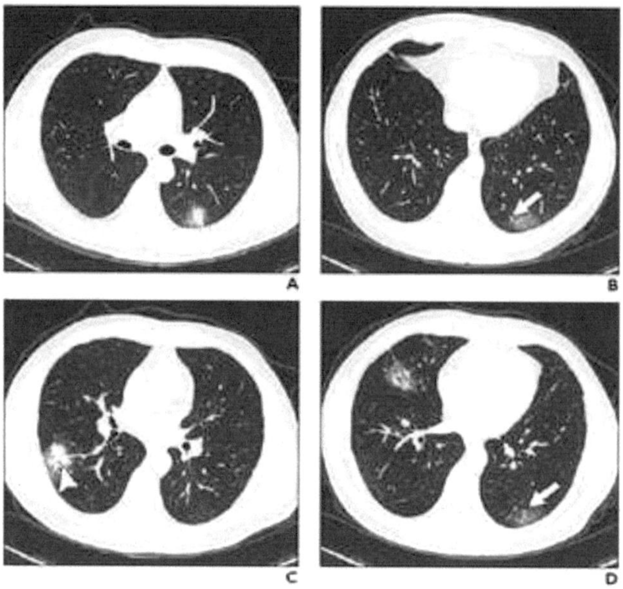


**Fig. (6).** A 37-year-old male patient presents with complaints of 38C fever and cough after a brief history of being in Wuhan. Bilateral multifocal GGO, bronchiectasis (C) and vascular enlargements (B, D) are seen on CT scans elicited on admission.

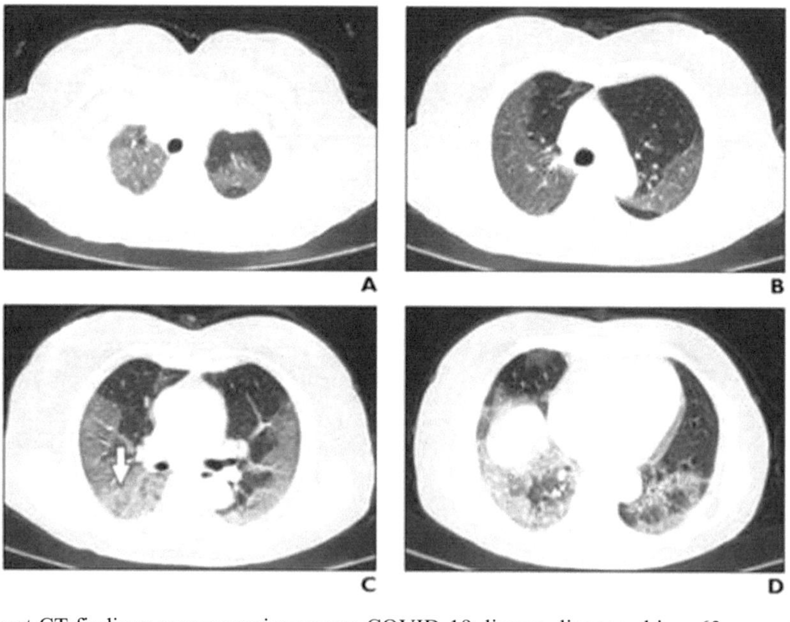


**Fig. (7).** Chest CT findings accompanying severe COVID-19 disease diagnosed in a 63-year-old woman in Wuhan. She presented with fever and cough. One day after admission, bilateral GGO and reticulation pattern is seen on CT images (CT involvement score 18).

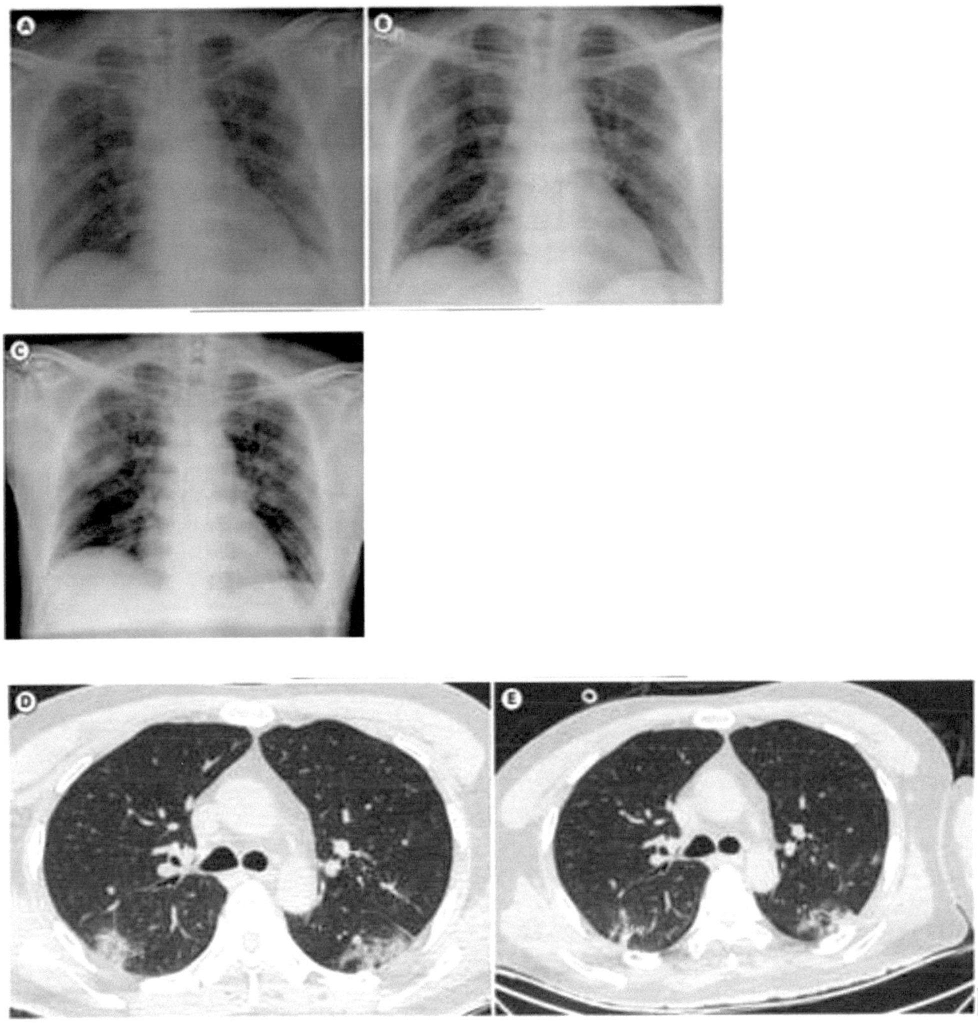

**Fig. (8). A.** Radiography on the 3rd day of the disease. **B.** 9th day, **C.** 15th day CXR. **D.** 9th day tomography. **E.** 15th day tomography.

## CONCLUSION

In summary, COVID-19 cases present with nonspecific clinical findings. Since epidemiological and clinical findings may be insufficient for diagnosis, laboratory and radiological findings are important adjuncts in diagnosis.

Identification of accurate biomarkers that can predict the severity and outcome of the disease is necessary to guide clinical care. Blood test analyses such as CRP, complete blood count (*e.g.*, sneutrophil/lymphocyte ratio, CD4/CD8 ratio), d-dimer, ferritin can be used as an alternative to RT-PCR to identify patients with

COVID-19 in countries with great shortages of RT-PCR reagents and / or specialist laboratories. These ancillary tests are also used as to support or refute the presumptive diagnoses of the clinicians, even if RT-PCR tests are readily available.

Radiological adjuncts are used both to screen the disease in suspected individuals, and also to highlight the severity of involvement in the respiratory tract. Both markers of blood chemistry and radiological adjuncts are also used to predict deterioration and follow the clinical course of the patients.

Typical CT findings are peripheral multifocal patch-like GGO and inferior / posterior lobe involvement. The greater the number and size of GGO, the more severe the disease. Thin-section CT and low-dose contrast-enhanced CT, if necessary, are recommended. If there is no finding in the CT, which can be obtained immediately in the suspect case, the patient can be sent home to be evaluated at regular intervals and to comply with the isolation recommendations, or if there are findings, the quarantine decision can be made more easily.

## REFERENCES

Acr.org (2020) *ACR recommendations for the use of chest radiography and computed tomography (CT) for suspected COVID-19 infection.*https://www.acr.org/Advocacy-and-Economics/ACR-Position-State

Buonsenso, D, Piano, A, Raffaelli, F, Bonadia, N, de Gaetano Donati, K & Franceschi, F (2020) Point-o--Care Lung Ultrasound findings in novel coronavirus disease-19 pnemoniae: a case report and potential applications during COVID-19 outbreak. *Eur Rev Med Pharmacol Sci,* 24, 2776-80. [PMID: 32196627]

Deeks, JJ, Dinnes, J, Takwoingi, Y, Davenport, C, Spijker, R, Taylor-Phillips, S, Adriano, A, Beese, S, Dretzke, J, Ferrante di Ruffano, L, Harris, IM, Price, MJ, Dittrich, S, Emperador, D, Hooft, L, Leeflang, MM & Van den Bruel, A Cochrane COVID-19 Diagnostic Test Accuracy Group (2020) Antibody tests for identification of current and past infection with SARS-CoV-2. *Cochrane Database Syst Rev,* 6, CD013652. [PMID: 32584464]

Du, S, Gao, S, Huang, G, Li, S, Chong, W, Jia, Z, Hou, G, Wáng, YXJ & Zhang, L (2020) Chest lesion CT radiological features and quantitative analysis in RT-PCR turned negative and clinical symptoms resolved COVID-19 patients. *Quant Imaging Med Surg,* 10, 1307-17. [http://dx.doi.org/10.21037/qims-20-531] [PMID: 32550139]

Elshazli, RM, Toraih, EA, Elgaml, A, El-Mowafy, M, El-Mesery, M, Amin, MN, Hussein, MH, Killackey, MT, Fawzy, MS & Kandil, E (2020) Diagnostic and prognostic value of hematological and immunological markers in COVID-19 infection: A meta-analysis of 6320 patients. *PLoS One,* 15, e0238160. [http://dx.doi.org/10.1371/journal.pone.0238160] [PMID: 32822430]

Henry, BM, de Oliveira, MHS, Benoit, S, Plebani, M & Lippi, G (2020) Hematologic, biochemical and immune biomarker abnormalities associated with severe illness and mortality in coronavirus disease 2019 (COVID-19): a meta-analysis. *Clin Chem Lab Med,* 58, 1021-8. [http://dx.doi.org/10.1515/cclm-2020-0369] [PMID: 32286245]

Huang, Y, Wang, S & Liu, Y (2020) A preliminary study on the ultrasonic manifestations of peripulmonary lesions of non-critical novel coronavirus pneumonia (COVID-19). *SSRN,* 3544750 [http://dx.doi.org/10.2139/ssrn.3544750]

Japanese National Institute of Infectious Diseases (2020) *Field Briefing: Diamond Princess COVID-19*

*Cases.*Https: // www.niid.go.jp/niid/en/2019-ncov-e/9417-covid-dp-fe-02.html

Khalili, N, Haseli, S & Iranpour, P (2020) Lung Ultrasound in COVID-19 Pneumonia: Prospects and Limitations. *Acad Radiol,* 27, 1044-5.
[http://dx.doi.org/10.1016/j.acra.2020.04.032] [PMID: 32444253]

Lei, J, Li, J, Li, X & Qi, X (2020) CT imaging of the 2019 novel coronavirus (2019-nCoV) pneumonia. *Radiology,* 295, 18.
[http://dx.doi.org/10.1148/radiol.2020200236] [PMID: 32003646]

Li, S, Liu, S, Wang, B, Li, Q, Zhang, H, Zeng, L, Ge, H, Ma, Q & Shen, N (2021) Predictive value of chest CT scoring in COVID-19 patients in Wuhan, China: A retrospective cohort study. *Respir Med,* 176, 106271.
[http://dx.doi.org/10.1016/j.rmed.2020.106271] [PMID: 33296777]

Lieveld, AWE, Azijli, K & Teunissen, BP (2020) Predictive value of chest CT scoring in COVID-19 patients in Wuhan, China: A retrospective cohort study. *Respir Med,* 176, 106271.

Liu, J, Liu, Y, Xiang, P, Pu, L, Xiong, H, Li, C, Zhang, M, Tan, J, Xu, Y, Song, R, Song, M, Wang, L, Zhang, W, Han, B, Yang, L, Wang, X, Zhou, G, Zhang, T, Li, B, Wang, Y, Chen, Z & Wang, X (2020) Neutrophil-to-lymphocyte ratio predicts critical illness patients with 2019 coronavirus disease in the early stage. *J Transl Med,* 18, 206.
[http://dx.doi.org/10.1186/s12967-020-02374-0] [PMID: 32434518]

Liu, Z, Long, W & Tu, M (2020) Lymphocyte subset (CD4+, CD8+) counts reflects the severity of infection and predict the clinical outcomes in patients with COVID-19. *J Infect,* 81, 318-56.

Mohammadi, A, Esmaeilzadeh, E, Li, Y, Bosch, RJ & Li, JZ (2020) SARS-CoV-2 detection in different respiratory sites: A systematic review and meta-analysis. *EBioMedicine,* 59, 102903.
[http://dx.doi.org/10.1016/j.ebiom.2020.102903] [PMID: 32718896]

Pallotto, C, Suardi, LR, Esperti, S, Tarquini, R, Grifoni, E, Meini, S, Valoriani, A, Di Martino, S, Cei, F, Sisti, E, Piani, F, Botta, A, Salomoni, E, Baragli, F & Blanc, P (2020) Increased CD4/CD8 ratio as a risk factor for critical illness in coronavirus disease 2019 (COVID-19): a retrospective multicentre study. *Infect Dis (Lond),* 52, 675-7.
[http://dx.doi.org/10.1080/23744235.2020.1778178] [PMID: 32543971]

Peng, Q-Y, Wang, X-T & Zhang, L-N Chinese Critical Care Ultrasound Study Group (CCUSG) (2020) Findings of lung ultrasonography of novel corona virus pneumonia during the 2019-2020 epidemic. *Intensive Care Med,* 46, 849-50. [Phan LT, Nguyen TV, Luong QC, *et al.* Importation and Human-to-Human Transmission of a Novel Coronavirus in Vietnam.].
[http://dx.doi.org/10.1007/s00134-020-05996-6] [PMID: 32166346]

Rouhezamin, MR & Haseli, S (2020) Diagnosing pulmonary thromboembolism in COVID-19: a stepwise clinical and imaging approach. *Acad Radiol,* 27, 896-7.
[http://dx.doi.org/10.1016/j.acra.2020.04.023] [PMID: 32331965]

Scialpi, M, Scialpi, S, Piscioli, I, Battista Scalera, G & Longo, F (2020) Pulmonary thromboembolism in critical ill COVID-19 patients. *Int J Infect Dis,* 95, 361-2.
[http://dx.doi.org/10.1016/j.ijid.2020.04.056] [PMID: 32339717]

Siddiqi, HK & Mehra, MR (2020) COVID-19 illness in native and immunosuppressed states: A clinical-therapeutic staging proposal. *J Heart Lung Transplant,* 39, 405-7.
[http://dx.doi.org/10.1016/j.healun.2020.03.012] [PMID: 32362390]

Sofia, S, Boccatonda, A, Montanari, M, Spampinato, M, D'ardes, D, Cocco, G, Accogli, E, Cipollone, F & Schiavone, C (2020) Thoracic ultrasound and SARS-COVID-19: a pictorial essay. *J Ultrasound,* 23, 217-21.
[http://dx.doi.org/10.1007/s40477-020-00458-7] [PMID: 32297175]

Tatum, D, Taghavi, S, Houghton, A, Stover, J, Toraih, E & Duchesne, J (2020) Neutrophil-to-Lymphocyte Ratio and Outcomes in Louisiana COVID-19 Patients. *Shock,* 54, 652-8.
[http://dx.doi.org/10.1097/SHK.0000000000001585] [PMID: 32554992]

Tsai, NW, Ngai, CW, Mok, KL & Tsung, JW (2014) Lung ultrasound imaging in avian influenza A (H7N9)

respiratory failure. *Crit Ultrasound J,* 6, 6.
[http://dx.doi.org/10.1186/2036-7902-6-6] [PMID: 24949191]

Wan, S, Yi, Q, Fan, S, Lv, J, Zhang, X, Guo, L, Lang, C, Xiao, Q, Xiao, K, Yi, Z, Qiang, M, Xiang, J, Zhang, B, Chen, Y & Gao, C (2020) Relationships among lymphocyte subsets, cytokines, and the pulmonary inflammation index in coronavirus (COVID-19) infected patients. *Br J Haematol,* 189, 428-37.
[http://dx.doi.org/10.1111/bjh.16659] [PMID: 32297671]

Wang, F, Nie, J, Wang, H, Zhao, Q, Xiong, Y, Deng, L, Song, S, Ma, Z, Mo, P & Zhang, Y (2020) Characteristics of peripheral lymphocyte subs *et al*teration in COVID-19 pneumonia. *J Infect Dis,* 221, 1762-9.
[http://dx.doi.org/10.1093/infdis/jiaa150] [PMID: 32227123]

Wang, W, Xu, Y, Gao, R, Lu, R, Han, K, Wu, G & Tan, W (2020) Detection of SARS-CoV-2 in Different Types of Clinical Specimens. *JAMA,* 323, 1843-4.
[http://dx.doi.org/10.1001/jama.2020.3786] [PMID: 32159775]

Warman, A, Warman, P & Sharma, A (2020) Characteristics of peripheral lymphocyte subs *et al*teration in COVID-19 pneumonia. *J Infect Dis,* 221, 1762-9.

Xia, W, Shao, J, Guo, Y, Peng, X, Li, Z & Hu, D (2020) Clinical and CT features in pediatric patients with COVID-19 infection: Different points from adults. *Pediatr Pulmonol,* 55, 1169-74.
[http://dx.doi.org/10.1002/ppul.24718] [PMID: 32134205]

Zhao, D, Yao, F, Wang, L, Zheng, L, Gao, Y, Ye, J, Guo, F, Zhao, H & Gao, R (2020) A Comparative Study on the Clinical Features of Coronavirus 2019 (COVID-19) Pneumonia With Other Pneumonias. *Clin Infect Dis,* 71, 756-61.
[http://dx.doi.org/10.1093/cid/ciaa247] [PMID: 32161968]

Zhou, F, Yu, T, Du, R, Fan, G, Liu, Y, Liu, Z, Xiang, J, Wang, Y, Song, B, Gu, X, Guan, L, Wei, Y, Li, H, Wu, X, Xu, J, Tu, S, Zhang, Y, Chen, H & Cao, B (2020) Clinical course and risk factors for mortality of adult inpatients with COVID-19 in Wuhan, China: a retrospective cohort study. *Lancet,* 395, 1054-62.
[http://dx.doi.org/10.1016/S0140-6736(20)30566-3] [PMID: 32171076]

Zu, ZY, Jiang, MD, Xu, PP, Chen, W, Ni, QQ, Lu, GM & Zhang, LJ (2020) Coronavirus Disease 2019 (COVID-19): A Perspective from China. *Radiology,* 296, E15-25.
[http://dx.doi.org/10.1148/radiol.2020200490] [PMID: 32083985]

# CHAPTER 7

# Cardiovascular Disease, Myocarditis, Infarctions, And COVID-19

**Abstract:** In the last centuries, cardiovascular diseases (CVD) have been the prominent cause of health impairment worldwide. Starting with the COVID-19 outbreak, which has become the predominant health issue all over the world since December 2019, this phenomenon has to be reassessed in many aspects. In a given patient, CVD results in a more serious clinical course of COVID-19 and a boosted risk of death. Additionally, both CVD and COVID-19 cause myocardial damage, which increases morbidity and mortality with a synergistic effect. It is also clear that cardiac patients (*i.e.*, CVD and others) are deprived of the usual healthcare services they receive due to the overcrowdedness and shift of hospital and pre-hospital medical services in the COVID-19 era. As we can contemplate that pandemics will not disappear quickly anytime soon, the health system will have to be reorganized completely. The purpose of this article is to reveal and seek solutions to the relationship between pandemics and heart disease and their impact on ordinary healthcare, along with CVD, myocardial damage, and other diseases caused by COVID-19.

**Keywords:** Acute myocardial infarction, Cardiovascular disease, Coronavirus, COVID-19, Diagnosis, Myocardial injury, Myocarditis, Treatment.

Cardiovascular disease (CVD) has been associated with viral infections or outbreaks for decades.It has been reported that approximately half of COVID-19 patients have CVD, and this rate increases to 70% in intensive care units (ICU) (Zhou *et al.*, 2020; Wang *et al.*, 2020). It is known that 50% of the cases with MERS infection in 2012 had DM and HT, and 30% had CVD (Badawi *et al.*, 2016).

## KEY FINDINGS FROM DIFFERENT DATABASE STUDIES

In the study which analyzed 5700 patients in New York; frequency of HT was reported as 56.6%, obesity 41.7%, DM 33.8%, CAD 11.1%, and CHF 6.9% (Richardson, 2020). In the study that included more than 72,000 patients in China, 12.8% hypertension, 5.3% DM, 4.2% CVD were found. The frequency of

Ozgur KARCIOGLU, Selman YENIOCAK and Mandana HOSSEINZADEH

comorbidity is similar in industrialized countries, except that the hypertension, metabolic disorders, and obesity rates are significantly higher than the far east, but the prevalence varies considerably.

When analyzing 22,254 patients who were screened with PCR tests between 5 March and 9 April in NYC, at least one comorbid disease was reported in about half of those with positive tests (46%) (Kalyanaraman Marcello *et al*, 2020). In the sample, 33% diabetes, 37% HT, 24% CVD, 11% CRF were noted. Among the hospitalized patients, 28% died. Male gender, age, DM, history of heart disease, presence of CRF are risk factors for both test positivity and death.

**CV Risk Factors that are Thought to Affect the Clinical Course of COVID-19:**

- Male gender,
- Advanced age,
- DM,
- Hypertension,
- Obesity,
- A history of cardiovascular or cerebrovascular disease,

In a case series from Detroit Suleyman *et al.* searched for independent risk factors for admission to intensive care units: being over the age of 60, male sex, HT, DM, CRF, severe obesity (BMI>= 40) and cancer were reported to be the ones (Suleyman *et al*, 2020). Smoking was also higher in hospitalized patients. Admissions due to dyspnea, tachypnea or hypoxia also increases the risk of hospitalization. Fever increases the likelihood of hospitalization but does not predict poor outcome in patients with COVID-19. Inflammatory markers were also found higher in those hospitalized in ED.

Respiratory failure developed in 74% of those hospitalized in ICU and MV was required in 81% among these. 25% of those hospitalized had to be transferred to ED. The majority of those who received MV under 40 years of age (62.5%) had severe obesity, while those who did not need MV were only 26%. Mortality in ICU was 40%, and 7% in all those hospitalized. 45.6% of those who require MV died of severe complications.

## ARE ETHNIC DIFFERENCES IMPORTANT FOR COVID-19?

Marcello *et al.* conducted a study which analyzed more than 22,000 patients in NYC, and reported that 26% of COVID-19s were black and 34% were Hispanic

(Kalyanaraman Marcello, 2020). They reported that comorbidities are more common in ethnic groups than others, but being black or Hispanic after adjustments is not directly related to positive PCR testing or death.

In another cohort reported from Louisiana, it is stated that blacks, which make up only 31% of the population, constitute 77% of the COVID-19 patients who are admitted into hospital, but being black is not an independent risk factor when confounding factors are excluded (Price-Haywood *et al*, 2020). 70.6% of the dead are black.

## HT AND COVID-19

In almost all studies analyzing the characteristics of patients with COVID-19, HT championed among the comorbidities in the given samples. In a study investigating the link of the existing diseases of patients with severe COVID-19 with clinical course in China, it was noted that being over 60 years old, male sex, CVD, HT, myocardial injury, and thrombocytopenia were associated with death (Hu *et al*, 2020). HT was detected in 29% of the dead, while it was found in only 9% in severe cases who survived (OR value for HT = 5.5). In the light of this information, the authors created a death prediction model.

### Death Relationship With Anti-HT Drugs:

Patients with COVID-19 from two locations in Italy were followed up for 24 days (Bravi *et al*, 2020). The average age of deceased patients was 79 and 71% were hypertensive, while 42% had CVD. No relationship has been established between using ACEI or ARB and severe illness or death. Important predictors for severe disease were being over the age of 70, male sex, DM, COPD and CVD. Of these, only age, male sex, and DM were predictors of very severe / lethal disease (Table **1**).

**Table 1. Logistic regression model predicting severe or very severe/lethal COVID-19 syndrome (grouped together, Model C) or very severe/lethal disease only (Model D), in the total sample (n = 1603) (Adapted from Bravi *et al*, 2020).**

| Variables | (C) Severe or Very Severe/ lethal OR (95% CI) | p | (D) Very Severe/ Lethal OR (95% CI) | p |
|---|---|---|---|---|
| Male gender | 1.76 (1.40–2.23) | <0.001 | 1.69 (1.20–2.37) | 0.003 |
| Age class, in years | - | | | |
| •<50 | 1 | - | 1 | - |
| •50–59.9 | 2.36 (1.68–3.32) | <0.001 | 3.92 (1.48–10.3) | 0.006 |
| •60–69.9 | 3.51 (2.43–5.07) | <0.001 | 11.4 (4.63–28.1) | <0.001 |
| •70–79.9 | 5.72 (3.81–8.58) | <0.001 | 16.5 (6.66–40.9) | <0.001 |

*(Table 1) cont.....*

| Variables | (C) Severe or Very Severe/ lethal OR (95% CI) | p | (D) Very Severe/ Lethal OR (95% CI) | p |
|---|---|---|---|---|
| •≥80 | 9.06 (6.04–13.6) | <0.001 | 27.1 (11.1–66.3) | <0.001 |
| Diabetes | 1.52 (1.05–2.18) | 0.025 | 1.58 (1.06–2.34) | 0.023 |
| Hypertension | 1.10 (0.82–1.47) | 0.5 | 1.39 (0.94–2.05) | 0.097 |
| Major cardiovascular diseases | 1.88 (1.32–2.70) | 0.001 | 1.05 (0.71–1.56) | 0.8 |
| Cancer | 1.26 (0.81–1.95) | 0.3 | 1.11 (0.67–1.82) | 0.7 |
| COPD | 1.88 (1.11–3.20) | 0.020 | 1.44 (0.84–2.47) | 0.2 |
| Renal disease | 1.58 (0.90–2.76) | 0.11 | 1.13 (0.64–1.99) | 0.7 |

The entry of SARS-CoV-2 into the cell using ACE2 receptors and subsequently causing damage to different cell, tissue and organ systems was illustrated in Fig. (**1**) .

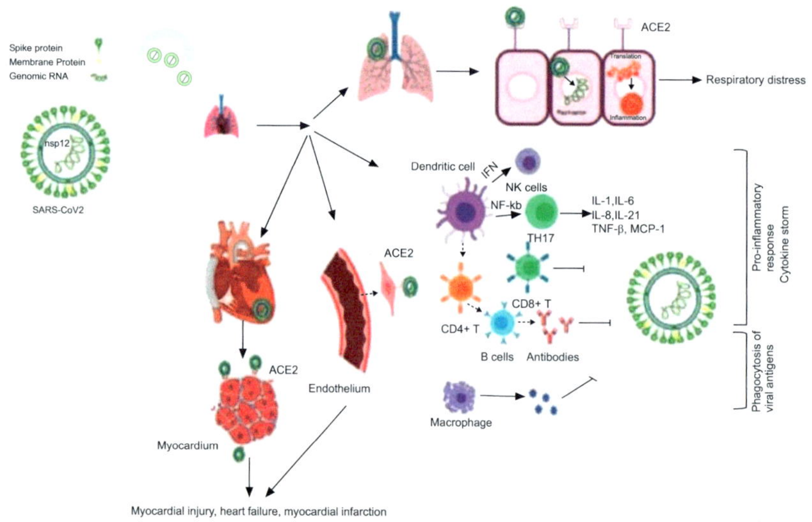


**Fig. (1).** Illustration depicting the entry of SARS-CoV-2 into the cell using ACE2 receptors and subsequently causing damage to different cell, tissue, and organ systems.

## Who is More Critical Among CVD + COVID-19?

Among 112 patients with CVD also diagnosed with COVID-19, lymphocyte count was significantly lower and CRP was significantly higher in the critical group than the others (Peng *et al*, 2020). BMI is higher, oxygenation index is low and lactic acid is higher in patients who die compared to survivors. The use of drugs such as ACE inhibitor, AT1RB is not different between the two groups.

Plasma IL-6 levels have also been reported to be higher in people with cardiac injury (Wang *et al*, 2020).

**Mechanisms that trigger myocardial damage in COVID-19:**

a. Severe systemic inflammatory stimulus - cytokine storm
b. Ischemia due to increased consumption or demand
c. Plaque rupture
d. Vascular inflammation

## MYOCARDIAL INJURY SEVERITY AND MORTALITY

Autopsy showed interstitial mononuclear inflammatory cell infiltration in the myocardium (Xu *et al*, 2020). Also, markers showing myocardial damage increase with COVID-19 (Xu *et al*, 2020; Guo *et al*, 2020; Shi *et al*, 2020). Shi *et al.* reported that myocardial damage was close to 20% in patients who died (Shi *et al*, 2020). Moreover, cardiac damage is the risk factor that affects mortality most and independently (hazard ratio: 4.26). Guo *et al.* reported that high troponin levels accompanied significantly increased mortality (Guo *et al*, 2020).

In the series of Guo *et al.*, which included 187 patients with COVID-19, they stated that there was a better clinical course in patients with CVD and no acute myocardial injury compared to those with both. For example, mortality in patients with fulminant myocarditis is between 40% and 70% (Caforio *et al*, 2013; Ammirati *et al*, 2019).

The relationship between the diagnosis of CVD, TnT levels and mortality rates in patients diagnosed with COVID-19 was studied by Guo *et al*, in 2020. The highest mortality is in the group with CVD and high TnT. B. The dynamic escalation of TnT and NT-proBNP levels in those who died and those who were discharged. Both TnT and NT-proBNP levels increased during the course of hospitalization in those who died, but no such dynamic changes of TnT or NT-proBNP levels were noted in survivors.

**How Much Myocardial Damage Occurs in COVID-19?**

In many studies,the myocardial damage has been reported to increase in parallel with the severity of the COVID-19 infection. He *et al.* demonstrated that more than half of the patients diagnosed with COVID-19 hospitalized in China in February 2020 had myocardial damage (He *et al*, 2020). This has been shown to have a direct affect in-hospital mortality (61% *vs.* 25%). In the study, levels of CRP and BNP were significantly higher (3 times or more) in those with myocardial damage than that of the others.

Chen *et al.* revealed that the disease is closely related to myocardial damage in their analysis on 150 COVID-19 cases (Chen *et al*, 2020). High levels of cTnI and the development of CHF have been disclosed as independent risk factors for myocardial damage.

## In Whom Does Myocardial Damage Occur and How Do We Identify It?

Myocardial damage is more common in older people with COVID-19 and those with increased TnT levels (Shi *et al*, 2020; Guo *et al*, 2020). Although TnT levels are normal in these patients, HT, CAD, CHF, and DM are more common than others.

While COVID-19 infects the alveoli in the lung and triggers obstruction in the small airways, it can also affect the vessels, causing damage to the heart, kidney and nervous system, intestines, and liver. For example, protein or blood cells may be detected in the urine in every second patient. It was also stated that hemodialysis was performed in 14% to 30% of the intensive care patients with COVID-19 in Wuhan. It is postulated that all this damage cannot be explained only by 'storming cytokines'.

In patients with COVID-19, death usually occurs from multiple organ failure, and it can be difficult to distinguish between myocardial damage and other organ failure syndromes. Myocardial damage occurs in patients with cardiac dysfunction and ventricular dysrhythmias.

Guo *et al.* reported that 28% of 187 COVID-19 patients had myocardial damage (Guo *et al*, 2020). He *et al.* raised the bar, and showed that 50% of 54 patients with COVID-19 diagnosed in China in February 2020 had myocardial damage (He *et al*, 2020).

Bansal *et al.* reported that acute cardiac damage was present in 8% to 12% of all COVID-19 cases as a result of the literature review (Bansal, 2020). Systemic inflammation and direct viral involvement contribute to cardiac injury. Presence of CVD and acute cardiac damage significantly accompany significant deterioration.

## Any Pathological Finding?

Yes. Interestingly, in autopsy cases died of COVID-19, incidence of SARS-Co--2 positivity in cardiac tissue as well as CD3+, CD45+, and CD68+ cells in the myocardium and gene expression of tumor necrosis growth factor α, interferon γ, chemokine ligand 5, as well as interleukin-6, -8, and -18 were identified (Lindner *et al*, 2020). Cardiac tissue from 39 consecutive autopsy cases were analyzed (median age: 85) SARS-CoV-2 could be documented in 24 of 39 patients (61.5%). Of note, there was no significant difference in regard to inflammatory cell infiltrates or leukocyte numbers per high power field between those with a diagnosis of COVID-19 and those without. These findings suggest that among individuals with COVID-19, overt myocarditis may not be identified in the acute phase, but the long-term consequences of this cardiac infection needs to be elucidated.

## Global View of Myocardial Infarction (STEMI / NSTEMI) After COVID-19

Due to the serious increase in COVID-19 cases all over the world, the health system is concerned that the "other" patients will be ignored when its focus has shifted and faces a serious healthcare burden.

Very interesting data are obtained from the world in this regard. In Hong Kong, Tam *et al.* shared data which indicated that the 'speed of care' was severely affected after COVID-19 in STEMI cases (Tam *et al*, 2020). In Hong Kong, there was a rapid increase in the duration of the ambulance reaching to the patient (Symptom onset to first medical contact) from 80-90 minutes to 318 minutes after the call. This raises a concern that healthcare system in the COVID-19 era may not be able to care for cardiac emergencies adequately due to the burden and chaos it brings to most institutions.

## Diagnostic Strategies:

In the pandemic period, invasive procedures necessitating close contact with the patient carry a high risk for disease transmission.Thus, additional non-invasive evaluation is required in the ED to verify the diagnosis, as STEMI cases can also be admitted with atypical symptoms and signs. In this way, both COVID-19 risk classification is made and the diagnosis is tried to be clarified in terms of STEMI. Myocardial wall movement deficits are evaluated by POCUS or bedside echocardiography. The diagnosis is clarified by clinical examination, ECG, laboratory (enzyme elevation), and imaging data. Coronary CT-angiography can be considered, for example, where ECG and echocardiography are vague and the patient is stable. Catheter laboratory activation should be considered immediately thereafter.

Myocarditis, which is more common in viral infections such that in the COVID-19 period, may also mimic STEMI. Among patients with COVID-19, death was found to be significantly more common in patients diagnosed with myocarditis.

## Treatment Strategy: PCI or Fibrinolysis?

The standard method for STEMI patients during the pandemic period will be the primary PCI within the appropriate time frame (Mahmud *et al*, 2020). In all cases, catheterization should be considered as a priority in the management of hemodynamic unstable patients. For this procedure, PPE should be fully worn and the intervention applied in a specially designed and adapted catheter laboratory. In the USA, the consensus document published with associations of cardiologists and emergency physicians stated that fibrinolytic-based strategies will be developed in cases where PCI cannot be implemented or the timing will not be correct (Mahmud *et al*, 2020).

Respiratory decompensation in intubated cases with severe COVID-19 in whom ARDS is also in the differential diagnosis should be evaluated on a case-by-case basis. There should be a critical assessment as to whether the patient will benefit from an invasive approach to have an impact on life expectancy.

### Did The Pandemic Affect Heart Attacks?

Yes, a lot. Italian researchers reported that the number of patients with STEMI or NSTEMI admitted to the catheter laboratory during the COVID-19 epidemic period decreased significantly, compared to the same period of the previous year (De Rosa, 2020). They found a total reduction of 48.4%, (26.5% in STEMI and 65% in NSTEMI) (P <0.001). The decrease in female patients with STEMI was more pronounced than in men (41.2% *vs.* 17.8%). Although the pandemic primarily affected Northern Italy, a similar decrease occurred in Southern and central Italy in a few weeks. STEMI case fatality rate boosted significantly with the pandemic compared to last year [risk ratio (RR) = 3.3, P <0.001]. Complications also increased (RR = 1.8, P = 0.009). This is an alarm finding in terms of public health and must be dealt with robust interventions.

## COVID-19 IS ASSOCIATED WITH CVD IN 5 DIFFERENT WAYS:

1. People who have previously been diagnosed with CVD have an increased risk of more severe disease and death when they are infected with COVID-19.
2. COVID-19 directly or indirectly causes CV complications. These are AMI, arrhythmias, myocarditis and VTE.
3. Medicines and other treatments for COVID-19 can damage CVS, as in hydroxychloroquine.
4. Patients may become susceptible to disease transmission for reasons such as going out to hospital for CV care, breaking a quarantine, *etc.*
5. The management, diagnosis and treatment of CVD may be delayed and the

clinical course may deteriorate due to the treatments and other problems in the pandemic environment (Table **2**).

**Table 2. The problems encountered in the pandemic process in the care of CVD emergencies and similar cases.**

| Problem Source | Description |
|---|---|
| **Reasons arising from the patient:** | Drug use and disruptions in follow-ups |
| | Inability to go to the hospital with the fear of COVID-19 |
| | Difficulties getting an appointment for examination or follow-up |
| | Difficulties in asking questions, consulting in urgent situations |
| | COVID-19-related problems experienced by the patients' caregiver or next of kin |
| **Causes arising from the hospital / physician:** | Disruptions such as changing the patient's permanent physician and care team, getting sick, death |
| | Material supply and problems in the arrangement of the catheter lab team |
| | Changes in interpretations in diagnosis and treatment protocols due to COVID-19 contamination concerns (such as fibrinolytic administration rather than PCI, keeping the patient free from interventions) |
| **System-related problems** | Failure to adequately protect the physician and the patient due to shortages in providing PPE |
| | Failure to provide the system organization and materials to initiate procedures/interventions safely |
| | Insufficiency in online systems to facilitate counseling, asking questions, *etc.* |
| | Underdeveloped home care systems |

## Case Report:

An obese black American woman in her 60s was admitted to ED with chief complaint of chest pain (Fig. **2**). She gives a medical history of coronary artery disease (had multiple stents), COPD (and smoking actively), pulmonary hypertension, and uncontrolled diabetes. (Adapted from Siddamreddy *et al*, 2020). Echocardiogram showed moderately reduced ejection fraction (EF) of 30-35%. Emergent left heart catheterization showed subtotal occlusion of her previous stent in the right coronary artery (RCA). She was treated with aspiration thrombectomy and a drug eluting stent placement. The patient was transferred to ICU after the stent placement and was initially placed on BIPAP followed by intubation due to worsening hypoxia. X-ray repeated at that time showed bilateral ground glass opacities (GGO) consistent with ARDS (Fig. **3**). She was started on HCQ along with azithromycin immediately and continued on MV with ARDS protocol. Her troponins peaked to 18 and then started to trend down.

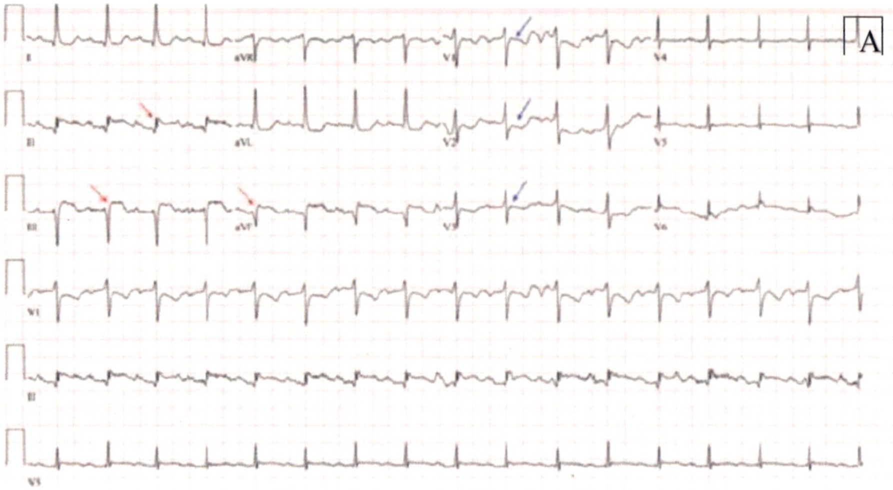


**Fig. (2).** (A/B). A. ECG revealed ST elevations (red arrow) in leads II, III, and aVF with reciprocal changes in V1, V2, V3 (blue arrow) which are interpreted to indicate acute inferior wall STEMI. B. Chest X-ray suggesting bilateral pulmonary edema, secondary to STEMI.

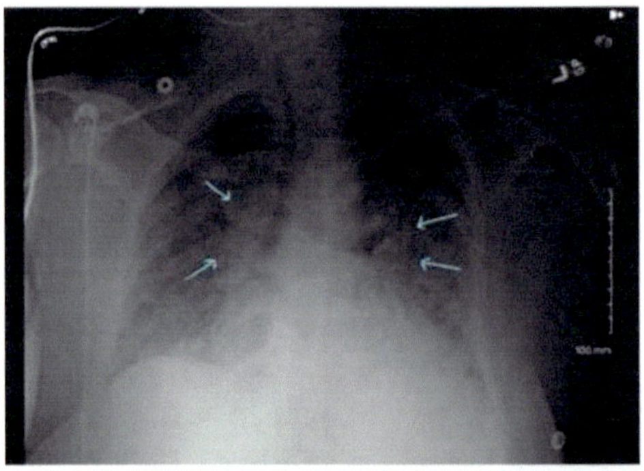

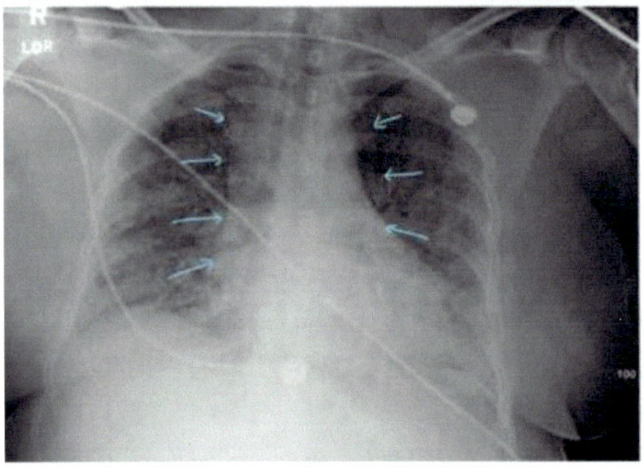

**Fig. (3).** Chest X-ray showing bilateral GGO with worsening aeration suggestive of ARDS (arrows).

## Damage Relationship with ACE2 Receptors:

The 'viral surface spike protein' or widely known 'S protein' binds to the ACE2 receptor, which is the entrance gate for the virus to enter the cell (Hoffman *et al*, 2020). There are also ACE2 receptors in various tissues and organs such as heart, vascular endothelium, lungs (type II alveolar cells) kidney, intestines (Zhao *et al*, 2020; Zhang *et al*, 2020; Tikellis *et al*, 2012). This is the rationale for the development of "multiorgan" failure in patients with COVID-19. It is also thought that the disease progresses more severely, since ACE2 receptors increase in smokers, hypertensive patients, and those diagnosed with heart failure.

## What Should Be Done?

Although it is understandable and necessary for the ambulance and emergency care system to pay special attention to suspected COVID cases, it is also vital that other patients in need of emergency care are not left behind. While adapting to the new challenging pandemic milieu, this point should be emphasized in training healthcare workers- EMS personnel, physicians, and nurses.

## COVID-19 and Myocardial Damage, Myocarditis

In the COVID-19 pandemic, which was ignited in China in December 2019 and gained prevalence mainly in Europe and America after March And April 2020, the patients mostly needed critical care due to bilateral pneumonia and respiratory failure. However, it is known that signs and symptoms consistent with myocarditis can ensue in a certain group of COVID-19 patients.

Myocarditis is an inflammation of myocardial tissue.The entity is triggered by exposure to infection, toxic effects, or autoimmune causes. Viruses, bacteria, fungi, autoimmune disease, and sometimes pharmacological agents can lead to myocarditis. There are cases that are symptomatic within hours while some are delayed to months.

It is reported at any age, but young people are inflicted more commonly. Its incidence has increased in the recent decades globally.

The most common agent is cardiotrophic viruses; Enteroviruses from the family of picornaviridae (*e.g.* Coxackie B virus), adenovirus (ADV), human herpes virus-6 (HHV6), parvovirus-B19 (PVB19) and cytomegalovirus (CMV). Apart from these, HIV, mumps, Epstein-Barr virus (EBV) coronaviruses (CoV) and influenza are also effective in selected cases. The pathophysiological mechanisms also vary depending on the causative agent. It can also be triggered by electric shock, hyperpyrexia, radiation.

Viral etiology has been reported to be between 37% and 77% in patients with myocarditis (Pankuweit *et al*, 2003; Kuhl *et al*, 2005). In patients with ejection fraction below 45%, viral etiology was found to be 42% (Marburg registry).

In a cohort of 100 patients recently recovered from COVID-19 infection, cardiac MRI revealed cardiac involvement in 78 patients (78%) and myocardial inflammation in 60 (60%), regardless of comorbid diseases, severity, and overall course of the acute illness (Fig. **4**) (Puntmann *et al*, 2020). The authors concluded that long-term cardiovascular outcomes need to be studied extensively.

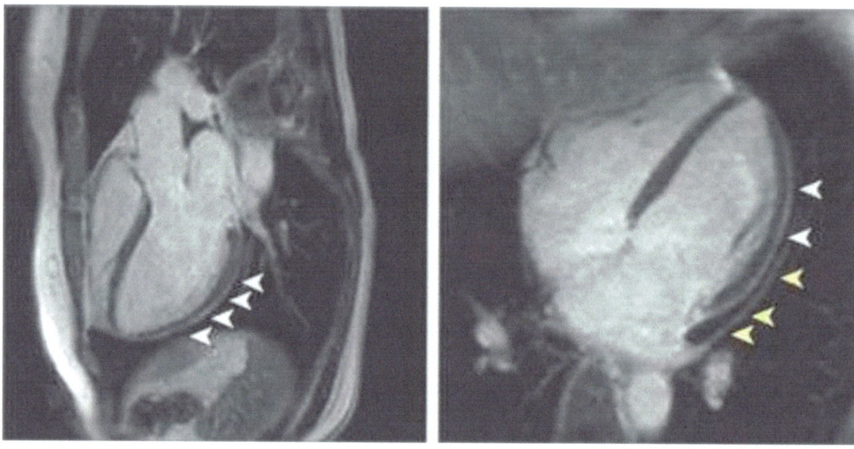

**Fig. (4).** Cardiac MRI of an elderly patient with elevated high-sensitivity troponin T level. Pericardial effusion and enhancement (arrowheads) and epicardial and intramyocardial enhancement (arrowheads) are remarkable (Adapted from Puntmann, 2020).

## *Fulminant Myocarditis (FM)*

### *Mechanism:*

Since cytokine storm is the leading pathophysiological mechanism especially in patients with multiple organ failure following COVID-19, development of FM is also suggested to be related to this inflammatory phenomenon (Chen *et al*, 2020; Wang *et al*, 2020). Patients with FM have a case fatality rate of 40% to 70%. FM should be given priority in the differential diagnosis and should be ruled out in patients with high levels of cTnI and BNP or newly ensued arrhythmia. When FM develops in the course of viral infection, treatment should be commenced early and expediently (Fig. **5**). Steroids, IV immunoglobulin, neuraminidase inhibitors, and active mechanical life support interventions, *e.g.* MV and intra-aortic balloon pulsation (IABP) may be required. ECMO and pacemaker insertions are also evaluated case by case basis.

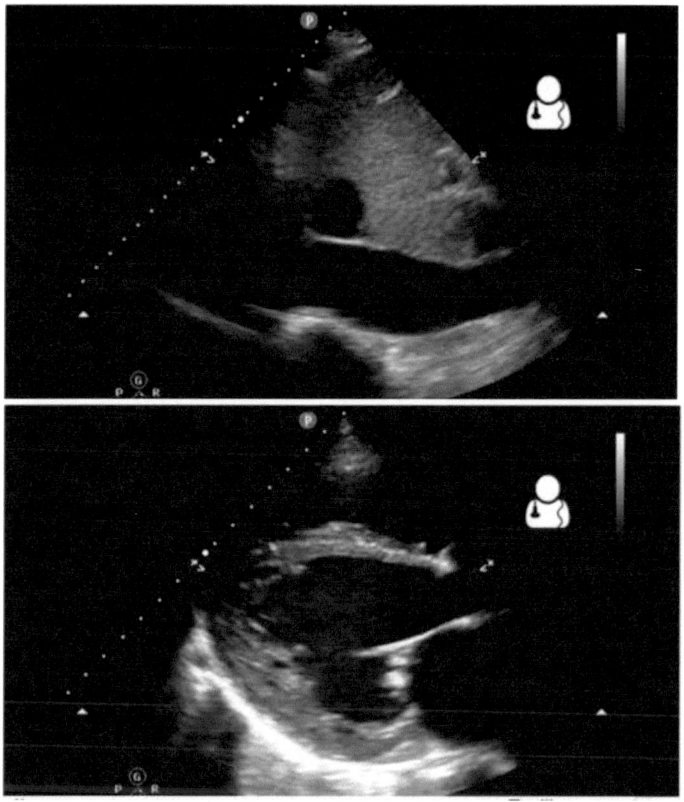

**Fig. (5).** (A/B). USG image of a patient with cardiogenic shock after acute viral myocarditis. Vena cavae turned into a wide and immobile channel. Edema and thickness are notable in the myocardium.

## *A Case with COVID-19 Myocarditis:*

A 63-year-old male in China was reported to have presented with signs of heart failure concurrent with elevated troponins. Sputum PCR test was positive for COVID-19 and negative for other viral factors and therefore the patient was diagnosed with COVID-19 myocarditis (Zeng *et al*, 2020). Heart failure was also confirmed by echocardiography, together with increased IL-6 levels. After antiviral treatment and mechanical life support, ejection fraction increased up to 68%, troponin levels decreased to normal. The patient eventually died on the 33$^{rd}$ day of hospitalization with secondary infection.

## *Symptoms and Signs in Myocarditis*

It may go undetected asymptomatic or mildly symptomatic for a certain time period. Rarely, it can progress rapidly to a severe HF, respiratory insufficiency, and death.

It can be evident with acute, subacute and chronic stages. In acute myocarditis, colds, flu-like syndrome, myalgia, diarrhea or similar complaints of the upper respiratory tract or gastrointestinal tract are noted initially. In days to weeks, complaints such that weakness, fatigue, shortness of breath, somatic chest pain, and palpitations can ensue.In cases with severe myocarditis, "classical triad" occurs as chest pain, arrhythmia, and heart failure.

In a small group of patients, signs of tachycardia, general moribund status, and tachypnea, which are not proportional to fever, can be seen. As a major complication, dilated cardiomyopathy (DCMP) develops in 16% of adults, and in almost half of the children.

On physical examination, tachycardia, softened S1, S3 gallop rhythm, mitral and/or tricuspid insufficiency/ murmurs, pericardial rub can be auscultated. It should be kept in mind that cardiac involvement can develop rapidly in a patient with COVID-19.

Myocarditis should also be considered in patients with rapidly developing 'idiopathic' DCMP, ventricular arrhythmia, shocky states, and AMI-like changes in their ECG despite normal coronary imaging.

### *Ancillary Studies*

CRP and BNP levels are reported to be significantly higher (3 times or more) in COVID-19 patients with myocardial damage than those without (He *et al*, 2020). ECG can reveal wide QRS, tachycardia and low voltage. It may also masquerade an AMI pattern. Delayed interventricular conduction may be noted. For example, right bundle branch block (RBBB) is remarkably common in Chagas myocarditis caused by Trypanosoma Cruzii. QRS expansion (> 120 msec) is a grave outcome indicator.

Cardiac enzymes, troponins may rise and are mostly proportional to severity of myocardial damage. However, it should be born in mind that myocarditis can be seen in patients with normal troponins.

**Imaging:** Doppler USG / echocardiogram and MRI are important diagnostic studies for these entities.

**USG / Echo:** Bedside echo / POCUS can be a life saver in those with rule-out pericarditis, especially in tamponade. Echocardiography can show global hypokinesia and regional wall motion abnormalities. Although the appearance of typical findings for bacterial endocarditis *e.g.*, vegetation can be diagnostic, its absence does not rule out the diagnosis. Duke criteria are an important guide in this regard (Table **3**).

**Table 3. Modified Duke Criteria.**

| |
|---|
| **A. Definitive infective endocarditis** |
| **+ Pathological criteria** |
| **- Demonstration of microorganisms in vegetative debris, intracardiac abscess or embolism by culture or histological examination** |
| **- Pathological confirmation of the presence of vegetation or intracardiac abscess with a histology indicative of active endocarditis** |
| **+ Clinical criteria** |
| **2 major criteria *or* 1 major and 3 minor criteria *or* 5 minor criteria** |
| **B. Possible infective endocarditis** |
| **+ 1 major + 1 minor criterion *or* + 3 minor criteria** |
| **C. Rule out criteria:** |
| **+ A strong alternative diagnosis which can explain the signs and symptoms that are thought to be related to endocarditis, *or*** |
| **+ Endocarditis symptoms and signs disappear with antibiotic treatment lasted for four days or less; *or*** |
| **+ No finding in favor of infective endocarditis in surgical or autopsy material in patients receiving antibiotic therapy** |

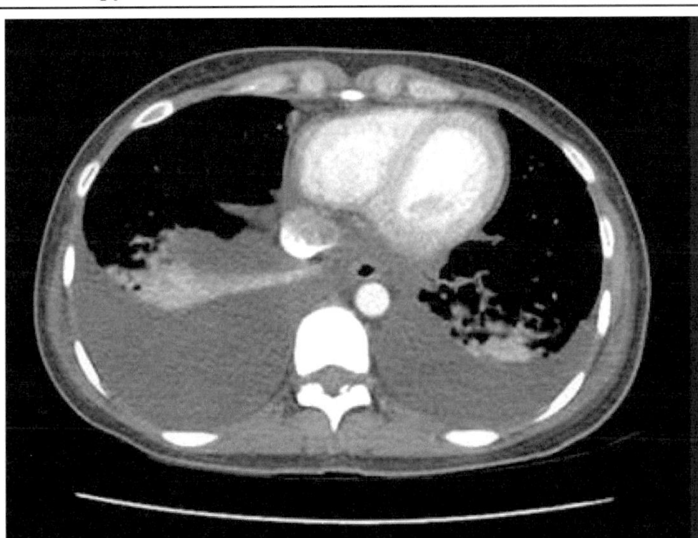

**Fig. (6).** CT image of an 35-year-old woman with pleural effusion and hepatitis. Thickening of the myocardium secondary to inflammatory edema is evident. The diagnosis is acute myocarditis.

In stable cases, chest X-ray / Telecardiogram is useful to rule out differential diagnoses. Pneumonia, pneumothorax, PTE should definitely be excluded, as these are in the list of differential diagnosis and also can develop as a complication of the disease sought for. Cardiomegaly / DCMP can ensue in patients with chronic pericarditis and myocarditis (Figs. **6** & **7**).

Table **4** shows signs and symptoms, diagnostic and therapeutic characteristics in myocarditis, endocarditis, and pericarditis.

**Table 4. Signs and symptoms, diagnostic and therapeutic characteristics in myocarditis, endocarditis, and pericarditis.**

| Disease | Endocarditis | Myocarditis | Pericarditis |
|---|---|---|---|
| **Symptoms** | Weakness/Malaise<br>Chest pain<br>Fever, chills, sweating, chills (high fever in bacterial origin)<br>Palpitation<br>Shortness of breath<br>Altered mental status<br>Signs& symptoms of septic / mycotic embolism | Weakness/Malaise<br>Chest pain<br>Mild fever, perspiration (High fever in bacterial / protozoal origin)<br>Complaints about heart failure: palpitations, shortness of breath, abdominal pain<br>Signs and symptoms of thromboembolism<br>Altered mental status | Weakness/Malaise<br>Chest pain (may decrease with leaning forward)<br>Pain on the back, neck, shoulder<br>Mild fever, perspiration<br>Palpitation<br>Dry cough<br>Shortness of breath, near-syncope (especially in tamponade)<br>Complaints of comorbid disease (RF, cancer, *etc.*) |
| **Finding** | Tachycardia, Gallop rhythm (S3)<br>Septic appearance<br>High fever Hypotension<br>Poor condition<br>Osler nodules, Janeway lesions | Tachycardia, Gallop rhythm (S3)<br>Mitral and / or tricuspid murmurs, Pericardial rub<br>Peripheral / scrotal edema,<br>Hypotension<br>Poor condition | Friction rub in auscultation<br>Poor peripheral perfusion<br>Tachycardia / tachyarrhythmias<br>Distended neck veins<br>Peripheral / scrotal edema,<br>Altered mental status in advanced cases / tamponade |
| **Lab** | ECG (not much useful)<br>Tachycardia is evident<br>CRP / ESR / leukocyte elevated | ECG: ST-T changes, wide QRS, tachycardia, low voltage<br>CRP / ESR / leukocyte elevated<br>Cardiac enzymes may rise<br>Endomyocardial biopsy / immunohistochemical examinations (PCR) | ECG: ST-T changes<br>CRP / ESR / leukocyte elevated<br>Cardiac enzymes may be elevated (in case of myopericarditis) |

*(Table 4) cont.....*

| Disease | Endocarditis | Myocarditis | Pericarditis |
|---|---|---|---|
| **Imaging recommendation and finding** | Chest X-ray to rule out pneumonia, HF<br>Echocardiography / POCUS (See Duke criteria)<br>CT or cardiac MRI in selected cases | Chest X-ray to rule out pneumonia, HF<br>Echocardiography / POCUS: Global hypokinesia, regional wall motion abnormalities<br>CT or cardiac MRI in selected cases | Chest X-ray to rule out pneumonia, HF (cardiomegaly only seen if fluid collection of more than 250 mL)<br>Echocardiography / POCUS: (normal does not rule out pericarditis)<br>Diastolic chamber collapse is diagnostic for tamponade.<br>CT or cardiac MRI |
| **Treatment** | Supportive therapy ($O_2$, fluid, rest) gets priority.<br>Combined antibiotic therapy<br>Agent-specific therapy (antibiotic, antiviral or antimycotic) | Supportive therapy ($O_2$, fluid, rest) gets priority.<br>Agent-specific therapy (antibiotic, antiviral or antimycotic) | Supportive therapy ($O_2$, fluid, rest) gets priority.<br>Agent-specific therapy (antibiotic, antiviral)<br>Ibuprofen or other NSAIDs<br>Colchicine can be added in recurrent cases<br>Pericardiectomy may be required in constrictive pericarditis<br>Dialysis is emergently performed in uremic pericarditis<br>**If findings of tamponade are present:** Right heart filling pressures should be augmented by administering IV fluids; perform pericardiocentesis or open pericardial window. |

## Management

Patients who are considered to have myocarditis should be hospitalized. They should be closely monitored with regard to HF, DCMP, arrhythmias, conduction disorders and TTEE. Exertion should be avoided during recovery. Fever should be treated, if any. Additional oxygen can be given in accord with the patient's condition. Fluid treatment may be required, but in case of HF, monitoring CVP and prevention of hypervolemia should be considered. Frequent assessments of the vena cavae would be an excellent guide fort his task. Water and salt restrictions are made when necessary.

Specific treatments are to be performed should specific myocarditis agents (Chagas, Lyme, Diphtheria, AIDS, echinococci or fungi) be identifed in selected cases.

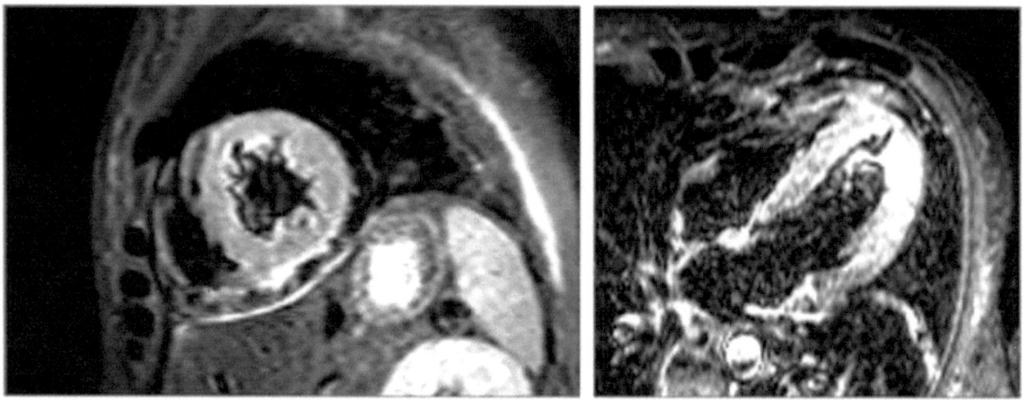

**Fig. (7).** (A/B). Diffuse myocardial signal hyperintensity in the ventricular walls in short axis (A) and 4-chamber images (B) with "short tau inversion recovery" (STIR) sequences. The findings are suggestive of interstitial edema secondary to myocardial inflammation.

In the presence of influenza epidemic, oseltamivir and similar antivirals should be commenced at the earliest period in case of a suspicion of myocarditis.

**IV immune globulins (IVIG):** Although IVIG are not indicated routinely, they can be useful in selected cases (Robinson *et al*, 2015).

**Specific haemodynamic treatments:** ECMO, IABP can be pleasing when started as early as possible in selected cases.

## THROMBOTIC EVENTS, BLEEDING, COAGULOPATHIES, AND COVID-19

**Thrombosis and thromboembolic events (TTEE) are in a two-way relationship with COVID-19:** A patient with TTEE can be infected with COVID-19, and a patient with COVID-19 can develop TTEE. Both bleeding and thrombosis cause significant morbidity in patients with COVID-19. Likewise, bleeding and thrombotic events are more common in patients who died after COVID-19 when compared to mild cases. Patients with high D-dimer levels have a significantly increased risk for TTEE, bleeding, critical illness, and death. Mean values of fibrinogen, ferritin, PCT are also higher in patients with thrombosis. In addition, the risk of pulmonary thromboembolism (PTE) is found to be higher in COVID-19 patients. Although it is reasonable to administer intensive anticoagulant prophylaxis, randomized studies are needed to estimate the benefit-to-harm ratio in this treatment.

The tendency to coagulopathy and TTEE appears to be a serious risk factor for admission to critical care and grave outcomes. Clinicians should be alert to notice the hallmarks of TTEE and also to take necessary measures for expedient management of this pathological process

Thrombosis and thromboembolic events (TTEE) are in a two-way relationship with COVID-19: A patient with TTEE can be infected with COVID-19, and a patient with COVID-19 can develop TTEE (Fig. **8**).

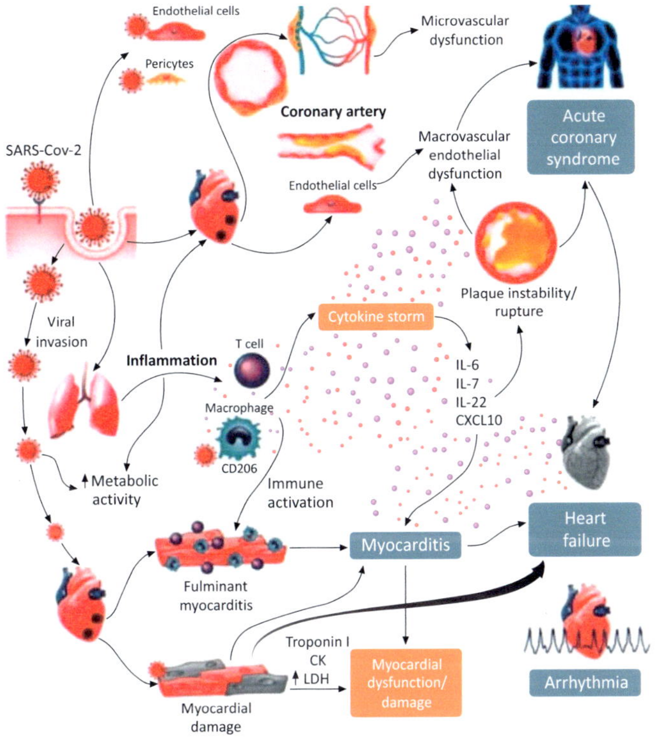


**Fig. (8).** The multifaceted interaction between SARS-CoV-2 is depicted in the figure.

## Cytokine-Mediated Alveolar Inflammation Triggers the Formation Of Microthrombi In The Pulmonary Vasculature, Which Can Culminate Into Thrombi Or Embolism In Severe Cases

Both bleeding and thrombosis cause significant morbidity in patients with COVID-19. Bleeding and thrombotic events are more common in patients who died after COVID-19 when compared to mild cases. Al-Samkari *et al.* investigated coagulopathy, bleeding, and thrombosis in 400 COVID-19 cases admitted into the hospital in multicenter recording studies (Al-Samkari *et al.*, 2020). There is 4.8% VTE / TTEE in the sample and a total of 9.5% thrombotic complication rate. A rate of 4.8% was observed for bleeding complications in the whole group. In critical patients, TTEE is noted in 7.6% and bleeding in 5.6%, in view of these bleeding rates.Although it is reasonable to administer intensive anticoagulant prophylaxis, randomized studies are a prerequisite to foresee the benefit-to-harm ratio in this treatment.

## Increased D-dimer, PT, aPTT, CRP, ESR, and PCT Levels Noted on Presentation were Found To Be Associated With Death In Covid-19 Patients (Al-Samkari *et al.*, 2020)

Patients with D-dimer level> 2,500 ng / mL have a significantly increased risk for TTEE, bleeding, critical illness, and death. (aOR for thrombosis, 6.79 (2.39-19.30), aOR for bleeding, 3.56 (1.01-12.66)] (Tables **5** and **6**).

**Table 5. Laboratory data showing increased risk for thrombosis.**

| |
|---|
| **D-dimer**> 2,500 ng / mL [aOR, 6.79 (2.39-19.30)], |
| **D-dimer**> 1000 ng / mL and <2,500 ng / mL [(aOR, 3.04 (1.26-7.31)], |
| **PLT**> 450 × 109 / L [aOR, 3.56 (1.27-9.97)], |
| **CRP**> 100 mg / L [aOR, 2.71 (1.26-5.86)], |
| **ESR**> 40 mm / h [aOR, 2.64 (1.07-6.51)]. |

**Table 6. Laboratory values which indicate increased risk for bleeding (Al-Samkari *et al*, 2020).**

| Variable | Level | Note- interpretation |
|---|---|---|
| **PLT** | **<150 x $10^9$ / L** [OR 2.90 (1.05-7.99)] | independent risk also for major bleeding |
| **D-dimer** | **> 2500 ng / mL,** [OR 3.56 (1.01-12.66)] | not for major bleeding |

The level of D-dimer taken on presentation is highly predictive for bleeding, VTE / TTEE, critical illness and death. Pulmonary thromboembolism (PTE) and COVID-19: Is the risk of PTE higher in COVID-19 than other viral syndromes?

## Additional Note: Mean Values Of Fibrinogen, Ferritin, Pct Are Also Higher In Patients With Thrombosis

Zhou *et al.* reported that advanced age, D-dimer level> 1 μg / mL, and high SOFA score on presentation increased the likelihood of in-hospital death (Zhou *et al*, 2020).

In patients with bleeding, higher rates of DIC, thrombocytopenia and hypofibrinogenemia were found when compared to the others.

Yes. French researchers compared COVID-19 patients with Influenza patients admitted with respiratory failure in ICU in 2019 with regard to PT. They reported that despite the higher frequency of CTPA in influenza patients in 2019, the rate of PTE was lower than that of COVID-19 patients (Poissy *et al*, 2020). In other words,the risk of PTE is found to be higher in COVID-19 patients.

In a Dutch study,the rate of diagnosis of VTE *via* CT angiogram and / or USG was 27% and arterial thrombotic events were 3.7% in patients hospitalized in ICUs in 3 hospitals (Klok *et al*, 2020). PTE has been reported as the most common thrombotic complication (n = 25, 81%). It is recommended that thrombosis prophylaxis and even high doses of heparin prophylaxis are given to COVID-19 patients (enoxaparin 40 mg BID).

The rate of thrombotic complications in ICU patients with COVID-19 infections increase as time passes through the first two weeks (Klok *et al*, 2020). The authors also listed the local protocols for thromboprophylaxis in Netherlands.

It has been revealed in a new study that 40% of patients hospitalized with COVID-19 in China have been categorized in the high-risk group for TTEE/VTE (Wang *et al*, 2020).

The tendency to coagulopathy and TTEE appears to be a serious risk factor that paves the way to critical care. A substantial percentage of critically ill patients admitted to the ICU had an increased likelihood for hypercoagulability and TTEE.

## Pathological Mechanism

Infection leads to endothelial dysfunction and hyperinflammatory medium. This increases thrombin formation and reduces fibrinolytic activity (Levi *et al*, 2017).

Hypoxia triggered by pneumonia increases thrombosis and therefore viscosity (Gupta *et al*, 2019). The microthrombi that obstruct pulmonary small vessels detected in the autopsies of COVID-19 patients support this opinion (Luo *et al*, 2020). As a result, fibrin deposits and microcirculation thrombosis appear to be the last step of the coagulation cascade in the alveolar and interstitial lung areas. This phase contributes to respiratory failure in COVID-19 cases.

In a large observational cohort study, Heparin was used in 1734 severe patients with COVID-19 (Ayerbe *et al*, 2020). Thromboprophylaxis was associated with lower mortality when the model was adjusted for age and gender, with OR (95% CI) 0.55 (0.37–0.82) p=0.003. This association remained significant when $O_2$ saturation 37°C were added to de model with OR 0.54 (0.36–0.82) p=0.003, and also when all the other drugs were included as covariates OR 0.42 (0.26–0.66) p<0.001.

**Case:** In Italy, a 50-year-old man presented with acute chest pain and exertion dyspnea eventually had respiratory failure worsening with PTE (Lorenzo, 2020). There is no thrombosis related medical history. There is a history of fever, weakness, and cough two weeks before admission. The home PCR test had been found positive and the patient was isolated at home. He recovered within 10 days without any medications. On the 13th day, she presented to the ED with sudden-onset dyspnea and chest pain. Hypoxic and hypocapnic respiratory failure were noted. Hypercoagulability has been demonstrated by thrombelastometry. Hemodynamics are stable. USG revealed DVT in the left tibial vein, and CTPA demonstrated left lobar, segmental and subsegmental PTE, and bilateral interstitial pneumonia. IgM and IgG tests are also positive for mycoplasma pneumonia.

The patient was treated with LMWH and azithromycin, hydroxychloroquine, and levofloxacin. After recovery, LMWH was discontinued and apixaban was started. He was discharged healthily after 10 days of hospitalization.

## Relationship of Laboratory Values And Clinical Course:

The most consistent clinical predictors in patients with COVID-19 are mild thrombocytopenia and elevated d-dimer levels (Fig. **9**). These two variables represent increased risk of admission to ICU and death (Lippi *et al*, 2020, Lippi *et al*, 2020).

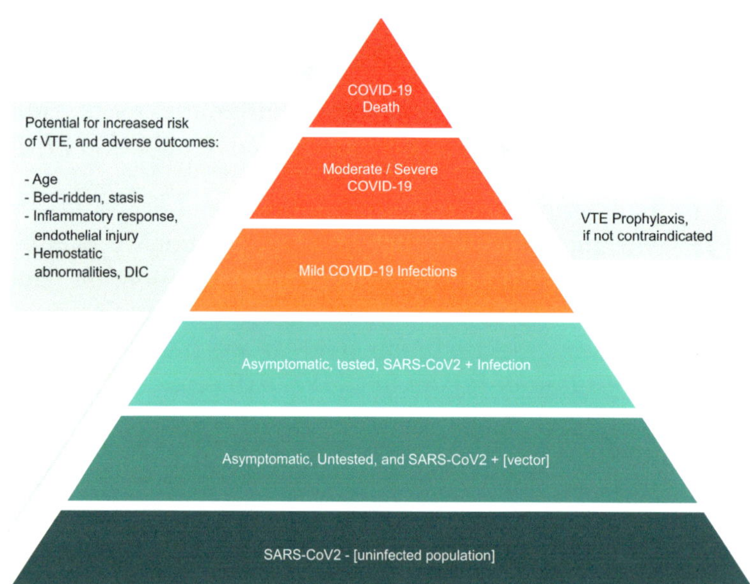


**Fig. (9).** Diagram showing changes of risk for VTE / PTE in Accord with the severity of COVID-19 (Bikdell *et al*, 2020).

Algorithm 1. Schematization of the recommended workflow in cases with severe COVID-19 (Adapted from Aryal *et al*, 2020).

As stated in the Swiss consensus report: "In ICU patients with high levels of d-dimer, severe inflammation, hepatic and/or renal failure findings, impending respiratory failure, administration of intermediate or therapeutic dose of LMWH or unfractionated heparin should be considered with respect to the risk of bleeding" (Algorithm 1) Casini *et al*, 2020).

## Do the Levels of Troponin and Bnp Predict the Severity of Covid-19?

Yes. This relationship has been disclosed in many studies (Lippi *et al*, 2020). However, troponin levels are elevated not only in COVID-19, but also in many diseases such as myocarditis, PTE, and AMI (Januzzi *et al*, 2020). Similarly, natriuretic peptides, such as BNP, are elevated in many entities, such as heart failure.

In 449 patients with severe COVID-19, coagulation tests, medications and findings on clinical follow-up were retrospectively analyzed (Tang *et al*, 2020). In multivariate analysis, D-dimer, prothrombin time and age were positively correlated with 28-day mortality and negatively with platelet counts. There is no significant difference regarding 28-day mortality between those who use heparin and those who do not. However, mortality was lower in heparin users in those with a SIC score of 4 and above (40.0% and 64.2%, $p = 0.029$) or in those with a D-dimer> 6 times higher than normal limits (32.8% and 52.4%, $p = 0.017$). The SIC score is shown in Table 7.

**Table 7. SIC score.**

| Variable | Score | Range |
|---|---|---|
| Platelet count ($x10^9$/L) | 1 | 100 to 150 |
| | 2 | <100 |
| PT-INR | 1 | 1,2 to 1,4 |
| | 2 | >1,4 |
| SOFA | 1 | 1 |
| | 2 | >2 |
| SIC-total score | >4 | - |

In a recent study, it was reported that TTEE were identified in 7.7% in 388 patients who were admitted to the ICU and approximately half of them were diagnosed within the first 24 hours (Lodigiani *et al*, 2020). In another series, the incidence of VTE was 25% (20/81) and 8 of the patients with VTE (40%) died (Cui *et al*, 2020). Age, lymphocyte count, activated partial thromboplastin time (aPTT) and D-dimer levels significantly differed between the group with VTE and those without. When 1.5 ug / mL was taken as the D-dimer cut off value to predict VTE, the sensitivity was 85%, specificity 88.5%, and negative predictive value (NPV) was 94.7%.

Literature findings and our experiences lead to the recommendation for thromboprophylaxis in all severe and critical COVID-19 patients admitted to the ED or ICU, and are strongly suggestive of increasing the prophylaxis towards high-prophylactic doses. Data favoring heparin for COVID-19 is sufficiently robust to justify urgent randomized controlled trials to determine the safety and effectiveness of this therapy.

## CONCLUSION

COVID-19 pandemic both causes CVD and is affected by it. Myocardial damage contributes to CVD-related mortality due to increased metabolic stress. During the diagnosis of COVID-19, myocardial damage should definitely be identified / excluded, and its management should be planned first. The inability of cardiac patients to receive the usual care they receive under pandemic conditions also threatens the public health. While it is understandable and necessary for the healthcare organization, including the ambulance personnel and emergency medical services, to pay special attention to suspected cases of COVID-19, it is also vital that other urgent patients are not left in the back row during ambulance calls. It is vital that hospital outpatient follow-ups are also designed to give the best possible ambulatory care to non-COVID-19 cases. In summary, while the health system provides optimal care for COVID-19, it should not ignore other patients in chronic and acute processes. While adapting to the new situation and pandemic, this point should be emphasized in team trainings.

## REFERENCES

Ammirati, E, Veronese, G, Brambatti, M, Merlo, M, Cipriani, M, Potena, L, Sormani, P, Aoki, T, Sugimura, K, Sawamura, A, Okumura, T, Pinney, S, Hong, K, Shah, P, Braun, Ö, Van de Heyning, CM, Montero, S, Petrella, D, Huang, F, Schmidt, M, Raineri, C, Lala, A, Varrenti, M, Foà, A, Leone, O, Gentile, P, Artico, J, Agostini, V, Patel, R, Garascia, A, Van Craenenbroeck, EM, Hirose, K, Isotani, A, Murohara, T, Arita, Y, Sionis, A, Fabris, E, Hashem, S, Garcia-Hernando, V, Oliva, F, Greenberg, B, Shimokawa, H, Sinagra, G, Adler, ED, Frigerio, M & Camici, PG (2019) Fulminant *versus* acute nonfulminant myocarditis in patients with left ventricular systolic dysfunction. *J Am Coll Cardiol,* 74, 299-311.
[http://dx.doi.org/10.1016/j.jacc.2019.04.063] [PMID: 31319912]

Aryal, MR, Gosain, R, Donato, A, Pathak, R, Bhatt, VR, Katel, A & Kouides, P (2020) Venous Thromboembolism in COVID-19: Towards an Ideal Approach to Thromboprophylaxis, Screening, and Treatment. *Curr Cardiol Rep,* 22, 52.
[http://dx.doi.org/10.1007/s11886-020-01327-9] [PMID: 32529517]

Ayerbe, L, Risco, C & Ayis, S (2020) The association between treatment with heparin and survival in

patients with Covid-19. *J Thromb Thrombolysis,* 50, 298-301.
[http://dx.doi.org/10.1007/s11239-020-02162-z] [PMID: 32476080]

Badawi, A & Ryoo, SG (2016) Prevalence of comorbidities in the Middle East respiratory syndrome coronavirus (MERS-CoV): a systematic review and meta-analysis. *Int J Infect Dis,* 49, 129-33.
[http://dx.doi.org/10.1016/j.ijid.2016.06.015] [PMID: 27352628]

Bansal, M (2020) Cardiovascular disease and COVID-19. *Diabetes Metab Syndr,* 14, 247-50.
[http://dx.doi.org/10.1016/j.dsx.2020.03.013] [PMID: 32247212]

Bikdeli, B, Madhavan, MV, Jimenez, D, Chuich, T, Dreyfus, I, Driggin, E, Nigoghossian, C, Ageno, W, Madjid, M, Guo, Y, Tang, LV, Hu, Y, Giri, J, Cushman, M, Quéré, I, Dimakakos, EP, Gibson, CM, Lippi, G, Favaloro, EJ, Fareed, J, Caprini, JA, Tafur, AJ, Burton, JR, Francese, DP, Wang, EY, Falanga, A, McLintock, C, Hunt, BJ, Spyropoulos, AC, Barnes, GD, Eikelboom, JW, Weinberg, I, Schulman, S, Carrier, M, Piazza, G, Beckman, JA, Steg, PG, Stone, GW, Rosenkranz, S, Goldhaber, SZ, Parikh, SA, Monreal, M, Krumholz, HM, Konstantinides, SV, Weitz, JI & Lip, GYH Global COVID-19 Thrombosis Collaborative Group, Endorsed by the ISTH, NATF, ESVM, and the IUA, Supported by the ESC Working Group on Pulmonary Circulation and Right Ventricular Function (2020) COVID-19 and Thrombotic or Thromboembolic Disease: Implications for Prevention, Antithrombotic Therapy, and Follow-Up: JACC State-of-the-Art Review. *J Am Coll Cardiol,* 75, 2950-73.
[http://dx.doi.org/10.1016/j.jacc.2020.04.031] [PMID: 32311448]

Bravi, F, Flacco, ME, Carradori, T, Volta, CA, Cosenza, G, De Togni, A, Acuti Martellucci, C, Parruti, G, Mantovani, L & Manzoli, L (2020) Predictors of severe or lethal COVID-19, including Angiotensin Converting Enzyme inhibitors and Angiotensin II Receptor Blockers, in a sample of infected Italian citizens. *PLoS One,* 15, e0235248.
[http://dx.doi.org/10.1371/journal.pone.0235248] [PMID: 32579597]

Caforio, AL, Pankuweit, S, Arbustini, E, Basso, C, Gimeno-Blanes, J, Felix, SB, Fu, M, Heliö, T, Heymans, S, Jahns, R, Klingel, K, Linhart, A, Maisch, B, McKenna, W, Mogensen, J, Pinto, YM, Ristic, A, Schultheiss, HP, Seggewiss, H, Tavazzi, L, Thiene, G, Yilmaz, A, Charron, P & Elliott, PM European Society of Cardiology Working Group on Myocardial and Pericardial Diseases (2013) Current state of knowledge on aetiology, diagnosis, management, and therapy of myocarditis: a position statement of the European Society of Cardiology Working Group on Myocardial and Pericardial Diseases. *Eur Heart J,* 34, 2636-2648, 2648a-2648d.
[http://dx.doi.org/10.1093/eurheartj/eht210] [PMID: 23824828]

Casini, A, Alberio, L, Angelillo-Scherrer, A, Fontana, P, Gerber, B, Graf, L, Hegemann, I, Korte, W, Kremer Hovinga, J, Lecompte, T, Martinez, M, Nagler, M, Studt, JD, Tsakiris, D, Wuillemin, W & Asmis, L (2020) Thromboprophylaxis and laboratory monitoring for in-hospital patients with COVID-19 - a Swiss consensus statement by the Working Party Hemostasis. *Swiss Med Wkly,* 150, w20247.
[http://dx.doi.org/10.4414/smw.2020.20247] [PMID: 32277760]

Chen, Q, Xu, L, Dai, Y, Ling, Y, Mao, J, Qian, J, Zhu, W, Di, W & Ge, J (2020) Cardiovascular manifestations in severe and critical patients with COVID-19. *Clin Cardiol,* 43, 796-802.
[http://dx.doi.org/10.1002/clc.23384] [PMID: 32562427]

Cui, S, Chen, S, Li, X, Liu, S & Wang, F (2020) Prevalence of venous thromboembolism in patients with severe novel coronavirus pneumonia. *J Thromb Haemost,* 18, 1421-4.
[http://dx.doi.org/10.1111/jth.14830] [PMID: 32271988]

De Rosa, S, Spaccarotella, C, Basso, C, Calabrò, MP, Curcio, A, Filardi, PP, Mancone, M, Mercuro, G, Muscoli, S, Nodari, S, Pedrinelli, R, Sinagra, G & Indolfi, C Società Italiana di Cardiologia and the CCU Academy investigators group (2020) Reduction of hospitalizations for myocardial infarction in Italy in the COVID-19 era. *Eur Heart J,* 41, 2083-8.
[http://dx.doi.org/10.1093/eurheartj/ehaa409] [PMID: 32412631]

Guo, T, Fan, Y, Chen, M, Wu, X, Zhang, L, He, T, Wang, H, Wan, J, Wang, X & Lu, Z (2020) Cardiovascular Implications of Fatal Outcomes of Patients With Coronavirus Disease 2019 (COVID-19). *JAMA Cardiol,* 5, 811-8.

[http://dx.doi.org/10.1001/jamacardio.2020.1017] [PMID: 32219356]

Gupta, N, Zhao, YY & Evans, CE (2019) The stimulation of thrombosis by hypoxia. *Thromb Res,* 181, 77-83.
[http://dx.doi.org/10.1016/j.thromres.2019.07.013] [PMID: 31376606]

He, XW, Lai, JS, Cheng, J, Wang, MW, Liu, YJ, Xiao, ZC, Xu, C, Li, SS & Zeng, HS (2020) [Impact of complicated myocardial injury on the clinical outcome of severe or critically ill COVID-19 patients]. *Zhonghua Xin Xue Guan Bing Za Zhi,* 48, 456-60.
[http://dx.doi.org/10.3760/cma.j.cn112148-20200228-00137] [PMID: 32171190]

Hoffmann, M, Kleine-Weber, H, Schroeder, S, Krüger, N, Herrler, T, Erichsen, S, Schiergens, TS, Herrler, G, Wu, NH, Nitsche, A, Müller, MA, Drosten, C & Pöhlmann, S (2020) SARS-CoV-2 Cell Entry Depends on ACE2 and TMPRSS2 and Is Blocked by a Clinically Proven Protease Inhibitor. *Cell,* 181, 271-280.e8.
[http://dx.doi.org/10.1016/j.cell.2020.02.052] [PMID: 32142651]

Hu, H, Yao, N & Qiu, Y (2020) Comparing Rapid Scoring Systems in Mortality Prediction of Critically Ill Patients With Novel Coronavirus Disease. *Acad Emerg Med,* 27, 461-8.
[http://dx.doi.org/10.1111/acem.13992] [PMID: 32311790]

Januzzi, JLn (2020) Troponin and BNP use in COVID-19. *Cardiology Magazine: American College of Cardiology.*

Kalyanaraman Marcello, R, Dolle, J & Grami, S (2020) Troponin and BNP use in COVID-19.*Cardiology Magazine: American College of Cardiology.*

Klok, FA, Kruip, MJHA, van der Meer, NJM, Arbous, MS, Gommers, DAMPJ, Kant, KM, Kaptein, FHJ, van Paassen, J, Stals, MAM, Huisman, MV & Endeman, H (2020) Incidence of thrombotic complications in critically ill ICU patients with COVID-19. *Thromb Res,* 191, 145-7.
[http://dx.doi.org/10.1016/j.thromres.2020.04.013] [PMID: 32291094]

Kühl, U, Pauschinger, M, Noutsias, M, Seeberg, B, Bock, T, Lassner, D, Poller, W, Kandolf, R & Schultheiss, HP (2005) High prevalence of viral genomes and multiple viral infections in the myocardium of adults with "idiopathic" left ventricular dysfunction. *Circulation,* 111, 887-93.
[http://dx.doi.org/10.1161/01.CIR.0000155616.07901.35] [PMID: 15699250]

Levi, M & van der Poll, T (2017) Coagulation and sepsis. *Thromb Res,* 149, 38-44.
[http://dx.doi.org/10.1016/j.thromres.2016.11.007] [PMID: 27886531]

Lindner, D, Fitzek, A, Bräuninger, H, Aleshcheva, G, Edler, C, Meissner, K, Scherschel, K, Kirchhof, P, Escher, F, Schultheiss, HP, Blankenberg, S, Püschel, K & Westermann, D (2020) Association of Cardiac Infection With SARS-CoV-2 in Confirmed COVID-19 Autopsy Cases. *JAMA Cardiol,* 5, 1281-5.
[http://dx.doi.org/10.1001/jamacardio.2020.3551] [PMID: 32730555]

Lippi, G & Favaloro, EJ (2020) D-dimer is associated with severity of coronavirus disease 2019 (COVID-19): a pooled analysis. *Thromb Haemost,* 120, 876-8.
[http://dx.doi.org/10.1055/s-0040-1709650] [PMID: 32246450]

Lippi, G, Lavie, CJ & Sanchis-Gomar, F (2020) Cardiac troponin I in patients with coronavirus disease 2019 (COVID-19): Evidence from a meta-analysis. *Prog Cardiovasc Dis,* 63, 390-1.
[http://dx.doi.org/10.1016/j.pcad.2020.03.001] [PMID: 32169400]

Lippi, G, Plebani, M & Henry, BM (2020) Thrombocytopenia is associated with severe coronavirus disease 2019 (COVID-19) infections: A meta-analysis. *Clin Chim Acta,* 506, 145-8.
[http://dx.doi.org/10.1016/j.cca.2020.03.022] [PMID: 32178975]

Lodigiani, C, Iapichino, G, Carenzo, L, Cecconi, M, Ferrazzi, P, Sebastian, T, Kucher, N, Studt, JD, Sacco, C, Bertuzzi, A, Sandri, MT & Barco, S Humanitas COVID-19 Task Force (2020) Venous and arterial thromboembolic complications in COVID-19 patients admitted to an academic hospital in Milan, Italy. *Thromb Res,* 191, 9-14.
[http://dx.doi.org/10.1016/j.thromres.2020.04.024] [PMID: 32353746]

Lorenzo, C, Francesca, B, Francesco, P, Elena, C, Luca, S & Paolo, S (2020) Acute pulmonary embolism in

COVID-19 related hypercoagulability. *J Thromb Thrombolysis,* 50, 223-6. [http://dx.doi.org/10.1007/s11239-020-02160-1] [PMID: 32474757]

Luo, W, Yu, H & Gou, J (2020) Clinical pathology of critical patient with novel coronavirus pneumonia (COVID-19). *Transplantation.* [http://dx.doi.org/10.1097/TP.0000000000003412] [PMID: 33122591]

Mahmud, E, Dauerman, HL, Welt, FGP, Messenger, JC, Rao, SV, Grines, C, Mattu, A, Kirtane, AJ, Jauhar, R, Meraj, P, Rokos, IC, Rumsfeld, JS & Henry, TD (2020) Management of acute myocardial infarction during the COVID-19 pandemic: A Consensus Statement from the Society for Cardiovascular Angiography and Interventions (SCAI), the American College of Cardiology (ACC), and the American College of Emergency Physicians (ACEP). *Catheter Cardiovasc Interv,* 96, 336-45. [http://dx.doi.org/10.1002/ccd.28946] [PMID: 32311816]

Pankuweit, S, Moll, R, Baandrup, U, Portig, I, Hufnagel, G & Maisch, B (2003) Prevalence of the parvovirus B19 genome in endomyocardial biopsy specimens. *Hum Pathol,* 34, 497-503. [http://dx.doi.org/10.1016/S0046-8177(03)00078-9] [PMID: 12792925]

Peng, YD, Meng, K & Guan, HQ (2020) Prevalence of the parvovirus B19 genome in endomyocardial biopsy specimens. *Hum Pathol,* 34, 497-503.

Poissy, J, Goutay, J, Caplan, M, Parmentier, E, Duburcq, T, Lassalle, F, Jeanpierre, E, Rauch, A, Labreuche, J & Susen, S Lille ICU Haemostasis COVID-19 Group (2020) Pulmonary Embolism in Patients With COVID-19: Awareness of an Increased Prevalence. *Circulation,* 142, 184-6. [http://dx.doi.org/10.1161/CIRCULATIONAHA.120.047430] [PMID: 32330083]

Price-Haywood, EG, Burton, J, Fort, D & Seoane, L (2020) Hospitalization and Mortality among Black Patients and White Patients with Covid-19. *N Engl J Med,* 382, 2534-43. [http://dx.doi.org/10.1056/NEJMsa2011686] [PMID: 32459916]

Puntmann, VO, Carerj, ML, Wieters, I, Fahim, M, Arendt, C, Hoffmann, J, Shchendrygina, A, Escher, F, Vasa-Nicotera, M, Zeiher, AM, Vehreschild, M & Nagel, E (2020) Outcomes of Cardiovascular Magnetic Resonance Imaging in Patients Recently Recovered From Coronavirus Disease 2019 (COVID-19). *JAMA Cardiol,* 5, 1265-73. [http://dx.doi.org/10.1001/jamacardio.2020.3557] [PMID: 32730619]

Richardson, S, Hirsch, JS, Narasimhan, M, Crawford, JM, McGinn, T, Davidson, KW, Barnaby, DP, Becker, LB, Chelico, JD, Cohen, SL, Cookingham, J, Coppa, K, Diefenbach, MA, Dominello, AJ, Duer-Hefele, J, Falzon, L, Gitlin, J, Hajizadeh, N, Harvin, TG, Hirschwerk, DA, Kim, EJ, Kozel, ZM, Marrast, LM, Mogavero, JN, Osorio, GA, Qiu, M & Zanos, TP the Northwell COVID-19 Research Consortium (2020) Presenting Characteristics, Comorbidities, and Outcomes Among 5700 Patients Hospitalized With COVID-19 in the New York City Area. *JAMA,* 323, 2052-9. [http://dx.doi.org/10.1001/jama.2020.6775] [PMID: 32320003]

Robinson, J, Hartling, L, Vandermeer, B & Klassen, TP (2015) Intravenous immunoglobulin for presumed viral myocarditis in children and adults. *Cochrane Database Syst Rev,* 5, CD004370. [http://dx.doi.org/10.1002/14651858.CD004370.pub3] [PMID: 25992494]

Shi, S, Qin, M, Shen, B, Cai, Y, Liu, T, Yang, F, Gong, W, Liu, X, Liang, J, Zhao, Q, Huang, H, Yang, B & Huang, C (2020) Association of cardiac injury with mortality in hospitalized patients with COVID-19 in Wuhan, China. *JAMA Cardiol,* 5, 802-10. [http://dx.doi.org/10.1001/jamacardio.2020.0950] [PMID: 32211816]

Siddamreddy, S, Thotakura, R, Dandu, V, Kanuru, S & Meegada, S (2020) Corona Virus Disease 2019 (COVID-19) Presenting as Acute ST Elevation Myocardial Infarction. *Cureus,* 12, e7782. [http://dx.doi.org/10.7759/cureus.7782] [PMID: 32337148]

Suleyman, G, Fadel, RA, Malette, KM, Hammond, C, Abdulla, H, Entz, A, Demertzis, Z, Hanna, Z, Failla, A, Dagher, C, Chaudhry, Z, Vahia, A, Abreu Lanfranco, O, Ramesh, M, Zervos, MJ, Alangaden, G, Miller, J & Brar, I (2020) Clinical Characteristics and Morbidity Associated With Coronavirus Disease 2019 in a Series of Patients in Metropolitan Detroit. *JAMA Netw Open,* 3, e2012270.

[http://dx.doi.org/10.1001/jamanetworkopen.2020.12270] [PMID: 32543702]

Tam, CF, Cheung, KS, Lam, S, Wong, A, Yung, A, Sze, M, Lam, YM, Chan, C, Tsang, TC, Tsui, M, Tse, HF & Siu, CW (2020) Impact of Coronavirus Disease 2019 (COVID-19) Outbreak on ST-Segment-Elevation Myocardial Infarction Care in Hong Kong, China. *Circ Cardiovasc Qual Outcomes,* 13, e006631.
[http://dx.doi.org/10.1161/CIRCOUTCOMES.120.006631] [PMID: 32182131]

Tang, N, Bai, H, Chen, X, Gong, J, Li, D & Sun, Z (2020) Anticoagulant treatment is associated with decreased mortality in severe coronavirus disease 2019 patients with coagulopathy. *J Thromb Haemost,* 18, 1094-9.
[http://dx.doi.org/10.1111/jth.14817] [PMID: 32220112]

Tikellis, C & Thomas, MC (2012) Angiotensin-Converting Enzyme 2 (ACE2) Is a Key Modulator of the Renin Angiotensin System in Health and Disease. *Int J Pept,* 2012, 256294.
[http://dx.doi.org/10.1155/2012/256294] [PMID: 22536270]

Wang, D, Hu, B, Hu, C, Zhu, F, Liu, X, Zhang, J, Wang, B, Xiang, H, Cheng, Z, Xiong, Y, Zhao, Y, Li, Y, Wang, X & Peng, Z (2020) Clinical Characteristics of 138 Hospitalized Patients With 2019 Novel Coronavirus-Infected Pneumonia in Wuhan, China. *JAMA,* 323, 1061-9.
[http://dx.doi.org/10.1001/jama.2020.1585] [PMID: 32031570]

Xu, Z, Shi, L, Wang, Y, Zhang, J, Huang, L, Zhang, C, Liu, S, Zhao, P, Liu, H, Zhu, L, Tai, Y, Bai, C, Gao, T, Song, J, Xia, P, Dong, J, Zhao, J & Wang, FS (2020) Pathological findings of COVID-19 associated with acute respiratory distress syndrome. *Lancet Respir Med,* 8, 420-2.
[http://dx.doi.org/10.1016/S2213-2600(20)30076-X] [PMID: 32085846]

Zeng, JH, Liu, YX, Yuan, J, Wang, FX, Wu, WB, Li, JX, Wang, LF, Gao, H, Wang, Y, Dong, CF, Li, YJ, Xie, XJ, Feng, C & Liu, L (2020) First case of COVID-19 complicated with fulminant myocarditis: a case report and insights. *Infection,* 48, 773-7.
[http://dx.doi.org/10.1007/s15010-020-01424-5] [PMID: 32277408]

Zhang, H, Penninger, JM, Li, Y, Zhong, N & Slutsky, AS (2020) Angiotensin-converting enzyme 2 (ACE2) as a SARS-CoV-2 receptor: molecular mechanisms and potential therapeutic target. *Intensive Care Med,* 46, 586-90.
[http://dx.doi.org/10.1007/s00134-020-05985-9] [PMID: 32125455]

Zhao, Y, Zhao, Z & Wang, Y (2020) Single-cell RNA expression profiling of ACE2, the putative receptor of Wuhan 2019-nCov. *Am J Respir Crit Care Med,* 202, 756-9.
[http://dx.doi.org/10.1164/rccm.202001-0179LE] [PMID: 32663409]

Zhou, F, Yu, T, Du, R, Fan, G, Liu, Y, Liu, Z, Xiang, J, Wang, Y, Song, B, Gu, X, Guan, L, Wei, Y, Li, H, Wu, X, Xu, J, Tu, S, Zhang, Y, Chen, H & Cao, B (2020) Clinical course and risk factors for mortality of adult inpatients with COVID-19 in Wuhan, China: a retrospective cohort study. *Lancet,* 395, 1054-62.
[http://dx.doi.org/10.1016/S0140-6736(20)30566-3] [PMID: 32171076]

# CHAPTER 8

# Gastrointestinal Signs and Symptoms in the Course of COVID-19

**Abstract:** Nausea/vomiting, diarrhea, abdominal pain, and ageusia are gastrointestinal (GI) symptoms commonly recorded in the pandemic. The gastrointestinal system (GIS) is important in diagnostic procedures screening for COVID-19. This chapter aims to highlight this important aspect of the course of COVID-19, with a special emphasis on diagnostic opportunities.

Many articles cited that GIS is closely related to COVID-19 in certain aspects. First of all, GI complaints and their severity show a strong correlation with the severity of the disease. Second, GI signs and symptoms are associated with higher AST and ALT and coagulation deficiencies. Patients with GI signs tend to have fever more frequently; however, they have a less severe course disease. Liver injury is seen more commonly in males and associated with lymphocytopenia, neutropenia. It has been observed that AST is associated with mortality in COVID-19. Inflammatory bowel diseases are not a high risk for COVID-19.

The objective of this chapter is to highlight the value of GI signs and symptoms in the evaluation of the patient suspected to have COVID-19 and to focus on the need to assess specific clues ruling in and out the disease.

**Keywords:** ACE2 receptors, Anal swab, COVID-19, Diagnosis, Fecal RNA, Gastrointestinal complaints, Inflammatory bowel diseases, Liver disease, Liver enzymes.

## INTRODUCTION

There is a considerable deficiency in diagnosing all patients suspected to have contracted the disease of COVID-19. Respiratory signs can lag behind others, *e.g.*, muscle aches, anosmia, dysgeusia, nausea, diarrhea, and other GI symptoms in many patients. An elaborate evaluation of the patient should comprise an examination of all systems to compose a whole picture.

Gastrointestinal system (GIS) does not champion among the systems damaged by the disease process of COVID-19. COVID-19 inflicted more than 55 million people around the world, officially causing more than 1.300.000 deaths in ten months. Dyspnea, fever, and dry cough are known to be recorded most commonly

**Ozgur KARCIOGLU, Selman YENIOCAK and Mandana HOSSEINZADEH**

in the verified patients, followed by muscle/joint pain, headache, nausea/vomiting, diarrhea, cerebrovascular symptoms, anosmia, *etc.*, with considerable variations between countries and regions, also showing temporal differences within the pandemic process.

Instead, GIS is important in diagnostic procedures in screening for COVID-19 in a given patient. SARS-CoV-2 RNA can be found throughout the GIS channel and thus in the feces in a longer time window than in the respiratory tract. The infection continues in faeces in cases with very few symptoms, even in asymptomatic ones. RNA positivity in GIS and faeces is both a diagnostic opportunity and indicates a dangerous situation for both healthcare workers carrying out procedures (*e.g.*, endoscopy, rectoscopy, digital rectal examination *etc.*) and also household members and the public, in regard to fecal-oral transmission.

GIS has been linked with COVID-19 also for patients with chronic disorders of GIS such that liver disease, inflammatory bowel diseases (IBD), and others.

This review aims to highlight this important aspect of the COVID-19 clinical course, with a special emphasis on diagnostic opportunities related to GIS.

## HOW IMPORTANT IS GIS IN THE PATHOPHYSIOLOGY OF THE VIRUS?

SARS-CoV-2 shows an affinity for every cell, which conveys ACE2 receptors. Since these receptors are abundant in GIS, these tissues can host the virus. The virus is excreted abundantly via faeces during acute illness, mostly in severe patients. Faecal-oral transmission occurs in 10% to 53% of patients. The most important aspect of GIS in the diagnosis of COVID-19 is that the RNA positivity in faeces continues much longer (up to 50 days) compared to the respiratory tract samples (maximum 14 days) (Cimolai 2020).

It is known that the SARS virus can be found in the feces / small intestine from the 7$^{th}$ day in animals, but the viruses placed directly in the stomach do not cause disease (Nagata, 2020). In specific relation to this, an interesting study revealed that viral RNA positivity was also evidenced in urban wastewater (Randazzo, 2020).

### Which GI Findings Do We Mention About?

GI findings are commonly recorded in patients with COVID-19, although they are not regarded as the so-called “main symptoms” (fever, shortness of breath, persistent dry cough). Abdominal pain, diarrhea, nausea, vomiting, loss of appetite and sense of taste (ageusia) are the most common GI complaints (Cheung, 2020). Although GI complaints are generally considered to be among the "atypical symptoms" in COVID-19 cases, they can represent an important adjunct to the main findings and help in the diagnosis of the disease. In rare cases, GI symptoms may ensue as the main complaint or finding on presentation to the hospital. Atypical or infrequent findings may also lead to difficult recognition of patients and longer hospital stay.

When 1141 cases were analyzed in the beginning period of the epidemic in China, it was reported that 183 (16%) presented with GI complaints (Luo, 2020). The most frequently reported among them were loss of appetite, nausea and vomiting, diarrhea and abdominal pain (Table **1**). As a rule, this group of patients had leukopenia, lymphopenia, increased CRP, and elevated liver enzymes, whereas the kidney function was normal. In 96% of cases, there was evidence of infection in chest tomography, so it was a severe group of patients.

**Table 1. Possible GI complaints in patients diagnosed with COVID-19 in order of frequency and laboratory findings primarily in patients presenting with GI complaint (Luo, 2020).**

| Complaints | Laboratory Findings |
|---|---|
| Loss of appetite,<br>Nausea<br>Vomiting<br>Diarrhea<br>Abdominal pain | Leukopenia (mean 2.7x 109 / L)<br>Lymphopenia (avg. 0.53x 109 / L)<br>CRP increase,<br>Liver enzyme elevation<br>Normal kidney functions |

Ghoshal *et al.* published a systematic review and cited that GI symptoms were found in the whole case pool at a rate of 17.6%, similar to that published by Luo *et al.* (Ghoshal, 2020). There are also studies reporting that patients with GI complaints have a worse clinical course.

Liang W *et al.* analyzed three studies to compare the incidences of signs and symptoms known to be the most common ones in patients with COVID-19 (Liang 2020, Chan 2020, Chen 2020, Huang 2020) (Table **2**). They noted that the incidence of leucopenia, fever, and diarrhea in the three studies showed a significant difference. Among these symptoms, diarrhea had the smallest p-value (p=0.016), suggesting that the criteria for diagnosing diarrhea may differ between hospitals. Therefore, clinicians may underestimate the value of this symptom in clinical practice, and it may affect the preliminary diagnostic accuracy. The authors concluded that the Bristol stool scale should be carefully collected in these patients. Healthcare workers should take caution when their patients complain of diarrhea to mitigate infection risks (Liang, 2020).

**Table 2. Intergroup comparison between three recent publications (Liang, 2020).**

| Characteristics | Huang *et al* (41 Cases) | Chan *et al* (6 Cases) | Chen *et al* (99 Cases) | Difference Between Groups (p value) |
|---|---|---|---|---|
| Age | 49.0 (17.0) | 46.2 (28.3) | 55.5 (17.7) | – |
| Sex (female) | 11/41 (27%) | 3 (50%) | 32 (32%) | 0.4591 |
| Comorbidity | 13/41 (32%) | 4 (67%) | 50 (51%) | 0.0818 |
| Fever | 40/41 (98%) | 5 (83%) | 82 (83%) | 0.0345* |
| Cough | 31/41 (76%) | 4 (67%) | 81 (82%) | 0.3829 |
| Diarrhoea | 1/38 (3%) | 2 (33%) | 2 (2%) | 0.016† |
| Shortness of breath/ difficulty in breathing | 22/40 (55%) | NA | 31 (31%) | – |
| Haemoptysis | 2/39 (5%) | NA | NA | – |
| Sputum production | 11/39 (28%) | 2 (33%) | NA | – |
| Myalgia or fatigue | 18/41 (44%) | 3 (50%)‡ | NA | – |
| Headache | 3/38 (8%) | NA | 8 (8%) | – |
| Leucopenia | 10/40 (25%) | 0 (0%) | 9 (9%) | 0.0443§ |
| Platelet count | 2/40 (5%) | 0 (0%) | NA | – |

- *Huang *vs* Chan: 0.2414; Chan *vs* Chen: 1.00; Huang *vs* Chen: 0.0235.
- †Huang *vs* Chan: 0.044; Chan *vs* Chen: 0.016; Huang *vs* Chen: 1.00.
- ‡ Symptom: generalized weakness.
- § Huang *vs* Chan: 0.3145; Chan *vs* Chen: 1; Huang *vs* Chen: 0.026.

In the study in which COVID-19 cases in Hubei were analyzed, respiratory symptoms were reported in the majority of the cases (89%), but every second patient complained of GI symptoms (Pan, 2020). Among the GI complaints, the most common ones were loss of appetite (78%), diarrhea (34%), vomiting (4%), abdominal pain (2%). It is interesting to note that in 3% of cases, presented with only GI complaints without respiratory symptoms.

GI complaints increase in parallel with the severity of the disease. Higher liver enzymes (AST and ALT), prolonged PT and monocytopenia were found in those with GI findings and complaints. Another important point is that patients with GI findings present later than those with respiratory complaints and thus, their recognition and management lag behind others.

Analyzing a series of 157 cases in two hospitals from Hubei, Cao *et al.* reported at least one GI complaint and/or finding at 40% of the sample (Cao, 2020). The most frequent loss of appetite (75%), nausea (33%) and diarrhea (40%) were recorded among the GI findings. There was no difference in terms of age, gender, comorbidities between those with and without GIS findings. Interestingly, those with GI signs and symptoms experience less severe disease (12.7% *vs*. 35.1%).

## Viral RNA Positivity in Faeces:

Coronaviruses have been found in faeces since 1980s. Although Rotaviruses and some Adenoviruses are famous in this regard, it is thought that up to 70% of "enteric viral particles" may be coronaviruses. It has been reported in many reports that viral RNA continues to exist in faecal samples until after the respiratory symptoms have been normalized. In a systematic review and meta-analysis, Parasa *et al.* reported that viral RNA shedding was detected in feces in 40.5% (95%CI, 27.4%-55.1%) of patients with COVID-19 (Parasa *et al.* 2020). Although only 12% of patients had GI manifestations of COVID-19, viral RNA shedding was detected in feces in 40.5% of the same population (Parasa *et al.* 2020).

Researchers from China pointed out that the positive rate of all stool samples tested was close to or reached 100% (Xu, 2020, Zeng, 2020, Xing, 2020, Hua, 2020, Liang, 2020). A majority of the patients (71%) were still positive for fecal RNA after the respiratory specimens turned negative. Furthermore, one-third of the patients were fecal nucleic acid-positive 15 days after a respiratory specimen was negative.

Cheung *et al.* reported that one-fourth of the patients with SARS-CoV-2 had GI symptoms and RNA was positive in nearly 40% of patients with diarrhea and only 8.7% in those without diarrhea (Cheung, 2020). Fever was present in 100% of the sample with GI complaints. In the meta-analytical study, 17.6% of patients have GI complaints, while the virus positivity in faeces is 48.1%.

## Prognosis and GI Symptoms in Adults:

There are few studies in regard to the relation of GI signs and symptoms and the outcome of COVID-19 cases. Nobel *et al.* conducted a retrospective comparative study including 278 patients with COVID-19, and 238 patients with fever and cough attributable to a common respiratory tract infection (Nobel *et al.*, 2020). The course of gastrointestinal symptoms was longer in those with COVID-19, but the mortality rate and rate of severe disease were lower in patients with GI symptoms than in those without such symptoms. Of note, among patients meeting criteria for COVID-19 testing, those with gastrointestinal symptoms were 70% more likely to test positive (Table **3**).

**Table 3. Rate of Positive or Negative COVID-19 Testing Based on Presence or Absence of Gastrointestinal Symptoms (Adapted from Nobel *et al.*, 2020).**

| Symptoms | COVID-19 Positive (N = 278) | COVID-19 Negative (N = 238) | *P* value |
|---|---|---|---|
| Any gastrointestinal symptoms | - | | **.04** |
| Present (n = 160) | 97 (61) | 63 (39) | - |
| Absent (n = 356) | 181 (51) | 175 (49) | - |
| Diarrhea [a] | - | | .14 |
| Present (n = 92) | 56 (61) | 36 (39) | - |
| Absent (n = 424) | 222 (52) | 202 (48) | - |
| Nausea/vomiting [a] | - | | .36 |
| Present (n = 109) | 63 (58) | 46 (42) | - |
| Absent (n = 407) | 215 (53) | 192 (47) | - |

(a: Frequency of symptom, with or without the other gastrointestinal symptoms; 51 patients had diarrhea only and 68 patients had nausea/vomiting only).

## Children and GI Complaints

In the early phase of the COVID-19 pandemic, there was a common misconception that children were not to catch the infection easily. As time passed, the figures of infected children have boosted worldwide. In children, it can be hard to discern the GI symptoms of COVID-19 from manifestations of other viral illnesses, drugs' side effects, and general nonspecific symptoms such as nausea and vomiting and diarrhea caused by the disturbance of gastrointestinal flora (Wang, 2020).

Analysis of 182 pediatric cases with a median age of 6 in China disclosed that the two most common complaints were fever and cough (43% to 44%, each) (Du H, 2020). GI symptoms were reported in 11% of cases, and mostly comprised of diarrhea, abdominal discomfort and vomiting.

## Pediatric Faecal Viral Positivity:

In the series consisting of 5 symptomatic and 5 asymptomatic 10 children in China, viral RNA positivity was not interrupted in 7 children after discharge of children diagnosed with COVID-19 (Du W, 2020). In respiratory samples, the median was 9 days, while the median was 34.4 days to return to negative in faeces. Researchers also reported that there was more RNA positivity in anal swabs than throat swabs and blood, even more markedly in the late period of the disease (Zhang, 2020).

## Inflammatory Bowel Diseases (IBD) and COVID-19

There are very few studies specific to this subject. It was reported that most of the COVID-19 cases (3/4) were female and the mean age was 52 (Taxonera, 2020). Two of three patients diagnosed with COVID-19 had to be admitted to the hospital. The most common complaint is diarrhea. Mean frequency of stool was around 5 times a day. The presenting symptom associated with COVID-19 is diarrhea in 5 patients (42%). Diarrhea can also be the only symptom in some patients (17%). It was reported that diarrhea was triggered by the initiation of HCQ or lopinavir / ritonavir in 4 cases in whom diarrhea was seen after admission to hospital.

In Spain, 6.2% incidence of COVID-19 have been reported in 1000 patients with IBD. Since this number is 6.6 in the general population, it is thought that IBD may have had a protective role. (OR = 0.74). The mortality rates associated with COVID-19 in patients with IBD do not differ from the general population. The standardized mortality risk is similar to the general population with 1/1000 people.

### Will We Change The Principles of Management?

There will be no essential change in the management because COVID-19 affects healthy people as well as those with other diseases (Mao, 2020, WHO; 2020). It is known that Anti-TNF used in the treatment of IBD can increase the risk of catching infection (Ford, 2013). It was also suggested to discontinue therapy with immunosuppressants and biological agents in COVID-19 cases (IOIBD, 2020, Rubin, 2020). Reporting a series from Milan, Fiorino *et al.* argued that discontinuation of medicines would be the wrong choice, instead, it would be more beneficial to continue, and it would be wise to delay commencement of de novo treatment in IBD patients without severe symptoms (Fiorino, 2020). There is no suggestion regarding discontinuation of steroids.

In conclusion, IBD does not convey a high risk per se for COVID and diarrhea requires attention as the most common complaint. Also, physicians should bear in mind that the patient may be diagnosed with COVID-19, even if the sole or main symptom is diarrhea in patients with IBD. Immunosuppressant agents should be discontinued.

## Hepatic Damage and COVID-19

Liver disease is recognized in many patients with COVID-19. Chronic liver disease (CLD) has been reported at a rate of 1.4% in some researches (Lei, 2020). The most common disease among them is hepatitis. In asymptomatic cases, mild liver damage with ALT, AST and GGT elevations can be noted in 10 to 50%. There may be a low degree of hyperbilirubinemia. The physician can notice this with yellow color in the sclerae and darkening in urine color. Mild liver damage does not require any specific treatment. Rarely, liver damage can lead to acute liver failure.

In a systematic review and meta-analysis, the pooled rate for AST levels outside reference ranges was 20% (95% CI, 15.3%-25.6%) of patients, and the pooled rate for increased ALT levels was 14.6% (95% CI, 12.8%-16.6%) of patients (Parasa *et al.* 2020). Elevations of AST, ALT, and total bilirubin and low levels of albumin were reportedly associated with severe COVID-19 (Parohan, 2020).

In a large meta-analysis involving more than 6,000 patients, researchers reported that abnormal liver function was recorded in 19% of the patients and elevated liver enzymes were associated with severe COVID-19 course (OR = 1.89 for ALT, 3.08 for AST) (Mao, 2020). Patients presenting with GI signs and symptoms were admitted to hospital later than those without GI symptomatology. Of note, this group carries a higher risk for ARDS (OR = 2.96) and poor prognosis.

In a retrospective multicenter study involving more than 5700 adult cases with COVID-19 pneumonia in Hubei, Lei *et al.* reported that AST is particularly closely related to mortality risk among all indicators of liver damage (Lei, 2020). Liver damage indicators are mostly associated with lymphopenia, neutropenia, and male sex. It is postulated that AST values should be monitored closely. Median AST levels in non-severe and severe COVID patients were 22 U / L and 31 U / L, respectively ($p < 0.001$).

In the APCOLIS (APASL COVID-19 Liver Injury Spectrum Study) (Sarin, 2020) the authors revealed that liver-related complications increased significantly with stage of LD. For example, a Child-Turcotte-Pugh score of 9 or more on admission was associated with high mortality in the course of COVID-19. A high mortality rate (43%) was notable in decompensated cirrhotic cases. High bilirubin and AST/ALT ratio is also a strong predictor of mortality of patients with CLD.

The mortality increased with SARS CoV2 infection significantly among cirrhotic patients than those without cirrhosis ($p < 0.001$) and with decompensation. The mortality is highest (43%) in the spectrum with onset of liver damage. Among cirrhosis those exposed to SARS CoV2 infection, the outcome is poor with Child-Turcotte-Pugh (CTP) score 9 or more [AUROC 0.94, sensitivity 86% and specificity of 94%, HR = 19.2 (95 CI 2.3–163.3), $p < 0.001$] (Sarin, 2020).

Hyperammonemia was detected in the examinations performed in two patients with intubation in a large cohort of COVID-19 due to delayed recovery from anesthesia (Honore, 2020). Both patients had severe diarrhea prior to hospitalization with COVID-19. The metabolic pattern was seen in EEG. They have responded to supportive therapy within 48-72 hours without any need for renal replacement therapy. Hyperammonemia due to acute LF should be distinguished in patients with severe diarrhea and having a poor clinical course.

On the other hand, there is a strong relationship between severe COVID-19 and LF. In a meta-analysis including more than 4K patients with COVID-19, LF was recorded in 22.8% (Samidoust, 2020). Liver damage is more frequent and more severe in severe patients than in mild ones.

## CONCLUSION

GIS complaints are seen very commonly (16% to 40%) in these patients, even after exclusion of loss of appetite. Those with GI signs have fever more commonly, while they experience milder disease course.

While RNA positivity in the GIS provides a major diagnostic opportunity, it also represents a dangerous situation for healthcare workers and the public in regard to fecal-oral transmission. Signs and symptoms related to the GIS was associated with COVID-19 in patients with chronic disorders such as liver disease and IBD.

RNA positivity for SARS-CoV-2 throughout the GIS channel and thus in the feces persists longer than in the respiratory tract, especially in late-presenting patients, even after discharge. There are also risks for nosocomial transmission and healthcare workers should have better protection in procedures such as endoscopy.

Patients with GIS signs and symptoms are admitted and hospitalized later than the patients with dyspnea. The presence and severity of GIS complaints show strong correlation with the severity of the disease. Those with GIS signs and symptoms have higher AST and ALT, and prolonged PT. Attention should be paid to the detection of fecal nucleic acids in most patients, particularly in children. Children with GI symptoms should be tested for the viral fecal nucleic acid. Fecal viral nucleic acid-negativity can be considered one of the discharge criteria.

While IBD per se does not pose a high risk for COVID-19, diarrhea is the most common complaint in these patients. The mortality of cirrhotic patients increased significantly with SARS CoV2 infection.

# REFERENCES

Cao, C, Chen, M, He, L, Xie, J & Chen, X (2020) Clinical features and outcomes of COVID-19 patients with gastrointestinal symptoms. *Crit Care,* 24, 340.
[http://dx.doi.org/10.1186/s13054-020-03034-x] [PMID: 32539863]

Chan, JF-W, Yuan, S, Kok, K-H, To, KK, Chu, H, Yang, J, Xing, F, Liu, J, Yip, CC, Poon, RW, Tsoi, HW, Lo, SK, Chan, KH, Poon, VK, Chan, WM, Ip, JD, Cai, JP, Cheng, VC, Chen, H, Hui, CK & Yuen, KY (2020) A familial cluster of pneumonia associated with the 2019 novel coronavirus indicating person-t--person transmission: a study of a family cluster. *Lancet,* 395, 514-23.
[http://dx.doi.org/10.1016/S0140-6736(20)30154-9] [PMID: 31986261]

Chen, N, Zhou, M, Dong, X, Qu, J, Gong, F, Han, Y, Qiu, Y, Wang, J, Liu, Y, Wei, Y, Xia, J, Yu, T, Zhang, X & Zhang, L (2020) Epidemiological and clinical characteristics of 99 cases of 2019 novel coronavirus pneumonia in Wuhan, China: a descriptive study. *Lancet,* 395, 507-13.
[http://dx.doi.org/10.1016/S0140-6736(20)30211-7] [PMID: 32007143]

Cheung, KS, Hung, IFN & Chan, PPY (2020) Gastrointestinal Manifestations of SARS-CoV-2 Infection and Virus Load in Fecal Samples From a Hong Kong Cohort: Systematic Review and Meta-analysis. *Gastroenterology,* S0016-5085, 30448-0.

Cimolai, N (2020) Features of enteric disease from human coronaviruses: Implications for COVID-19. *J Med Virol,* 92, 1834-44.
[http://dx.doi.org/10.1002/jmv.26066] [PMID: 32462689]

Du, H, Dong, X & Zhang, JJ (2020) Clinical Characteristics of 182 Pediatric COVID-19 Patients With Different Severities and Allergic Status. *Allergy.* [Online ahead of print.].
[http://dx.doi.org/10.1111/all.14452] [PMID: 32524611]

Du, W, Yu, J & Liu, X (2020) Persistence of SARS-CoV-2 virus RNA in feces: A case series of children. *J Infect Public Health,* S1876-0341, 30491-.

Fiorino, G, Allocca, M, Furfaro, F, Gilardi, D, Zilli, A, Radice, S, Spinelli, A & Danese, S (2020) Inflammatory Bowel Disease Care in the COVID-19 Pandemic Era: The Humanitas, Milan, Experience. *J Crohn's Colitis,* 14, 1330-3.
[http://dx.doi.org/10.1093/ecco-jcc/jjaa058] [PMID: 32211765]

Ford, AC & Peyrin-Biroulet, L (2013) Opportunistic infections with anti-tumor necrosis factor-α therapy in inflammatory bowel disease: meta-analysis of randomized controlled trials. *Am J Gastroenterol,* 108, 1268-76.
[http://dx.doi.org/10.1038/ajg.2013.138] [PMID: 23649185]

Ghoshal, UC, Ghoshal, U & Dhiman, RK (2020) Gastrointestinal and Hepatic Involvement in Severe Acute Respiratory Syndrome Coronavirus 2 Infection: A Review. *J Clin Exp Hepatol,* 10, 622-8.
[http://dx.doi.org/10.1016/j.jceh.2020.06.002] [PMID: 32837095]

Honore, PM, Barreto Gutierrez, L, Kugener, L, Redant, S, Attou, R, Gallerani, A & De Bels, D (2020) Liver injury without liver failure in COVID-19 patients: how to explain, in some cases, elevated ammonia without hepatic decompensation. *Crit Care,* 24, 352.
[http://dx.doi.org/10.1186/s13054-020-03088-x] [PMID: 32546201]

Hua, C-Z, Miao, Z-P, Zheng, JS, Huang, Q, Sun, QF, Lu, HP, Su, FF, Wang, WH, Huang, LP, Chen, DQ, Xu, ZW, Ji, LD, Zhang, HP, Yang, XW, Li, MH, Mao, YY, Ying, MZ, Ye, S, Shu, Q, Chen, EF, Liang, JF, Wang, W, Chen, ZM, Li, W & Fu, JF (2020) Epidemiological features and viral shedding in children with SARS-CoV-2 infection. *J Med Virol,* 92, 2804-12.
[http://dx.doi.org/10.1002/jmv.26180] [PMID: 32542750]

Huang, C, Wang, Y, Li, X, Ren, L, Zhao, J, Hu, Y, Zhang, L, Fan, G, Xu, J, Gu, X, Cheng, Z, Yu, T, Xia, J, Wei, Y, Wu, W, Xie, X, Yin, W, Li, H, Liu, M, Xiao, Y, Gao, H, Guo, L, Xie, J, Wang, G, Jiang, R, Gao, Z, Jin, Q, Wang, J & Cao, B (2020) Clinical features of patients infected with 2019 novel coronavirus in Wuhan, China. *Lancet,* 395, 497-506.

[http://dx.doi.org/10.1016/S0140-6736(20)30183-5] [PMID: 31986264]

IOIBD *IOIBD Update on COVID-19 for Patients with Crohn's Disease and Ulcerative Colitis.* https://www.ioibd.org/ioibd-update-oncovid19-for-patients-with-crohns-disease-andulcerative-colitis/(2020)

Lei, F, Liu, YM, Zhou, F, Qin, JJ, Zhang, P, Zhu, L, Zhang, XJ, Cai, J, Lin, L, Ouyang, S, Wang, X, Yang, C, Cheng, X, Liu, W, Li, H, Xie, J, Wu, B, Luo, H, Xiao, F, Chen, J, Tao, L, Cheng, G, She, ZG, Zhou, J, Wang, H, Lin, J, Luo, P, Fu, S, Zhou, J, Ye, P, Xiao, B, Mao, W, Liu, L, Yan, Y, Liu, L, Chen, G, Li, H, Huang, X, Zhang, BH & Yuan, Y (2020) Longitudinal association between markers of liver injury and mortality in COVID-19 in China. *Hepatology,* 72, 389-98.
[http://dx.doi.org/10.1002/hep.31301] [PMID: 32359177]

Liang, W, Feng, Z, Rao, S, Xiao, C, Xue, X, Lin, Z, Zhang, Q & Qi, W (2020) Diarrhoea may be underestimated: a missing link in 2019 novel coronavirus. *Gut,* 69, 1141-3.
[http://dx.doi.org/10.1136/gutjnl-2020-320832] [PMID: 32102928]

Luo, S, Zhang, X & Xu, H (2020) Don't Overlook Digestive Symptoms in Patients With 2019 Novel Coronavirus Disease (COVID-19). *Clin Gastroenterol Hepatol,* 18, 1636-7.
[http://dx.doi.org/10.1016/j.cgh.2020.03.043] [PMID: 32205220]

Mao, R, Qiu, Y, He, JS, Tan, JY, Li, XH, Liang, J, Shen, J, Zhu, LR, Chen, Y, Iacucci, M, Ng, SC, Ghosh, S & Chen, MH (2020) Manifestations and prognosis of gastrointestinal and liver involvement in patients with COVID-19: a systematic review and meta-analysis. *Lancet Gastroenterol Hepatol,* 5, 667-78.
[http://dx.doi.org/10.1016/S2468-1253(20)30126-6] [PMID: 32405603]

Nagata, N, Iwata, N, Hasegawa, H, Sato, Y, Morikawa, S, Saijo, M, Itamura, S, Saito, T, Ami, Y, Odagiri, T, Tashiro, M & Sata, T (2007) Pathology and virus dispersion in cynomolgus monkeys experimentally infected with severe acute respiratory syndrome coronavirus via different inoculation routes. *Int J Exp Pathol,* 88, 403-14.
[http://dx.doi.org/10.1111/j.1365-2613.2007.00567.x] [PMID: 18039277]

Nobel, YR, Phipps, M, Zucker, J, Lebwohl, B, Wang, TC, Sobieszczyk, ME & Freedberg, DE (2020) etal. Gastrointestinal symptoms and coronavirus disease 2019: a case-control study from the United States. *Gastroenterology,* 159, 373-375.e2.
[http://dx.doi.org/10.1053/j.gastro.2020.04.017] [PMID: 32294477]

Pan, L, Mu, M, Yang, P, Sun, Y, Wang, R, Yan, J, Li, P, Hu, B, Wang, J, Hu, C, Jin, Y, Niu, X, Ping, R, Du, Y, Li, T, Xu, G, Hu, Q & Tu, L (2020) Clinical Characteristics of COVID-19 Patients With Digestive Symptoms in Hubei, China: A Descriptive, Cross-Sectional, Multicenter Study. *Am J Gastroenterol,* 115, 766-73.
[http://dx.doi.org/10.14309/ajg.0000000000000620] [PMID: 32287140]

Parasa, S, Desai, M, Thoguluva Chandrasekar, V, Patel, HK, Kennedy, KF, Roesch, T, Spadaccini, M, Colombo, M, Gabbiadini, R, Artifon, ELA, Repici, A & Sharma, P (2020) Prevalence of Gastrointestinal Symptoms and Fecal Viral Shedding in Patients With Coronavirus Disease 2019: A Systematic Review and Meta-analysis. *JAMA Netw Open,* 3, e2011335.
[http://dx.doi.org/10.1001/jamanetworkopen.2020.11335] [PMID: 32525549]

Parohan, M, Yaghoubi, S & Seraji, A (2020) Liver injury is associated with severe coronavirus disease 2019 (COVID-19) infection: A systematic review and meta-analysis of retrospective studies. *Hepatol Res,* 50, 924-35.
[http://dx.doi.org/10.1111/hepr.13510] [PMID: 32386449]

Randazzo, W, Truchado, P, Cuevas-Ferrando, E, Simón, P, Allende, A & Sánchez, G (2020) SARS-CoV-2 RNA in wastewater anticipated COVID-19 occurrence in a low prevalence area. *Water Res,* 181, 115942.
[http://dx.doi.org/10.1016/j.watres.2020.115942] [PMID: 32425251]

Rubin, DT, Feuerstein, JD, Wang, AY & Cohen, RD (2020) AGA Clinical Practice Update on Management of Inflammatory Bowel Disease During the COVID-19 Pandemic: Expert Commentary. *Gastroenterology,* 159, 350-7.
[http://dx.doi.org/10.1053/j.gastro.2020.04.012] [PMID: 32283100]

Samidoust, P, Samidoust, A, Samadani, AA & Khoshdoz, S (2020) Risk of hepatic failure in COVID-19 patients. A systematic review and meta-analysis. *Infez Med,* 28 (Suppl. 1), 96-103.
[PMID: 32532945]

Sarin, SK, Choudhury, A, Lau, GK, Zheng, MH, Ji, D, Abd-Elsalam, S, Hwang, J, Qi, X, Cua, IH, Suh, JI, Park, JG, Putcharoen, O, Kaewdech, A, Piratvisuth, T, Treeprasertsuk, S, Park, S, Wejnaruemarn, S, Payawal, DA, Baatarkhuu, O, Ahn, SH, Yeo, CD, Alonzo, UR, Chinbayar, T, Loho, IM, Yokosuka, O, Jafri, W, Tan, S, Soo, LI, Tanwandee, T, Gani, R, Anand, L, Esmail, ES, Khalaf, M, Alam, S, Lin, CY, Chuang, WL, Soin, AS, Garg, HK, Kalista, K, Batsukh, B, Purnomo, HD, Dara, VP, Rathi, P, Al Mahtab, M, Shukla, A, Sharma, MK & Omata, M APASL COVID Task Force, APASL COVID Liver Injury Spectrum Study (APCOLIS Study-NCT 04345640) (2020) Pre-existing liver disease is associated with poor outcome in patients with SARS CoV2 infection; The APCOLIS Study (APASL COVID-19 Liver Injury Spectrum Study). *Hepatol Int,* 14, 690-700.
[http://dx.doi.org/10.1007/s12072-020-10072-8] [PMID: 32623632]

Taxonera, C, Sagastagoitia, I, Alba, C, Mañas, N, Olivares, D & Rey, E (2020) 2019 novel coronavirus disease (COVID-19) in patients with inflammatory bowel diseases. *Aliment Pharmacol Ther,* 52, 276-83.
[http://dx.doi.org/10.1111/apt.15804] [PMID: 32359205]

Wang, JG, Cui, HR, Tang, HB & Deng, XL (2020) Gastrointestinal symptoms and fecal nucleic acid testing of children with 2019 coronavirus disease: a systematic review and meta-analysis. *Sci Rep,* 10, 17846.
[http://dx.doi.org/10.1038/s41598-020-74913-0] [PMID: 33082472]

*World Health Organization Q&A on coronaviruses (COVID-19).* https://www.who.int/news-room/q-a-detail/q-a-coronaviruses

Xing, Y, Ni, W, Wu, Q, Li, W, Li, G, Wang, W, Tong, J, Song, X, Wong, GWK & Xing, Q (2020) Dynamics of faecal SARS-CoV-2 in infected children during the convalescent phase. *J Infect,* 81, 318-56.
[http://dx.doi.org/10.1016/j.jinf.2020.03.049] [PMID: 32283149]

Xu, Y, Li, X, Zhu, B, Liang, H, Fang, C, Gong, Y, Guo, Q, Sun, X, Zhao, D, Shen, J, Zhang, H, Liu, H, Xia, H, Tang, J, Zhang, K & Gong, S (2020) Characteristics of pediatric SARS-CoV-2 infection and potential evidence for persistent fecal viral shedding. *Nat Med,* 26, 502-5.
[http://dx.doi.org/10.1038/s41591-020-0817-4] [PMID: 32284613]

Zhang, T, Cui, X, Zhao, X, Wang, J, Zheng, J, Zheng, G, Guo, W, Cai, C, He, S & Xu, Y (2020) Detectable SARS-CoV-2 viral RNA in feces of three children during recovery period of COVID-19 pneumonia. *J Med Virol,* 92, 909-14.
[http://dx.doi.org/10.1002/jmv.25795] [PMID: 32222992]

Zhang, W, Du, R-H, Li, B, Zheng, XS, Yang, XL, Hu, B, Wang, YY, Xiao, GF, Yan, B, Shi, ZL & Zhou, P (2020) Molecular and serological investigation of 2019-nCoV infected patients: implication of multiple shedding routes. *Emerg Microbes Infect,* 9, 386-9.
[http://dx.doi.org/10.1080/22221751.2020.1729071] [PMID: 32065057]

# CHAPTER 9

# Is Our Psychology Affected By the Pandemic? How?

**Abstract:** We are facing a *de novo* global crisis that we have never faced after World War II. During the pandemic period, there is an increased and uncontrollable level of 'information pollution' compared to the past, especially in social media and other mass media. This increases the stress load on people. Developing adverse emotional, physical, or cognitive responses that arise in response to the effects of the COVID-19 pandemic is viewed as a normal reaction to one's environment. Anxiety, depression, and delirium can ensue as a pathological and extreme persistent response to these stimuli.

During the pandemic period, it is normal to feel down as you get information about it. In fact, worrying during this process is a necessary reaction to protect ourselves and is a normal emotional response. Self-awareness and recognition of the psychological and physical responses getting out of control to decide to get help from professionals are crucial.

**Keywords:** Anxiety, Cognitive responses, COVID-19, Delirium, Depression, Emotional responses, Pandemic, Psychology, Stress.

## WHAT ARE STRESS REACTIONS? WHAT CAN WE DO?

Stress is an emotional, physical, and cognitive response in which your usual general harmony is disturbed by the emergence of new conditions.

We are facing a *de novo* global crisis that we have never faced after World War II. Although it seems partially comparable to the AIDS and swine flu pandemics, it should be considered normal for people to be psychologically affected after an event that affects the world extensively, in many aspects (*e.g.*, public health and socioeconomically).

## WHY ARE WE STRESSED DURING THIS PERIOD?

During the pandemic era, there is an increased and uncontrollable level of 'information pollution' compared to the past, especially in social media and other mass media . This increases the stress load on people . If there is a lack of

**Ozgur KARCIOGLU, Selman YENIOCAK and Mandana HOSSEINZADEH**

“reliable” information on any subject, the human brain is ready to fill in the gaps with bad scenarios, which increases anxiety.

The feeling that something bad will happen to a person or his loved ones (his children, parents, spouse, siblings) which will be difficult to prevent, is the most prominent source of anxiety in the world. The danger of life causes the 'flight or fight' response, which is our most primitive reflex. Considering that both “escaping” from the virus and “fighting” in a reasonable and effective way involve difficulties, it is quite understandable that anxiety is high in the masses worldwide. On the contrary, it will be abnormal for you to remain unresponsive to a situation that threatens your life.

## ADVERSE EMOTIONAL, PHYSICAL, OR COGNITIVE RESPONSES THAT ARISE IN RESPONSE TO THE EFFECTS OF THE COVID-19 PANDEMIC INCLUDE

- Fear and anxiety for the health of yourself, offspring and next of kin (anxiety),
- Feeling excessive fear / anxiety about being stigmatized and infecting others,
- Feeling tense and overwhelmed, anxiety and fear of ordinary situations,
- Feeling constantly sad, depressed, and tearful,
- Decreased interest in enjoyable activities,
- A change in sleep patterns; difficulty falling asleep, nightmares,
- Increased appetite, A boost in chronic health problems,
- Persistent and repetitive negative thoughts that you cannot control,
- Difficulty to concentrate,
- Memory weakness,
- Physical symptoms: Increase in heart rate (pulse), stomach cramps / discomfort, weakness, tiredness

If we summarize the negative effects of these situations on the individual

- Feeling hopeless in general,
- Being detached from close people or social environment,
- To be anxious about entering public spaces,
- Being unable to relax, always feeling tense
- Increasing use of alcohol, cigarette, and other substances

Patients hospitalized for covid-19 have additional stressors

- Not being able to see the staff and communicate easily due to personal protective equipment
- Social isolation – relatives/loved ones are unable to visit
- The negative effects of noise, alarms, rushing in ED and ICUs
- Hearing about or witnessing other patients or deaths on a mechanical ventilator
- Anxiety about not getting adequate care because of shortage of personnel, and/or equipment

Pearl: The development process of our perceptions in the pandemic. When news of disasters and images of dying people come, people first enter the fear phase. Then there is the area of learning, and finally maturation on the issue. These areas may not be separated by clear lines, but may overlap each other. Although it is not possible to pass through these areas very quickly without digestion, healthier transitions can be achieved with information and solidarity among people and staying in an area too long can be prevented.

## COVID-19 and our Psychology: What do the Researchers Say?

In a national-scale study investigating how the psychological state of the people was afflicted by the COVID-19 pandemic in China, it was reported that 35% of people were negatively affected (Qiu *et al*, 2020). The responses of more than 52,000 subjects were analyzed, and severe distress was found in 5.1% of the cases. In the regression analysis, female gender, advanced age (especially over 60 years old), high education level, being a migrant worker, living in Hubei where the disease affected the society more intensely than most places, are significantly associated with high psychological strain.

In the study started on January 31, it was observed that the level of stress decreased as time passed, and even decreased to the lowest level with the Lantern Festival on February 8. It is thought that this is related to the adequate level of medical resources and support throughout the country and activities regarding public awareness. Therefore, it was postulated that "psychological first aid" and the coordination of measures taken were important during the pandemic period, and programs specific to women, the elderly and migrant workers should also be carried out.

## SARS-CoV and Psychiatric Syndromes:

There are few studies, meta-analyzes or systematic reviews with high level of evidence regarding psychological disturbances occurring in the course of COVID-

19 and other SARS-CoV diseases. Rogers *et al.* analyzed 65 studies and 7 preprint findings (Rogers *et al*, 2020).

They stated that in the course of SARS in 2002, mania and psychosis associated with both steroid treatment and the disease itself occurred at a rate of 0.7% in the whole affected population. High rates of psychiatric findings were noted during the recovery period of SARS-CoV diseases:

- insomnia 12.1%,
- anxiety 12.3%,
- irritability 12.8%,
- memory impairment 18.9%,
- weakness-fatigue was seen at the rate of 19.3%.
- posttraumatic stress disorder 32.2%,
- depression is as high as 14.9%.

When the COVID-19 patients were examined specifically, findings suggestive of delirium were found at a high rate, especially in ICU patients: 69% agitation and 21% altered mental status were recorded

In preprint-level studies in China, it has been pointed out that there is a need for psychological interventions in addition to antiviral and other treatments in patients who are kept in isolation wards or hospitalized for COVID-19 pneumonia. HAMA and HAMD (Hamilton anxiety and depression scales) scores of patients hospitalized due to COVID-19 are higher than other patients with pneumonia (Yang *et al*, 2020).

Kong *et al.* evaluated 144 patients diagnosed with COVID-19 and reported that anxiety and depression were encountered with very high frequencies of 35% and 28%, respectively (Kong *et al*, 2020).

## COVID-19 and Dealing with Stress

With the COVID-19 pandemic, the important thing as a result of our changing living conditions is recognition of how to cope with stress. First of all we need to know; before the epidemic, we couldn't control everything in our lives; now we cannot control either.

Groups most likely to overreact to stress

- The elderly and the groups at high risk of infected by COVID-19 and having severe diseases because of chronic comorbid diseases.
- Children and adolescents.
- Healthcare workers who help and care for patients or suspects with COVID-19.
- Those who lost a relative or loved one due to illness.
- People with psychological problems, including substance abuse, especially those diagnosed with Obsessive-Compulsive Disorder (OCD) and those with anxiety disorders.

**Coping with Stress**

The vast majority of our worries and concerns are related to the future and most of them do not come true. We can neither blame ourselves nor strive to change things that are beyond our control.

Modern life drives us to anxious thoughts. Considering generations ago, levels of anxiety were also very low, as there was no such advanced technology.

Recommendations for minimizing the effects during the pandemic period

- **Take a break:** It is wrong if anything takes too long hours, such as reading, watching movies, surfing the internet. You should find ways for taking breaks when prompted by your body and mind.
- **Take care of your body:** it will benefit yourself to exercise, to eat well and to get enough sleep, to stay away from alcohol and drugs.
- **Do something that will distract you:** Always keep yourself busy with things that are different from what you do every time. it will be very useful, especially to produce, to create and learn new things.
- **Connect with people:** Talk to people you trust and love, stay connected.

What kind of activities are good for you?

Productive activities are always better than doing nothing or passively watching TV, or surfing in the internet. It will be very good for mental health to grow flowers in pots or gardens, to write memories by keeping a diary, to develop ourselves further and to try to write poems, stories, if there is a possibility and talent, to produce pictures or music. These types of activities are also very useful in getting your sleep back on track.

If we can get the stress response right and control it positively, stress is necessary to some extent, without any harm to the body. additional tips can be listed as follows:

- If we obtain information from reliable sources, we will be relieved of the worry of information pollution.
- Social media is known to increase anxiety in general. Evaluate how much time you spend in SM.
- Watching news should also be minimized. You can watch it at certain times, for example, at most twice a day.
- Remember that keeping rhythm, singing, and dancing accompanied by music has a soothing effect on your mood.
- It is useful to wander outside as much as possible by creating an opportunity.
- It will be beneficial for people who have to stay at home but cannot go outside to acquire hobbies and occupations to keep them busy.
- Exercise as much as possible. By increasing the amount of oxygen that circulates to the brain, sports strengthen the memory and increases brain performance. It also helps reduce unhappiness and tension by increasing the secretion of endorphins. Moreover, when we do sports, we become more rested, energetic, and calm. It also improves our sleep quality and allows us to cope with stress more easily.
- Practicing breathing exercises and learning the right breathing techniques reduce the negative reactions we give to the source of stress and help us cope with stress more easily.

You should consider what you can do to protect yourself and those around you. The following two questions may lead us to a more solution-oriented approach:

“What can I control?”

“Which methods have helped me cope with the challenges I have faced in the past?

**What's on The Flip Side?**

An excessive perception of threat can trigger an overtly defensive reflex. For example, an epidemic can precipitate over-meticulous thinking. People who take acceptable measures are not at higher risk for disease than those who take extreme precautions. Nobody will benefit from running from room to room with a cloth soaked in bleach.

Avoid alcohol, smoking, drugs, and medication. Similarly, foods and drinks containing caffeine can be harmful. Because the half-life of caffeine is 6 hours, if you drank a cup of coffee at 16:00 in the evening, half of the caffeine you drink at 22:00 will still be circulating in your bloodstream.

## Awareness of Emotions

During the pandemic period, it is normal to feel bad as you get information about it. In fact, worrying during this process is a necessary reaction to protect ourselves and is a normal emotional response. We can think of this as a person walking on the railway feeling scared and anxious when he hears the sound of the train, the opposite will be a more problematic situation. However, if anxiety is more than necessary, it impairs the immune system, so anxiety is something that should be dealt with. First of all, it is very important that we accept that this process is temporary. No pandemics has lasted to eternity and none will do.

Do not neglect to contact people you think may be anxious or you know live alone. This will not only make you feel good, but also help those people cope with their anxiety and worry.

A wise approach may be to focus on other activities. For example, if we spend time on our hobbies in bad times, we will feel better. Apart from that, doing sports and being in motion increases the level of endorphins known as happiness hormones in our body, making it easier for us to feel happy. When you feel that your anxiety is getting too high, it is important to share your feelings with your loved ones.

One of the suggested ways to deal with stress is art and humor. When faced with difficulties, life will always find a way out. Art has always been a part of this life energy, resistance, and activism. Nothing changes when we worry, so let us choose to laugh as much as we can instead of worry. However, let us be careful that the subject of art or humor is not particularly related to the pandemic at this time. Although it seems to instantly relax us, it may be possible to increase negative stress symptoms afterwards, as it will constantly remind us of the pandemic and the stress it creates.

## It is Normal To Be In A Bad Mood From Time To Time. So When Will We Wonder If We Are Depressed?

Depression is one of the most misused terms in the public. In its simplest definition, it is a continuous state of unhappiness and sadness. Although the condition of a person who has lost a relative is similar to depression, it differs from depression with a significant improvement over time. It is more common in women and elderly people. The good thing is; it has a very favorable response to treatment after the correct diagnosis. It should also be known that depressed people often have anxiety disorder.

After epidemics similar to COVID-19 such as SARS and MERS, depression was detected in 15% of patients within a few months, and anxiety disorder was found in 15%. Post-traumatic stress disorder (PTSD) can be up to 30%. We can see depression in all age groups. Prolonged weakness and fatigue have been reported in about 19%.

The following symptoms should last at least two weeks to be diagnosed with depression:

- Feeling constantly sad, depressed, and pessimistic
- Loss of interest and pleasure in activities that were previously done lovingly,
- Sexual dysfunctions (sexual reluctance, arousal disorder, inability to have orgasm, erectile dysfunction in men, pelvic contractions in women, premature ejaculation / inability to ejaculate),
- Difficulty falling asleep, waking up frequently or sleeping excessively,
- Feeling worthless and guilty,
- Loss of concentration and difficulty making decisions,
- Slowness in speech and movements,
- Constant weakness-tiredness,
- Change in appetite; *i.e.* overeating or lack of appetite,
- Frequent thinking about death and suicidal / self-harming tendency.

**Social Relations**

Although we have to keep distance from other people due to the pandemic, this distance is only a physical distance. On the contrary, it is clear that we are in a period in which social solidarity should be emphasized. In fact, the more active we keep our social relationships, the quicker and easier we can overcome stressful times.

- Share it. Tell other people about the music you listen to, the movies you have watched, the places you've visited before, the games you've played.
- Getting ideas from friends or consultants for your projects or lessons helps you focus on the job and enjoy working.

## Try not to Disturb your Routine and Sleep Patterns

Experts recommend that we continue our routine no matter what. Sleeping and waking up at a certain time, doing productive work positively affect our mental health. It is beneficial to maintain sleep patterns. For example, "going to sleep in the morning" for watching movies *etc.* in the night will have a detrimental effect on your psychology as it will disrupt your schedule the next day.

If you sleep well, 'Growth hormone' is released when you fall asleep. In this way, your muscle and bone strength increases, protein metabolism is regulated, and aging is also delayed.

## Do Hobbies Work?

Yes, definitely. If you have not adopted a specific hobby, try to find a hobby that you can fondly get involved in.

- Once upon a time you have complained about the lack of time, remember? You were sorry for the books you could not read and the movies you could not watch. Now this is your time.
- You now have time to spare for your wishes such as learning a new language, starting painting, and learning how to cook.
- You can spare time for delayed tasks such as clearing your diaries, notes, arranging the balcony, dealing with something to be repaired.
- You can do many things like learning sign language, puzzles, watching documentaries, researching history, *etc.*

## What Does Physical Activity Bring us?

It is known that there is a close relationship between physical activity such as regular sports and mental health. Try to do whatever is good for you to recover your motivation for life. Light or moderate exercise decreases the cortisone (stress) hormone. This way, you will feel better.

Along with regular exercise, the hormone called irisin is also released regularly. This hormone protects brain cells from injury and aging, as well as allowing you to lose weight.

Remember that even when you are at home, you can find many ways to stimulate your body, *e.g.*, organizing your study room, playing games, or exercising with the kids.

## Bias and Stigmatization

- **Stigmatization:** Attitudes and behaviors triggered by the rigid thoughts in our mind that can harm the subjected individual from time to time by causing loss of social status and / or discrimination in individuals for certain reasons, resulting in multiple negative experiences such as stress, decreased self-esteem, mood disorders and depression, deterioration in social adaptation and reduced compliance with treatment. In the past, it has been debated extensively for homosexuality and diseases such as the plague and AIDS.
- COVID-19 is a widespread public health problem affecting many people around the world, regardless of ethnicity, gender, and age. Remember that you or someone around you may also be diagnosed with COVID-19 and could be among those who received treatment and / or recovered. In brief, stigmatization is a threat to public welfare and should be avoided explicitly.
- Individuals who are being treated with a diagnosis of COVID-19 should be careful not to use stigmatizing expressions such as "case", "Covid" or "victim".

## CONCLUSION

During the pandemic period, it is normal to feel bad as you get information about it. In fact, worrying during this process is a necessary reaction to protect ourselves.

As in the ancient Turkish saying "Flood goes, sand and mud remains", epidemics will somehow end, but it is inevitable to have various permanent effects on the human organism. In addition to the damages to physiological structure *i.e.*, effects such as pneumonia, fever and pain; the loss of loved ones and socioeconomic damage to the society also have short and long term effects on our psychological well-being. The direct effect of the disease on the nervous system and brain also creates changes on psychology. Self-awareness and recognition of the psychological and physical responses getting out of control to decide getting help from professionals is crucial. Staying at home due to quarantine, being sick and staying in the hospital will also directly injure the mood. Maintenance of health against all these effects and returning to a happy, productive life can be achieved through conscious interventions such as individual activities, physical activity, hobbies, and being together with our loved ones, along with social solidarity. In addition, it will be inevitable for the person to get professional help when he / she cannot cope on his own.

## REFERENCES

Bavel, JJV, Baicker, K, Boggio, PS, Capraro, V, Cichocka, A, Cikara, M, Crockett, MJ, Crum, AJ, Douglas, KM, Druckman, JN, Drury, J, Dube, O, Ellemers, N, Finkel, EJ, Fowler, JH, Gelfand, M, Han, S, Haslam, SA, Jetten, J, Kitayama, S, Mobbs, D, Napper, LE, Packer, DJ, Pennycook, G, Peters, E, Petty, RE, Rand,

DG, Reicher, SD, Schnall, S, Shariff, A, Skitka, LJ, Smith, SS, Sunstein, CR, Tabri, N, Tucker, JA, Linden, SV, Lange, PV, Weeden, KA, Wohl, MJA, Zaki, J, Zion, SR & Willer, R (2020) Using social and behavioural science to support COVID-19 pandemic response. *Nat Hum Behav,* 4, 460-71. [http://dx.doi.org/10.1038/s41562-020-0884-z] [PMID: 32355299]

Kong, X, Zheng, K & Tang, M (2020) Prevalence and factors associated with depression and anxiety of hospitalized patients with COVID-19. *medRxiv.* preprint

Qiu, J, Shen, B, Zhao, M, Wang, Z, Xie, B & Xu, Y (2020) A nationwide survey of psychological distress among Chinese people in the COVID-19 epidemic: implications and policy recommendations. *Gen Psychiatr,* 33, e100213.
[http://dx.doi.org/10.1136/gpsych-2020-100213] [PMID: 32215365]

Rogers, JP, Chesney, E & Oliver, D (2020) Psychiatric and neuropsychiatric presentations associated with severe coronavirus infections: a systematic review and meta-analysis with comparison to the COVID-19 pandemic. *Lancet Psychiatry,* S2215-0366, 30203-0.

Yang, L, Wu, D & Hou, Y (2020) Analysis of psychological state and clinical psychological intervention model of patients with COVID-19. *medRxiv.* preprint

# CHAPTER 10

# COVID-19 and Our Brain: What's New?

**Abstract:** We all recognize the typical signs and symptoms of COVID-19 (fever, shortness of breath, persistent non-productive cough). Less common symptoms are headaches, confusion (talking nonsense), numbness/hypoesthesia, seizure (convulsions), vomiting, loss of smell (anosmia), and sense of taste (ageusia). It can be noted that this group of symptoms consisted mostly of neurological complaints. COVID-19 causes CNS damage with various mechanisms. For example, anosmia or hyposmia is seen quite frequently among individuals even with mild COVID-19. Therefore, physicians should be alert in noting nervous system-related symptoms and findings that can be seen in the course of COVID-19.

**Keywords:** ACE2 receptors, Ageusia, Anosmia, Confusion, Cognitive disorders, COVID-19, Headache, Neurology, Pandemic.

## INTRODUCTION

Medical community and healthcare workers have a huge knowledge base on the disease, which directly inflicted more than 27 million people in the world and killed nearly 900,000 people in September 2020. Now we all recognize the typical signs and symptoms of COVID-19 (fever, shortness of breath, persistent non-productive cough). Less common symptoms are headaches, confusion (talking nonsense), numbness/hypoesthesia, seizure (convulsions), vomiting, loss of smell (anosmia), and sense of taste (ageusia). It can be noted that this group of symptoms consisted mostly of neurological complaints (Table **1**).

**Case 1** A 24-year-old Japanese male without any history of travel abroad is admitted to the hospital with chief complaints of headache, fever, and malaise. Flu tests are negative, and he was sent home. He goes to another clinic with worsening head and throat pain three days later. X-ray and blood tests are normal. Four days later, he is unconscious and found drowning in his vomitus at home. He has seizures in the ambulance. There is edema in the brain CT in the ED. COVID-19 swabs are also negative. In the CSF sample obtained *via* lumbar puncture, COVID is positive. The physicians interpreted that the virus invades the brain.

**Ozgur KARCIOGLU, Selman YENIOCAK and Mandana HOSSEINZADEH**

**Table 1. Nervous system-related symptoms and findings that can be seen in the course of COVID-19.**

| Acute Cerebrovascular (cv) Signs and Symptoms | Acute-onset Speech Disorder, Confusion, Uni/or Bilateral Weakness on The Limbs (paralysis). |
|---|---|
| Intracranial infection signs and symptoms: | headache, seizures, altered mental status |
| Muscle damage signs and symptoms: | myalgia, weakness, fatigue, |
| Other neural signs and symptoms: | Neuralgias and abnormal sensations (hyperalgesia or hypoesthesia). |

The triad of fever, persistent dry cough, and shortness of breath or dyspnea on exertion should be the principal features to look for in the triage of any suspected patient. The number of patients with atypical or rare symptoms mentioned above were reported in some studies, albeit in small numbers. It can be thought that such findings are seen in only a small minority, but many clinicians think these findings are important adjuncts since they can lead to different points of view in diagnosis and treatment.

In a multidisciplinary multicenter registration study conducted in the UK, 153 patients who were admitted with COVID-19-related neurological complaints and/or findings were identified (Varatharaj *et al*, 2020). The mean age of COVID-19 cases admitted with neuropsychiatric complications was 71, and 62% presented with CVA and 31% with altered mental status. 23% of the patients with altered mental status were diagnosed with nonspecific encephalopathy and 18% with encephalitis. Others are new (92%) or old (8%) psychiatric diagnoses. Most of the patients with CVA (82%) are over 60 years old.

Treatments may have to change in the presence of CNS signs. For example, many drugs do not pass the invisible obstacle, which we call the 'blood-brain barrier', so it does not affect brain cells. Therefore, physicians should take it into account if the target of the treatment includes the CNS.

In a publication from Wuhan, CNS findings were recorded in 36% of 214 patients with COVID-19 hospitalized in three hospitals (Mao *et al*, 2020). Among these, muscle aches, headache, dizziness, and confusion have been reported most frequently. These can be seen in other viral infections, especially in the elderly. In a smaller group, there is stroke, prolonged seizure, loss of taste and anosmia. An interesting point is that cases with headache showed symptoms days before fever and cough.

Loss of taste sensation was reported in 5.6% and anosmia was reported in 5.1% of cases. In European series, higher rates are given. We should add that these findings are more common in mild-to-moderate cases. In a multicenter study involving mild to moderate patients in Europe, these percentages are 88% and 85.6%, respectively. (International Federation of Oto-Rhino-Laryngological Societies (YO-IFOS) (Lechien *et al*, 2020). Myelitis, prolonged seizures, encephalopathy, meningitis are cited in anecdotal reports.

## HOW CAN COVID-19 AFFECT THE BRAIN AND NERVOUS SYSTEM?

In the 2002-2003 SARS epidemic with a 10% fatality rate, SARS virus genome was found in the brain in 8 of the autopsy cases (Gu *et al*, 2005). The authors investigating its mechanisms reported that the virus was located in the brain after the instillation of SARS-CoV to the nose in genetically modified mice. More interestingly, the virus has traveled through the olfactory nerve (olfactory nerve) as it enters the brain/. After passing to the brain, SARS-CoV spread rapidly, causing the death of animals. The genetic cousin of this virus, SARS-CoV-2, also enters the cells with ACE2 receptors in this way.

### Hypoxic Damage

This is thought to cause neurological damage in patients with COVID-19 who have experienced severe respiratory failure.

### Hematogenous Spread

Although hematogenous spread of other viruses to SSS *via* impaired blood-brain barrier is well established, more information is needed on SARS-CoV-2 in this issue.

### ACE2 and Neurological Damage

ACE2 receptors are important because these are structures that SARS-CoV-2 viruses have to bind to before entrance to the cell. Other coronaviruses and influenza viruses can also use the same gate. Abnormally elevated blood pressure in the course of infection by binding to these receptors can lead to intracranial bleeding. The same mechanism explains the deterioration of the blood-brain barrier in this infection (Baig *et al*, 2020).

## WHAT KIND OF DAMAGE DOES COVID-19 CAUSE IN THE BRAIN?

Helms *et al.* analyzed 58 COVID-19 patients treated in ICU due to ARDS in France (Helms *et al*, 2020). Neurological findings were noted in 8 (14%) of patients with a median age of 63 during intensive care. Agitation was detected in the majority of patients when neuromuscular blocking agents were discontinued (40/58, 69%). Diffuse corticospinal tract findings and Babinski positivity were found in 2/3 of the patients. In the majority of 13 patients who received MRI, bilateral frontotemporal hypoperfusion was found in all 11 patients with perfusion images. Although no stroke was found clinically in any patient, minor stroke was recognized in 2 asymptomatic patients. All 7 patients with CSF analysis were RT-PCR negative for COVID.

COVID-19 causes CNS damage with three main mechanisms (Azim *et al*, 2020):

**a. Hypoxic injury** Pneumonia results in cerebral edema associated with respiratory failure.

**b. Immune-mediated damage** Macrophage and complement activation triggered by cytokine storm results in DIC and multiorgan failure.

**c. Cerebrovascular injury** Factors such as increased intravascular pressure, thrombocytopenia, elevated D-dimer through ACE2 receptor activation increase the risk of intracranial hemorrhage.

Combined with the information in other studies, it is thought that COVID-19 can lead to various nervous system findings such as altered mental status, loss of taste and sensations, seizures, strokes, and neuroimmunological damages.

## WHAT KINDS OF NEUROLOGICAL SIGNS AND SYMPTOMS DO COVID-19 CAN BE EVIDENT?

**Headache** It was reported in 6.5% of a large series in Beijing (Tian *et al*, 2020). This rate is in the range of 6-8% in Wuhan (Li *et al*, 2020). Chen *et al*. reported that headache was noted in both groups at a rate of 10% and 12% and did not show a significant difference in the study comparing the deceased and survived patients following a diagnosis of COVID-19 (Chen *et al*, 2020).

Thrombosis and stroke the peripheral nervous system is also affected by SARS-COV. Axonal neuropathy is observed 2-3 weeks after the onset of the disease (Tsai *et al*, 2004, Zochodne, 2004).

Pain compatible with neuritis was recorded as 8.9% in the series reported by Mao *et al*. (Mao *et al*, 2020).

**Myopathies** Fatigue and weakness are encountered in ¼ to half of COVID-19 cases (Huang *et al*, 2020).

**Myalgia** Muscle pain is detected in more than 1/3 of the cases (Yang *et al*, 2020).

Elevations of muscle enzymes and creatine kinase are also seen in a similar rate. However, muscle pathology detected by EMG has not been reported. Rhabdomyolysis has just been shown in anecdotal reports.

## DOES IT HAVE LONG-TERM EFFECTS ON THE CNS?

Yes. Because if writers ask such a question, it should be yes.

### Immune Damage

It has been discussed for years that neurological problems occurring in the course of viral infection act *via* the immune system (Klein *et al*, 2017). It has also been reported that the severity of neurological findings in the course of COVID-19 is associated with SIRS findings, and early administration of anti-inflammatory agents reduce this (Mehta *et al*, 2020). The fact that interleukin (IL) -6 level, which is the most important component of cytokine storm, is directly related to the severity of COVID-19 infection also supports this (Wan *et al*, 2020). It is also thought that activation of immune cells (macrophages, microglia, astrocytes) in the brain causes chronic neurological damage.

To date, knowledge about whether COVID-19 causes long-term CNS damage is insufficient, and it can be clarified *via* well-designed studies spanning a wide time frame. However, considering both stroke and immunological injuries, it can be said that a trend in this direction may arise.

## EFFECTS OF COVID-19 ON PEOPLE WITH NEUROLOGICAL DISORDERS

We have little information on how patients with a history of CVA/stroke were affected by COVID-19. Aggarwal *et al.* conducted a systematic review on the data of 6 studies and stated that 1% to 6% of patients with COVID-19 developed stroke, and the probability of experiencing severe COVID-19 in these cases was found to be 2.5 times higher than others (Aggarwal *et al*, 2020).

In a series reported from Wuhan, it was written that patients who were hospitalized with COVID-19 developed a 5% stroke (11 in 221 people) (Li *et al*, 2020). The youngest patient is 55 years old. In this series, stroke mostly affected women and elderly people (mean age: 52 whole group, *versus* 72 years in the stroke group). In this study, CRP and d-dimer levels were found to be higher in patients who had suffered from COVID-19 after stroke (CRP: mean 51 *versus* 12 mg/L and D-dimer: 6.9 *versus* 0.5 mg/L). Antiplatelet therapy and anticoagulation may be required. A high mortality rate of 38% has been reported in patients developing stroke in the course of COVID-19.

In the light of current information, it can be postulated that the patients who have had a stroke are in the high-risk group in terms of COVID-19, and that treatment should be more careful and aggressive.

## DOES COVID-19 INCREASE THE RISK OF STROKE?

Yes. In the Netherlands, a total of 31% of the patients had thrombosis and thromboembolic events (TTEE) complications in 3 hospitals, and stroke / CVA was found in 3% of cases (Klok *et al*, 2020). When patients with TTEE are examined, 27% of cases have venous and 3.7% of cases have arterial thrombosis. In other words, approximately 90% of thrombotic events involve the venous system. Pulmonary thromboembolism (PTE) is the most common TTEE in the course of COVID-19.Coagulopathy appears as an independent predictive factor for TTEE, with PT extending beyond 3 seconds or PTT longer than 5 seconds. Mao *et al.* reported a 2.4% stroke in the series in Wuhan (Mao *et al*, 2020).

In Iran, a 12-year-old child experienced weakness and speech disorder (dysarthria) on the right side following a seizure and viral nucleic acid was detected both in RT-PCR from throat swab and in the cerebrospinal fluid sample (Mirzaee *et al*, 2020). MR imaging showed obstruction in the left middle cerebral artery in the brain. It is an interesting phenomenon for both occurring in a child and that stroke being almost the first manifestation of COVID-19.

In the USA, stroke has been reported also in the young and those with a milder course of COVID-19 (Oxley *et al*, 2020). In the two-week period between March 23 and April 7, 2020, five patients were reportedly diagnosed with CVA in New York. They are all younger than 50 years of age with signs of severe large vessel occlusion. Only one of them had a previous history of stroke. When the data in these small groups are examined, it is thought that COVID-19 increases the risk of stroke, but it is obvious that more studies are needed to extrapolate this finding.

## MANY PATIENTS MENTION LOSS OF SMELL / TASTE

**Anosmia or hyposmia** A small number of autopsies of the deceased with COVID-19 were also examined in the brain. Researchers have reported that coronaviruses involved the brain tissue. At least in severe cases, the virus is thought to cross the blood-brain barrier.

In a large literature review, sudden onset loss of or decrease in smelling sensation was observed in 80% of COVID-19 cases and this was accompanied by a great loss of taste sensation (Sedaghat *et al*, 2020). In one of every four patients, these findings appeared as the first complaint. Generally, complaints improved within a few weeks. The authors stated that the questioning for this finding could increase our ability to make COVID-19 diagnosis.

In a study in patients with COVID-19 of various clinical courses were analyzed in detail in Korea, it was reported that as much as one-fifth of the patients remained asymptomatic from exposure to admission (Kim *et al*, 2020). Hyposmia was quite frequent among individuals with mild COVID-19, but fever was not. More than one-fifth of the patients complained of hyposmia, and a great majority of these patients (90%) had accompanying symptoms such as hypogeusia, nasal congestion or rhinorrhea. It is noted that this finding is more common in women and young patients than others. In more than half of the patients, two findings (problems with taste and smell) are combined. The findings disappeared in an average of 7 days, within a maximum of 3 weeks. A more interesting point is that anosmia occurs in mild cases rather than severe cases.

According to preliminary data, 30 to 50% of cases with COVID-19 had olfactory damage. Anosmia or hyposmia is one of the first findings. Approximately 1/8 of the severe cases, loss of taste and smell sensations appeared before other findings. The American Ear-Nose-Throat Academy has suggested that anosmia and ageusia be included in the primary list to seek for in these patients (Xydakis *et al*, 2020; Giacomelli *et al*, 2020).

Interestingly, olfactory nerve damage in mice is not associated with severe brain involvement. In other words, those with loss of smell seem to stop the disease there. It is not known exactly whether this is repeated in humans. Because unlike genetically modified mice, human olfactory nerve cells do not have an ACE2 receptor. In new studies, it is primarily evaluated that the virus targets the nasal mucosa cells and the like adjacent to the olfactory nerve, thereby preventing the nerve from sensing the smell.

It has been reported that the sudden loss of sense of smell and taste in workers in healthcare or other risky sector is frequently the leading finding in the course of COVID-19 and should be considered as a starting point for further examinations (Lechner *et al*, 2020). This becomes such an important finding that the authors have suggested that it is necessary to investigate the reduction of smell and taste using special and advanced tests and scales.

## IS THERE AN ASSOCIATION BETWEEN ANOSMIA AND RESPIRATORY FAILURE?

Roman *et al*. put forth that respiratory failure in severe COVID-19 cases was a neurological consequence of invasion through the first cranial nerve (olfactory nerve) to the rhinencephalon and brainstem (Roman *et al*, 2020). It has been suggested that cytokine storm triggers acute hemorrhagic necrotizing encephalitis.

It is postulated that SARS-COV-2 has neurogenic properties like other coronaviruses, and this is largely the reason for anosmia reaching the nasal mucosa through ACE2 receptors during disease transmission (Lechien *et al*, 2020). Since it is known that nasal congestion and rhinorrhea are very rare, the presence of the virus in the olfactory bulb causes this. Then, almost half of the patients' defense mechanisms overcome the virus. In some of the remainder, the virus reaches the brain and rhinencephalon *via* the olfactory nerve and through the transneuronal route, from there to the brainstem, and triggers the process leading to fatal respiratory failure. As Bagheri reported, this mechanism explains the worsening of breathing without significant dyspnea (Bagheri *et al*, 2020). These points are open to debate in the near future.

## DOES COVID-19 TRIGGER BRAIN TISSUE INFLAMMATION (ENCEPHALITIS)?

Yes, if not very often. Ye *et al.* published a case with COVID-19 encephalitis (Ye *et al*, 2020).

To interpret the course of this patient, it can be thought that generalized inflammation and immune system response caused brain edema, which caused waxing-and-waning mentation. Rapid improvement after mannitol and antiviral treatment also supports this idea. This case is a good example of self-limiting encephalitis in the course of SARS-CoV-2 infection.

A young male patient from Turkey was reported recently. 25-year old man without any comorbid diseases displayed SARS-CoV-2 positivity in the CSF ( https://www.hurriyet.com.tr/gundem /turkiyede-ilk-kez-bir-hastanin--eyin-omurilik -sivisinda-koron avirus-tespit-edildi-41536199). Other frequent reasons of persistent fever and seizures were ruled out in the management of the patient and finally the virus was detected in the CSF elicited *via* LP with a high index of suspicion of COVID-19. He responded well to treatment with favipiravir.

It has been pointed out for a long time that coronaviruses pass through the olfactory nerve to the brain starting from the early stage of the disease and complete the course within 7 days (Desforges *et al*, 2019).

While these are happening in the CNS, the virus is generally also attached to the respiratory epithelium, heart, and kidneys through the ACE2 receptors and inflicted the damage. This is also what sparked coagulopathy (Helms *et al*, 2020). Widespread involvement of the vascular endothelium facilitates coagulation and generation of microthrombi. Cardiovascular and cerebrovascular thrombosis and TTEE are also triggered *via* this mechanism.

**Case 3** Meningeal irritation is marked in the patient who was admitted to the emergency department with fever, dyspnea, and impaired consciousness. The patient was COVID-19 positive with RT-PCR, and the first brain CT was normal. Leukopenia and lymphopenia were noted. The COVID-19 test performed in CSF following LP is negative. BOS opening pressure is 220 mmHg. PaO2 / FiO2 ratio is 240. Mannitol infusion has also been added to supportive therapy. Within three weeks, the patient regained consciousness and ground-glass opacities in his chest CT improved. He was discharged in 4 weeks.

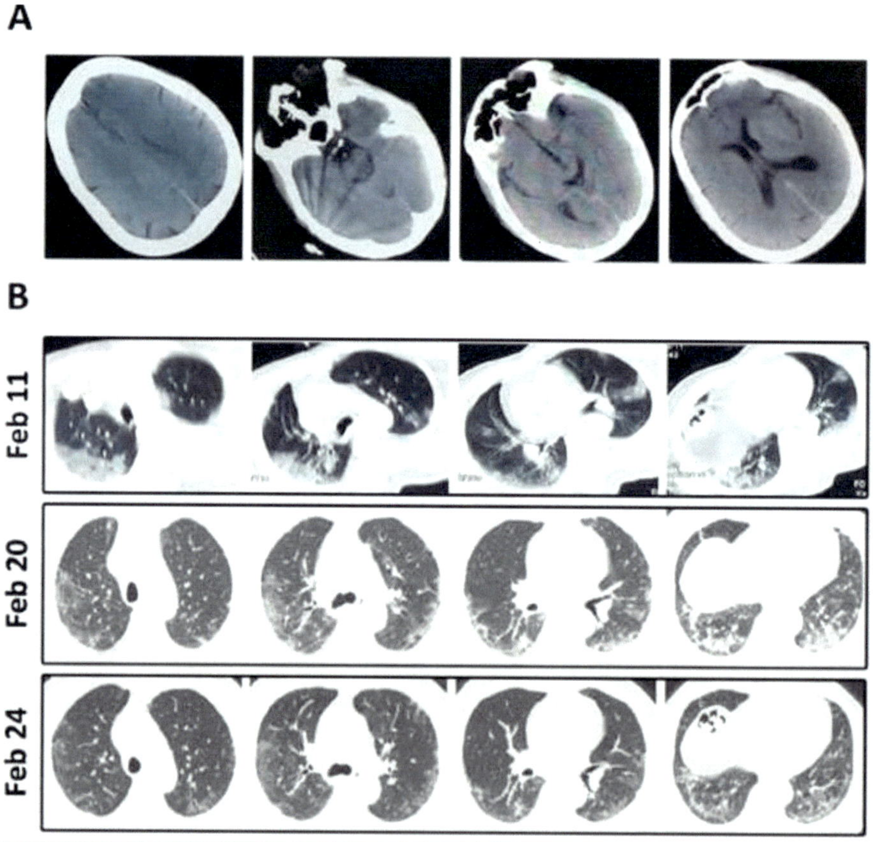

## WHAT ARE THE TREATMENT METHODS AFTER COVID-19 INFLICTS THE CNS?

Supportive therapy and certain antiviral agents for COVID-19 are the mainstay therapies in patients with encephalitis. In patients with severe brain edema that augments intracranial pressure, mannitol can be added with caution.

One of the main messages; acutely altered mental status in the patient should prompt further investigation for COVID-19. Otherwise, there may be delays in diagnosis which can be subject to litigation, as these leading findings will mean skipping, ignoring, and continuing to spread the virus. It is thought that CNS is affected by direct or indirect inflammation as a direct result of immune system response.

It has also been reported that doing LP more frequently and easily will facilitate COVID-19 research in patients with neurological findings.

## CONCLUSION

In conclusion, it is apparent that patients mostly face serious neurological impairment in the COVID-19 process. Coronaviruses affect the CNS, but together with the immune system response, persistent signs of infection, as a result of these, appear in constellations of neurological diseases. CNS involvement is mostly seen as a result of inflammatory and metabolic processes in the elderly who have had severe illness. It is also established that viruses invaded CNS *via* the transneural route. Still, an explanation of the high mortality could be the direct attack of the virus on the CNS.

It will be wise to question those with a presumptive diagnosis of COVID-19 with special regard to headache, changes in mental status, paresthesia, anosmia and ageusia. In those with positive signs, a CSF examination and, advanced imaging such as CT or MRI will be warranted, especially if there are concurrent systemic findings.

Another important point is that the patients' reluctance to refer to the hospital with neurological findings during the pandemic process, and being deprived of the support they receive normally due to isolation. These issues may cause delay or under-treatment, which may worsen the disease course. Both public and healthcare professionals need additional training on these subjects in the pandemic period.

## REFERENCES

Aggarwal, G, Lippi, G & Michael Henry, B (2020) Cerebrovascular disease is associated with an increased disease severity in patients with Coronavirus Disease 2019 (COVID-19): A pooled analysis of published

literature. *Int J Stroke,* 15, 385-9.
[http://dx.doi.org/10.1177/1747493020921664] [PMID: 32310015]

Azim, D, Nasim, S, Kumar, S, Hussain, A & Patel, S (2020) Neurological Consequences of 2019-nCoV Infection: A Comprehensive Literature Review. *Cureus,* 12, e8790.
[http://dx.doi.org/10.7759/cureus.8790] [PMID: 32601577]

Bagheri, SH, Asghari, A & Farhadi, M (2020) Coincidence of COVID-19 epidemic and olfactory dysfunction outbreak in Iran. *medRxiv Prepr.*

Baig, AM, Khaleeq, A, Ali, U & Syeda, H (2020) Evidence of the COVID-19 Virus Targeting the CNS: Tissue Distribution, Host-Virus Interaction, and Proposed Neurotropic Mechanisms. *ACS Chem Neurosci,* 11, 995-8.
[http://dx.doi.org/10.1021/acschemneuro.0c00122] [PMID: 32167747]

Chen, T, Wu, D, Chen, H, Yan, W, Yang, D, Chen, G, Ma, K, Xu, D, Yu, H, Wang, H, Wang, T, Guo, W, Chen, J, Ding, C, Zhang, X, Huang, J, Han, M, Li, S, Luo, X, Zhao, J & Ning, Q (2020) Clinical characteristics of 113 deceased patients with coronavirus disease 2019: retrospective study. *BMJ,* 368, m1091.
[http://dx.doi.org/10.1136/bmj.m1091] [PMID: 32217556]

Desforges, M, Le Coupanec, A, Dubeau, P, Bourgouin, A, Lajoie, L, Dubé, M & Talbot, PJ (2019) Human Coronaviruses and Other Respiratory Viruses: Underestimated Opportunistic Pathogens of the Central Nervous System? *Viruses,* 12, 14.
[http://dx.doi.org/10.3390/v12010014] [PMID: 31861926]

Giacomelli, A, Pezzati, L, Conti, F, Bernacchia, D, Siano, M, Oreni, L, Rusconi, S, Gervasoni, C, Ridolfo, AL, Rizzardini, G, Antinori, S & Galli, M (2020) Self-reported Olfactory and Taste Disorders in Patients With Severe Acute Respiratory Coronavirus 2 Infection: A Cross-sectional Study. *Clin Infect Dis,* 71, 889-90.
[http://dx.doi.org/10.1093/cid/ciaa330] [PMID: 32215618]

Gu, J, Gong, E, Zhang, B, Zheng, J, Gao, Z, Zhong, Y, Zou, W, Zhan, J, Wang, S, Xie, Z, Zhuang, H, Wu, B, Zhong, H, Shao, H, Fang, W, Gao, D, Pei, F, Li, X, He, Z, Xu, D, Shi, X, Anderson, VM & Leong, AS (2005) Multiple organ infection and the pathogenesis of SARS. *J Exp Med,* 202, 415-24.
[http://dx.doi.org/10.1084/jem.20050828] [PMID: 16043521]

Helms, J, Kremer, S, Merdji, H, Clere-Jehl, R, Schenck, M, Kummerlen, C, Collange, O, Boulay, C, Fafi-Kremer, S, Ohana, M, Anheim, M & Meziani, F (2020) Neurologic Features in Severe SARS-CoV-2 Infection. *N Engl J Med,* 382, 2268-70.https://www.hurriyet.com.tr/gundem/turkiyede-ilk-kez-bir-hast-nin-beyin-omurilik-sivisinda-koronavirus-tespit-edildi-41536199
[http://dx.doi.org/10.1056/NEJMc2008597] [PMID: 32294339]

Huang, C, Wang, Y, Li, X, Ren, L, Zhao, J, Hu, Y, Zhang, L, Fan, G, Xu, J, Gu, X, Cheng, Z, Yu, T, Xia, J, Wei, Y, Wu, W, Xie, X, Yin, W, Li, H, Liu, M, Xiao, Y, Gao, H, Guo, L, Xie, J, Wang, G, Jiang, R, Gao, Z, Jin, Q, Wang, J & Cao, B (2020) Clinical features of patients infected with 2019 novel coronavirus in Wuhan, China. *Lancet,* 395, 497-506.
[http://dx.doi.org/10.1016/S0140-6736(20)30183-5] [PMID: 31986264]

Kim, GU, Kim, MJ, Ra, SH, Lee, J, Bae, S, Jung, J & Kim, SH (2020) Clinical characteristics of asymptomatic and symptomatic patients with mild COVID-19. *Clin Microbiol Infect,* 26, 948.e1-3.
[http://dx.doi.org/10.1016/j.cmi.2020.04.040] [PMID: 32360780]

Klein, RS, Garber, C & Howard, N (2017) Infectious immunity in the central nervous system and brain function. *Nat Immunol,* 18, 132-41.
[http://dx.doi.org/10.1038/ni.3656] [PMID: 28092376]

Klok, FA, Kruip, MJHA, van der Meer, NJM, Arbous, MS, Gommers, DAMPJ, Kant, KM, Kaptein, FHJ, van Paassen, J, Stals, MAM, Huisman, MV & Endeman, H (2020) Incidence of thrombotic complications in critically ill ICU patients with COVID-19. *Thromb Res,* 191, 145-7.
[http://dx.doi.org/10.1016/j.thromres.2020.04.013] [PMID: 32291094]

Laurendon, T, Radulesco, T, Mugnier, J, Gérault, M, Chagnaud, C, El Ahmadi, AA & Varoquaux, A (2020)

Bilateral transient olfactory bulb edema during COVID-19-related anosmia. *Neurology,* 95, 224-5. [http://dx.doi.org/10.1212/WNL.0000000000009850] [PMID: 32444492]

Lechien, JR, Chiesa-Estomba, CM, De Siati, DR, Horoi, M, Le Bon, SD, Rodriguez, A, Dequanter, D, Blecic, S, El Afia, F, Distinguin, L, Chekkoury-Idrissi, Y, Hans, S, Delgado, IL, Calvo-Henriquez, C, Lavigne, P, Falanga, C, Barillari, MR, Cammaroto, G, Khalife, M, Leich, P, Souchay, C, Rossi, C, Journe, F, Hsieh, J, Edjlali, M, Carlier, R, Ris, L, Lovato, A, De Filippis, C, Coppee, F, Fakhry, N, Ayad, T & Saussez, S (2020) Olfactory and gustatory dysfunctions as a clinical presentation of mild-to-moderate forms of the coronavirus disease (COVID-19): a multicenter European study. *Eur Arch Otorhinolaryngol,* 277, 2251-61. [http://dx.doi.org/10.1007/s00405-020-05965-1] [PMID: 32253535]

Lechner, M, Chandrasekharan, D & Jumani, K (2020) Olfactory and gustatory dysfunctions as a clinical presentation of mild-to-moderate forms of the coronavirus disease (COVID-19): a multicenter European study. *Eur Arch Otorhinolaryngol,* 277, 2251-61.

Li, Y, Li, M, Wang, M, Zhou, Y, Chang, J, Xian, Y, Wang, D, Mao, L, Jin, H & Hu, B (2020) Acute cerebrovascular disease following COVID-19: a single center, retrospective, observational study. *Stroke Vasc Neurol,* 5, 279-84.
[http://dx.doi.org/10.1136/svn-2020-000431] [PMID: 32616524]

Mao, L, Jin, H, Wang, M, Hu, Y, Chen, S, He, Q, Chang, J, Hong, C, Zhou, Y, Wang, D, Miao, X, Li, Y & Hu, B (2020) Neurologic Manifestations of Hospitalized Patients With Coronavirus Disease 2019 in Wuhan, China. *JAMA Neurol,* 77, 683-90.
[http://dx.doi.org/10.1001/jamaneurol.2020.1127] [PMID: 32275288]

Mehta, P, McAuley, DF, Brown, M, Sanchez, E, Tattersall, RS & Manson, JJ HLH Across Speciality Collaboration, UK (2020) COVID-19: consider cytokine storm syndromes and immunosuppression. *Lancet,* 395, 1033-4.
[http://dx.doi.org/10.1016/S0140-6736(20)30628-0] [PMID: 32192578]

Mirzaee, SMM, Gonçalves, FG, Mohammadifard, M, Tavakoli, SM & Vossough, A (2020) Focal Cerebral Arteriopathy in a Pediatric Patient with COVID-19. *Radiology,* 297, E274-5.
[http://dx.doi.org/10.1148/radiol.2020202197] [PMID: 32484418]

Oxley, TJ, Mocco, J, Majidi, S, Kellner, CP, Shoirah, H, Singh, IP, De Leacy, RA, Shigematsu, T, Ladner, TR, Yaeger, KA, Skliut, M, Weinberger, J, Dangayach, NS, Bederson, JB, Tuhrim, S & Fifi, JT (2020) Large-Vessel Stroke as a Presenting Feature of Covid-19 in the Young. *N Engl J Med,* 382, e60.
[http://dx.doi.org/10.1056/NEJMc2009787] [PMID: 32343504]

Román, GC, Spencer, PS, Reis, J, Buguet, A, Faris, MEA, Katrak, SM, Láinez, M, Medina, MT, Meshram, C, Mizusawa, H, Öztürk, S & Wasay, M WFN Environmental Neurology Specialty Group (2020) The neurology of COVID-19 revisited: A proposal from the Environmental Neurology Specialty Group of the World Federation of Neurology to implement international neurological registries. *J Neurol Sci,* 414, 116884. [http://dx.doi.org/10.1016/j.jns.2020.116884] [PMID: 32464367]

Sedaghat, AR, Gengler, I & Speth, MM (2020) Olfactory Dysfunction: A Highly Prevalent Symptom of COVID-19 With Public Health Significance. *Otolaryngol Head Neck Surg,* 163, 12-5.
[http://dx.doi.org/10.1177/0194599820926464] [PMID: 32366160]

Tian, S, Hu, N, Lou, J, Chen, K, Kang, X, Xiang, Z, Chen, H, Wang, D, Liu, N, Liu, D, Chen, G, Zhang, Y, Li, D, Li, J, Lian, H, Niu, S, Zhang, L & Zhang, J (2020) Characteristics of COVID-19 infection in Beijing. *J Infect,* 80, 401-6.
[http://dx.doi.org/10.1016/j.jinf.2020.02.018] [PMID: 32112886]

Tsai, LK, Hsieh, ST & Chao, CC (2004) Characteristics of COVID-19 infection in Beijing.*J Inf Secur,* 80, 401-6.doi.org/10

Varatharaj, A, Thomas, N, Ellul, MA, Davies, NWS, Pollak, TA, Tenorio, EL, Sultan, M, Easton, A, Breen, G, Zandi, M, Coles, JP, Manji, H, Al-Shahi Salman, R, Menon, DK, Nicholson, TR, Benjamin, LA, Carson, A, Smith, C, Turner, MR, Solomon, T, Kneen, R, Pett, SL, Galea, I, Thomas, RH & Michael, BD CoroNerve Study Group (2020) Neurological and neuropsychiatric complications of COVID-19 in 153 patients: a UK-

wide surveillance study. *Lancet Psychiatry,* 7, 875-82.
[http://dx.doi.org/10.1016/S2215-0366(20)30287-X] [PMID: 32593341]

Wan, SX, Yi, QJ & Fan, SB (2020) Neurological and neuropsychiatric complications of COVID-19 in 153 patients: a UK-wide surveillance study. *The Lancet Psychiatry,* 7, 875-2.

Xydakis, MS, Dehgani-Mobaraki, P, Holbrook, EH, Geisthoff, UW, Bauer, C, Hautefort, C, Herman, P, Manley, GT, Lyon, DM & Hopkins, C (2020) Smell and taste dysfunction in patients with COVID-19. *Lancet Infect Dis,* 20, 1015-6.
[http://dx.doi.org/10.1016/S1473-3099(20)30293-0] [PMID: 32304629]

Yang, X, Yu, Y, Xu, J, Shu, H, Xia, J, Liu, H, Wu, Y, Zhang, L, Yu, Z, Fang, M, Yu, T, Wang, Y, Pan, S, Zou, X, Yuan, S & Shang, Y (2020) Clinical course and outcomes of critically ill patients with SARS-CoV-2 pneumonia in Wuhan, China: a single-centered, retrospective, observational study. *Lancet Respir Med,* 8, 475-81.
[http://dx.doi.org/10.1016/S2213-2600(20)30079-5] [PMID: 32105632]

Ye, M, Ren, Y & Lv, T (2020) Clinical course and outcomes of critically ill patients with SARS-CoV-2 pneumonia in Wuhan, China: a single-centered, retrospective, observational study. *Lancet Respir Med,* 8, 475-81.

Zochodne, DW (2004) SARS, SIRS, and neurological disease. *Arch Neurol,* 61, 1647-8.
[http://dx.doi.org/10.1001/archneur.61.11.1647] [PMID: 15534173]

# CHAPTER 11

# COVID-19 Pneumonia and ARDS: The Real Killer?

**Abstract:** Pneumonia and its major complication, acute respiratory distress syndrome (ARDS), are the outstanding causes of morbidity and mortality attributed to the SARS-CoV-2. Angiotensin-converting enzyme 2 (ACE2) receptor is commonly found in the alveolar cells of the lung, causing common respiratory symptoms in COVID-19. In addition, the development of respiratory failure, ARDS, and the need for a mechanical ventilator is precipitated by an undertreated pneumonia. ARDS is a condition associated with many disease processes, which causes reduced lung compliance and severe hypoxemia. For early diagnosis and treatment, attention should be paid to the risk of developing ARDS in patients whose disease duration lasts for longer than one week.

**Keywords:** ARDS, COVID-19, COVID-19 pneumonia, Critical care, Hypoxia, Mechanical ventilation , Pandemic, Pneumonia, Respiratory failure.

## DEFINITION

SARS-CoV-2 binds to the angiotensin-converting enzyme 2 (ACE2) receptor with S protein to enter the cells. Binding of the virus with host cell receptors is an important step for the mechanism of infection. This receptor is commonly found in the alveolar cells of the lung, causing common respiratory symptoms in COVID-19 (Fig. **1**). Although less common, cardiovascular pathologies are also thought to be caused by the virus binding to the ACE-2 receptor in myocardial cells (Li *et al*., 2020).

Pneumonia and its major complication, acute respiratory distress syndrome (ARDS), are the outstanding causes of morbidity and mortality attributed to the virus.

Although the spark of the epidemic is thought to be ignited in a seafood market that sold live animals, person-to-person transmission has become the main form of transmission as the pandemic progressed. According to current evidence, SARS-CoV-2 is transmitted primarily through droplets and close personal

**Ozgur KARCIOGLU, Selman YENIOCAK and Mandana HOSSEINZADEH**

contact. Airborne propagation was not reported in many researches as much as it was thought before. For example, environmental contamination in the ICU with SARS-CoV-2 was found to be lower than in the wards (Ong SWX *et al*., 2020). The use of mechanical ventilation or high-flow nasal oxygen was not associated with greater surface contamination.

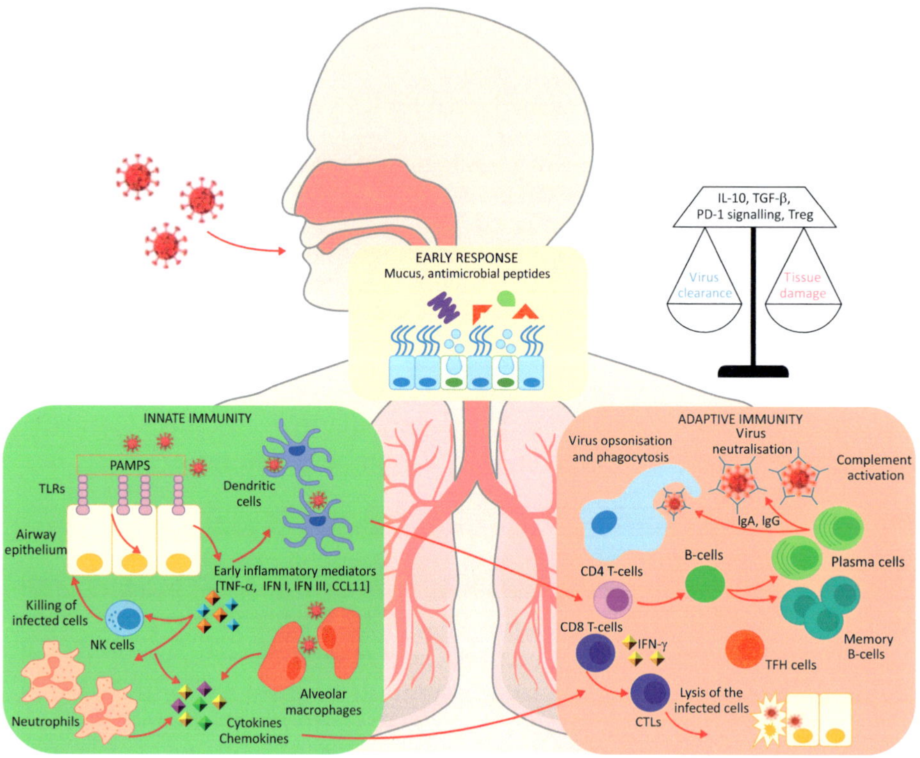


**Fig. (1).** The lungs are among the primary routes for environmental substances and pathogens to enter the host tissues. The early protection response to viruses includes mucus, surfactants, and antiviral peptides that can prevent entry to the respiratory epithelia that have a key role in triggering the immune response by recognizing viral components. These cellular sensors start a series of stimuli precipitating the upregulation of the inflammatory response (Adapted from Ong CWM *et al*., 2020)

However, there is a risk of airborne transmission in conditions that cause direct aerosolization such as endotracheal intubation, bronchoscopy, manual ventilation (bagging), bringing the patient to the prone position, non-invasive mechanical ventilation, tracheostomy, and cardiopulmonary resuscitation. (WHO, 2020). The highest contagiousness is around the initial phase after the symptoms begin; it continues by decreasing from a few days to a few weeks. The effect of the exact viral RNA load required for SARS -CoV2 propagation is uncertain. (CDC, 2020)

## CLINICAL FEATURES

Although the development of symptoms takes an average of 5 to 6 days after infection, it can be delayed for 14 days in some cases. The viral load of SARS-CoV-2 is predominantly detected in the upper airways (nose and mouth, hypopharynx) after being infected, till three days after the initial symptoms (Pan *et al.*, 2020). On the other hand, infected persons have a potential of contagiousness starting from one to three days before the symptoms (Wei We, 2020)

Although the symptoms of COVID-19 vary substantially; the most common complaints are (CDC 2020).

- fever (83-99%),
- cough (59-82%),
- fatigue (44-70%),
- anorexia (40-84%),
- shortness of breath (31-40%),
- sputum (28-33%)
- myalgia (11-35%).

- Headache, confusion, rhinorrhea, sore throat, hemoptysis, vomiting, and diarrhea are reported but less common (<10%).
- In the presence of advanced age and comorbidity, fever, pain, and respiratory symptoms may be delayed.
- Some patients can present with an atypical clinic.

  Anosmia, ageusia, which develops before the onset of respiratory symptoms, has been reported. (CDC 2020)

  According to the 'New Coronary Virus Infection Pneumonia Diagnosis and Treatment Program' guide prepared by the China National Health Commission, COVID-19 patients were classified as mild, moderate, severe, and critical according to their clinical status (Table **1**).

Findings may be detected in the lung imaging before the onset of symptoms. However; younger patients are less likely to develop viral pneumonia.

It was found in studies conducted that the average duration of dyspnea is between 5 and 8 days in patients with severe disease. The duration of ARDS varies between 8-12 days, and the average ICU hospitalization period varies between 10-12 days. (Huang C, 2020; Wang D, 2020)

Among all patients admitted to the hospital, 26% to 32% of patients are admitted to ICU, and the mortality rate varies between 39% to72% among patients admitted to ICU. Mean length of stay in survivors is 10 to 13 days. (CDC, 2020).

**Table 1. Clinical characteristics as a basis for classification of COVID-19 patients**

| Clinical Classification | Features |
|---|---|
| Mild | Clinical symptoms present,<br>No findings on imaging. |
| Moderate | Fever and respiratory symptoms are present,<br>Findings on imaging (opacity, consolidation) |
| Severe | Respiratory distress, RR≥ 30 beats / min,<br>Oxygen saturation <93% or<br>Presence of any of the findings of $PaO_2$ / $FiO_2 \leq 300$ mmHg<br>If there is> 50% progression in the imaging findings or<br>within 24-48 hours, the clinical status should also be considered severe. |
| Critical | Respiratory failure and development of need for mechanical ventilator,<br>- Development of shock or organ failure in need of ICU care |

## DIAGNOSIS

The clinical diagnosis of suspicious cases is established by the combination of epidemiological, clinical, laboratory and thorax CT findings. Standard diagnostic method used; oropharyngeal swab is a real-time polymerase chain reaction (RT-PCR) performed to detect viral nucleotides from samples obtained by nasopharyngeal swab, bronchoalveolar lavage, and tracheal aspirate. (CDC, 2020) However, studies have shown that RT-PCR has 60% to 71% sensitivity in detecting the SARS-CoV2 virus, despite high specificity (Ai *et al*, 2020; Fang Y *et al*, 2020). This means that low viral load at the time of the test may lead to failure to yield highly accurate results from the test. However, it is put forward that thorax CT diagnoses COVID-19 with 5% to 98% sensitivity, which will help correct false negative results of RT-PCR. Both the chest radiography and primary findings in thorax CT are compatible with atypical and viral pneumonia. (Bai *et al*, 2020).

Although the sensitivity of chest X-ray is lower than thorax CT, it is recommended as the ‘initial’ imaging modality (Wong HYF *et al*, 2020). There is an ongoing debate on this issue, for example, Radiology Societies do not recommend CXR to be used as an initial screening tool to diagnose COVID-19 pneumonia. Portable graphs are recommended to minimize contamination (ACR, 2020). The radiology is insensitive in the mild clinical condition or early stage of the disease. Most symptoms can be detected 10 to 12 days after the onset of symptoms. The most common findings are airspace opacities, consolidation, and ground glass opacities (Hafiz *et al*, 2020). The distribution is predominantly bilateral, dominant in the peripheral and basal regions. Unlike parenchymal abnormalities, pleural effusion is rare (3%) (Wong HYF, 2020). However, CXR is not sensitive enough to identify GGOs which are a main finding for COVID-19 pneumonia (ACR, 2020). CXR can oversee important pulmonary lesions that can be detected in CT images (Fig. **2**). In the Consensus statement of the Fleishner Association published on April 7, it was proposed to use the chest radiography to evaluate disease progression and to exclude alternative diagnoses (bacterial superinfection, pneumothorax, pleural effusion) (Figs. **3a** & **3b**).

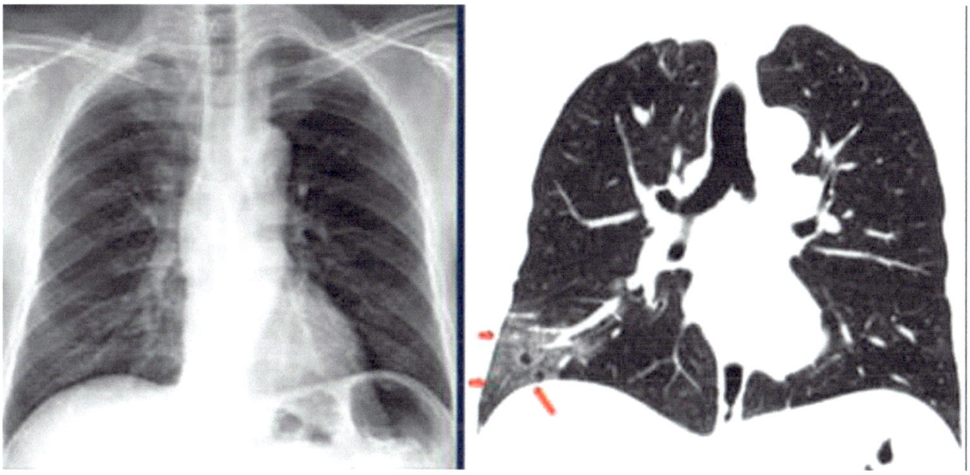

**Fig. (2).** Thorax CT is more sensitive than chest x-ray in imaging lesions. In thorax CT, ground glass opacities in the lower right lobe are not noticed on the simultaneous radiograph (red arrow).

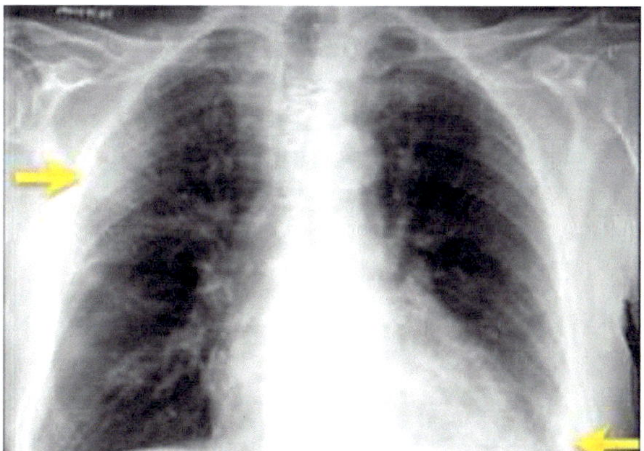

**Fig. (3a).** Chest radiography can be useful in monitoring the disease. When the COVID-19 patient was admitted to the hospital, the chest film was normal. Bilateral consolidations were detected on the radiograph of the patient, who was under mechanical ventilation 4 days later.

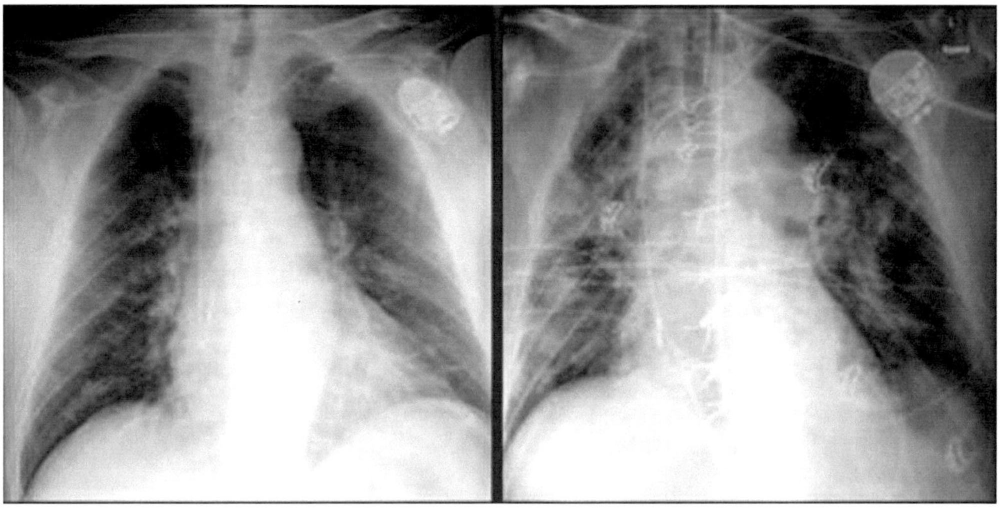

**Fig. (3b).** On the radiography of the patient diagnosed with COVID-19, who is 83 years old with known heart failure, pulmonary hypertension and atrial fibrillation, ground glass opacities and consolidation are seen in the right upper lobe and lower left lobe.

Asymptomatic carriers of COVID19 are estimated to be 18% to 33% of all infected cases. It was remarkable that 54% of asymptomatic cases diagnosed with COVID-19 on the 'Diamond Princess' vessel may have pneumonia in CT (Mizumoto *et al*, 2020).

Within four days after the emergence of complaints, CT is not sensitive as an initial test, as CT may be normal in 50% of patients. After these first days, sensitivity of CT increases (Kovacs *et al.*, 2020).

## THE MOST COMMON CT FINDINGS ON PRESENTATION (ADAPTED FROM PAN *ET AL*, 2020)

- Ground glass opacity (GGO) 88%
- Bilateral involvement 88%
- Posterior distribution 80%
- Peripheral distribution 79%
- Consolidation 32%

Tips on pneumonia in CT:

- The most common involvement is detected in the lower lobes, followed by the middle lobes.
- Combination of the consolidation and GGO at the time of admission can be seen in a distinct group of cases; predominantly in the elderly population.

- Bronchiectasis, septal thickening, pleural thickness, and subpleural involvement are among the findings mostly seen in the advanced stages of the disease.
- Although pleural effusion, pericardial effusion, lymphadenopathy, cavitation, halo sign, pneumothorax are rare findings, they are usually indicative of the progression of the disease.
- CT images of other viral pneumonia can mostly masquerade COVID-19.

In the first months of the pandemics, the Radiological Society of North America (RSNA), Society of Thoracic Radiology, the American College of Radiology issued a consensus statement to standardize reporting language in hospitals (Table **2**).

**Table 2. The Radiological Society of North America (RSNA), Society of Thoracic Radiology, the American College of Radiology issued a consensus statement that categorizes the CT appearance of COVID-19 into four categories for the standard reporting language (Adapted from Simpson, *et al.*, 2020)**

| Typical View | Intermediate | Atypical View | Negativity Criteria for Pneumonia |
|---|---|---|---|
| Bilateral, peripheral GGOs +/- consolidation or 'crazy paving' pattern | Absence of typical CT findings AND | Absence of typical and intermediate appearance AND | Absence of GGO or consolidation indicates that there is no COVID-19 finding in CT. |
| Multifocal GGO, irregularly rounded or 'crazy paving' pattern | Multifocal, diffuse, perihilar or unilateral GGO and consolidation without round and peripheral distribution | Isolated lobar and segmental consolidation without GGO | - |
| "Reverse halo sign" or other signs of organized pneumonia | Few and small GGOs without round and peripheral distribution | Separate small nodules (*e.g.*, centrilobular nodules, "budding tree" view) | - |
| - | - | Lung cavitation | - |
| - | - | Pleural effusion, interlobular septal thickening | - |

Stages of pneumonia: In a study of COVID-19 patients who had improved after the disease, thorax CT findings were followed and categorized in different stages of the disease. Findings from the early period of the disease to the healing period were depicted in the Table **3** (Pan *et al*, 2020).

**Table 3. Staging of COVID-19 according to thorax CT findings**

| Stage | Key Findings |
|---|---|
| **Early Stage (0-2 days)** | 17%: CT normal<br>42%: single lobe involvement<br>75%: GGO<br>42%: consolidation<br>42%: multifocal lung opacity<br>54%: peripheral distribution predominant<br>25% Crazy-paving pattern |
| **Middle Stage (5-13 days)** | Peak Lung involvement;<br>New and increased lung consolidation (47%) and higher bilateral and multilobar involvement rate (76%)<br>82%: GGO<br>Development of Crazy Paving (53%) |
| **Advanced Stage (9-13 days)** | 90% consolidation is the main imaging finding<br>71%: GGOs tend to decrease when compared to previous stages<br>19% Crazy-paving pattern |
| **Convalescence (> 14 days)** | consolidation (75%) is going to heal and absorbed without any crazy-paving pattern |

Thorax CT can be used for imaging disease progression and alternative diagnoses (bacterial superinfection, viral pneumonia, acute heart failure (myocardial injury due to COVID-19, development of pleural effusion)). (Rubin *et al*, 2020). It was also found that the increase in the GGO detected in chest CT in a short term follow-up (24-48 hours) was related to deterioration in the outcome.

In a study to evaluate the severity of COVID-19 pneumonia using the Thorax CT severity scoring scale previously developed for SARS (Yang R *et al*, 2020):

18 segments of both lungs are divided into 20 regions.
- Opacity ratios in chest CT images were evaluated subjectively in 20 lung areas using a system that was established upon receiving 0, 1, and 2 scores based on less than 50%, equal or more than 50% of each area. CT severity scoring was defined as the sum of scores ranging from 0 to 40 points in the 20 lung segments.
Serious and critical cases were grouped as 'severe', and the rest were assigned in the 'mild' disease group.
It was found that the severity score of CT was higher in the severe disease group and detected severe disease at a cut-off point of 19.5 points with a sensitivity of 83.3% and 94% specificity (Yang R *et al*, 2020).
In a recent study to describe the relationship between COVID-19 mortality and chest CT scan findings obtained at the time of admission, Abbasi *et al.* showed that mortality was significantly higher in patients with higher CT severity score even after adjustment for clinical, demographics and laboratory parameters (Table **4**) (Abbasi *et al*, 2020).

**Table 4. CT severity score is a major predictor of disease severity in COVID-19 (Adapted from Abbasi *et al*, 2020)**

| CT Findings | | Overall (n = 262) | Survivors (n = 206) | Deceased (n = 56) | P value |
|---|---|---|---|---|---|
| CT severity score | | 8 (6–12) | 7.5 (6–11) | 14.5 (10–21) | **<0.001** |
| Parenchymal infiltrate | GGO | 67 (25.6) | 56 (27.2) | 11 (19.6) | 0.26 |
| | Consolidation | 79 (30.1) | 65 (31.6) | 14 (25) | |
| | GGO and consolidation | 116 (44.3) | 85 (41.3) | 31 (55.4) | |
| RSNA pattern | Typical | 143 (54.6) | 113 (54.9) | 30 (53.6) | 0.81 |
| | Indeterminate | 81 (30.9) | 62 (30.1) | 19 (33.9) | |
| | Atypical | 38 (14.5) | 31 (15) | 7 (12.5) | |
| Bilateral | | 253 (96.6) | 198 (96.1) | 55 (98.2) | 0.39 |
| Longitudinal distribution | Upper zone | 21 (8) | 16 97.8) | 5 (8.9) | 0.23 |
| | Middle zone | 38 (14.5) | 33 (16) | 5 (8.9) | |
| | Lower zone | 100 (38.2) | 82 (39.8) | 18 (32.1) | |
| | Random | 103 (39.3) | 75 (36.4) | 28 (50) | |
| Axial distribution | Peripheral | 101 (38.5) | 90 (43.7) | 11 (19.6) | 0.094 |
| | Central | 4 (1.5%) | 4 (1.9) | 0 (0) | |
| | Diffuse | 131 (50) | 91 (44.2) | 40 (71.4) | |
| | Random | 26 (9.9) | 21 (10.2) | 5 (8.9) | |
| Number of involved lobes | - | 5 (5–5) | 5 (5–5) | 5 (5–5) | 0.36 |
| Round infiltrate | - | - | - | - | - |
| Halo sign | - | 19 (7.3) | 17 (8.3) | 2 (3.6) | 0.18 |
| Reverse halo sign | - | 26 (9.9) | 21 (10.2) | 5 (8.9) | 0.78 |
| Crazy paving | - | 77 (29.4) | 54 (26.2) | 23 (41.1) | **0.03** |
| Architectural distortion | - | 150 (57.3) | 131 (63.6) | 19 (33.9) | **<0.001** |
| Parenchymal lines | - | 93 (35.5) | 85 (41.3) | 8 (14.3) | **<0.001** |
| Pleural effusion | - | 26 (9.9) | 19 (9.2) | 7 (12.5) | 0.47 |
| Lymphadenopathy | - | 6 (2.3) | 3 (1.5) | 3 (5.4) | 0.11 |
| Pleural thickening | - | 30 (11.5) | 26 (12.6) | 4 (7.1) | 0.49 |
| Pericardial effusion | - | 1 (0.4) | 0 (0) | 1 (1.3) | – |

**Case examples:** Figs. **4** - **7** provide case scenarios and corresponding radiological appearances of COVID-19 pneumonia. Various imaging manifestations at different stages may be related to the distinct pathological mechanism of viral pneumonia, which initially affects terminal bronchioles and surrounding pulmonary parenchyma, and then infiltration of the pulmonary lobules and finally widespread alveolar damage (Figs. **4** - **7**).

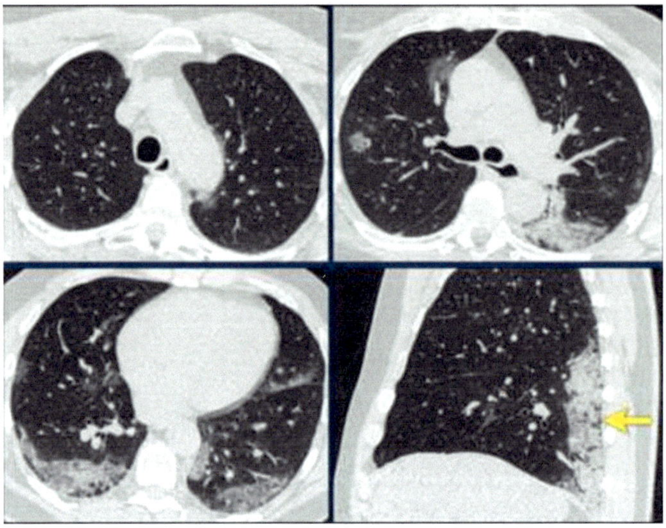

**Fig. (4).** A 59-year-old male patient presented with fever and non-productive cough lasting for 1 week. PCR test was negative. In thorax CT taken due to clinical suspicion; GGO and consolidation were noted in the posterior segments of the lower lobe. RT-PCR turned out to be positive 2 days later.

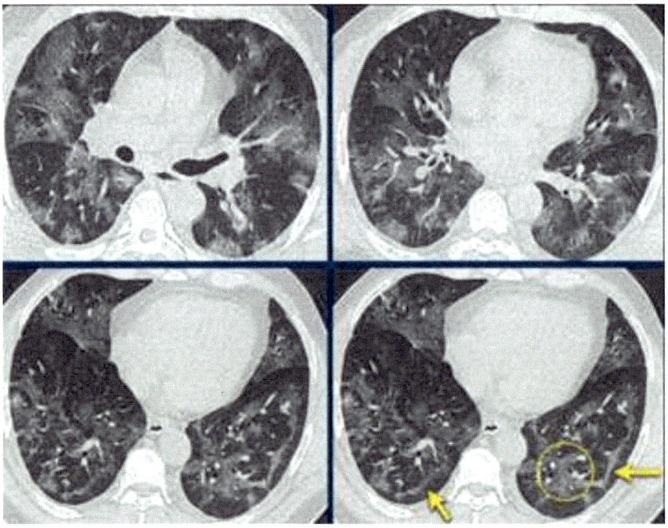

**Fig. (5).** A 49-year-old male presented with fever and cough. His oxygen saturation was low on pulse oximetry. On CT, bilateral GGOs, the fibrotic band (indicated with arrow, dilated vascular structure in the involved area (circle) were evaluated as COVID-19 late phase finding.

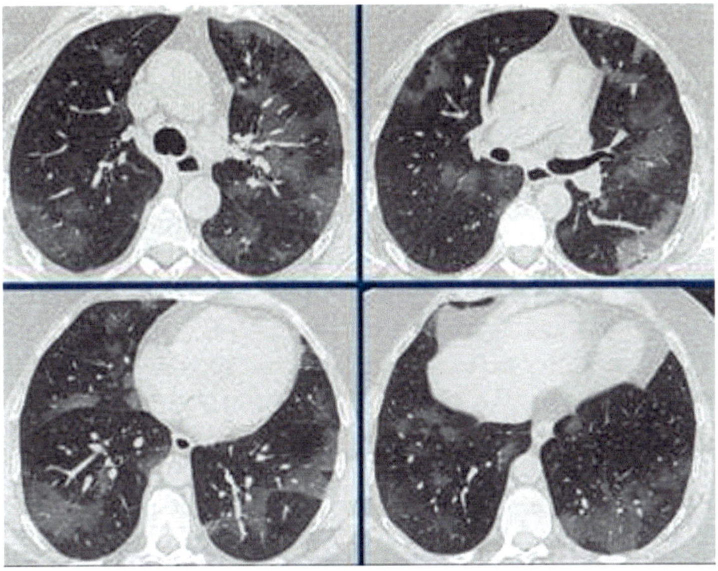

**Fig. (6).** A 59-year-old female patient presented with fever that has been lasting for 10 days and a cough for 5 days. Her $O_2$ saturation is 89%, the respiratory rate is 30 / min. Widespread ground glass image was present without consolidation. The images were reported as early stage COVID-19.

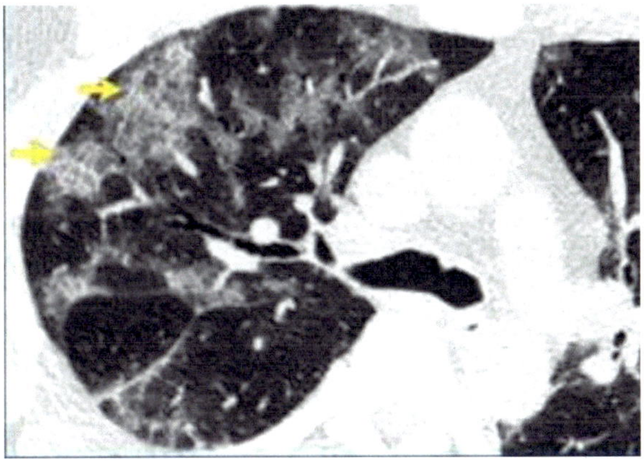

**Fig. (7).** Finding known as 'Crazy Paving'. GGOs with thickened interlobular and intralobular lines can be identified.

**Chest Ultrasound (CUSG)** is not recommended to be used as a standard diagnostic test because it cannot clearly distinguish between bacterial and viral pneumonia and between pulmonary edema and pneumonia. Nonetheless, its bedside use (POCUS) is recommended to be used to evaluate pleural effusion, pneumothorax, calculate pulmonary fluid load and adjust MV settings, especially in patients undergoing mechanical ventilation (MV) (Revel, 2020). CT should be employed whenever the clinician is not sure for the diagnosis, and ruling out an important diagnosis is not impossible with this test.

## DIFFERENTIAL DIAGNOSES

Thorax CT detects viral pneumonia in up to 90-95% of the instances. In contrast, the low sensitivity of the RT-PCR test (the test may need to be repeated two or three times) and the number of people waiting for the test to detect SARS-CoV-2 causes many patients not to be recognized in a timely manner and miss the chance of early treatment. As explained above; the severity of the lung lesions is closely related to clinical symptoms. This reflects the importance of thorax CT in the preliminary screening of COVID-19. However, it is difficult to distinguish COVID-19 pneumonia from influenza AB, cytomegalovirus (CMV), respiratory syncytial virus (RSV), Severe Acute Respiratory Syndrome (SARS-CoV), Middle East Respiratory Syndrome (MERS-CoV) and other viral and bacterial agents just using thoracic CT images (Table **5**) (Shi *et al*, 2020; Dai *et al*, 2020).

## OTHER SITUATIONS TO BE DISTINGUISHED

- HSV Pneumonia: Pleural effusion is often present in immunocompromised patients
- Cryptogenic organized pneumonia
- Chronic eosinophilic pneumonia (CEP)
- Rheumatoid arthritis-associated pneumonia; other connective tissue diseases (SLE, scleroderma)
- "Crazy paving" finding is predominant: Pulmonary alveolar proteinosis should also be considered.

**Table 5. Characteristic features of COVID-19, other viral pneumonias, and bacterial pneumonia. Clinicians can use these clues to distinguish the entities from each other**

| | **COVID-19** | **Other Viral Pneumonias** | **Bacterial Pneumonia** |
|---|---|---|---|
| **Pathogens** | SARS-CoV-2 | A and B type Influenza viruses, parainfluenza virus, CMV, adenovirus, RSV | Bacteria (streptococci *etc.*), mycoplasmae and chlamydiae |
| **Initial symptoms** | In most cases, fever, and dry cough, in some cases, diarrhea. | High fever, cough, sore throat, muscle pain, *etc.* | Nasal congestion, rhinorrhea, *etc.*, mild in most cases |
| **History of exposure to COVID-19** | Exposure to epidemic regions (may be obsolete after May 2020), mostly men aged 40-60 | Widespread in winter and spring, children, but less common in adults or community | widespread in winter, children, and community |

*(Table 5) cont.....*

| | COVID-19 | Other Viral Pneumonias | Bacterial Pneumonia |
|---|---|---|---|
| **Laboratory** | Positive RT-PCR result, normal or low leukocyte count, lymphopenia, and high serum CRP level | Influenza A and B viruses, positive PCR results for identification of parainfluenza virus, cytomegalovirus, adenovirus, and respiratory syncytial virus; lymphocytosis | High leukocyte count, high erythrocyte sedimentation rate (ESR) and markedly elevated CRP level |
| **Chest CT** | **Early stage:** GGO **Middle stage:** Multiple GGO, consolidations, crazy paving pattern. **Advanced stage:** diffuse exudative lesions, "white lung" view | Interstitial inflammation, reticular patterns or multiple fibrous lines, localized pulmonary edema and / or atelectasis | Bronchial/ lobar pneumonia, bronchial wall thickening, centrilobular nodules, multiple consolidations mainly inflicting lung parenchyma |

## SERUM ANTIBODY DETECTION

Specific antibodies are produced following SARS-CoV-2 infection. Serum antibody detection methods include colloidal gold immunochromatography, ELISA, chemoluminescence immunoassay, *etc*. Specific lgG antibody titers in the recovery phase or positive serum specific lgM ($\geq$ 4 times higher than in the acute phase) can be used as diagnostic criteria for suspected patients with negative nucleic acid detection in the follow-up. The viral load gradually decreases with increasing serum antibody levels. (Liang *et al*, 2020).

## LABORATORY FINDINGS

Complete blood count, CRP, procalcitonin (PCT), kidney and liver function tests, cardiac enzyme, arterial blood gas, LDH values should be evaluated in relation with CXR. Blood cultures should be taken before antibiotherapy, if any.

The white blood cells counts may vary substantially in patients with COVID-19. Lymphopenia is the most commonly reported CBC abnormality, but leukopenia, leukocytosis and lymphopenia have also been reported. High ferritin levels are common and high aminotransferase (AST) levels have also been described. (Wang D *et al*, 2020; Bajema *et al*, 2020)

At admission, many patients with pneumonia have normal serum PCT levels; however, those who require ICU care are more likely to have higher PCT levels. It appears to be valuable for early risk stratification and ruling out bacterial coinfection in COVID-19 patients on presentation. (Guan *et al*, 2020). Monitoring of PCT has been suggested to assess secondary infections and more serious disease conditions such as sepsis and/or septic shock.

High D-dimer levels and more severe lymphopenia have been associated with mortality. (Chen *et al*, 2020).

The neutrophil to lymphocytes ratio (NLR) may be an indicator of cytokine storms, with increased NLR due to elevated cytokine levels, and also an indicator of severe outcomes.

## RISK FACTORS FOR SEVERE DISEASE

General (Adapted from WHO, 2020)

- Advanced age: Severe disease can occur in healthy individuals of any age, but it occurs predominantly advanced age and those with medical comorbidities.
- Home care patients
- Male gender
- Comorbidities (Zhou *et al*, 2020 )
    - Cardiovascular Disease
    - Diabetes Mellitus
    - Hypertension
    - Chronic Lung Diseases
    - Cancer
    - Immunosuppression
    - Chronic Kidney Disease
    - Obesity (BMI ≥40)

      Clinical and laboratory findings of the patients with severe disease (Adapted from Wu *et al*, 2020)
- Sepsis, shock signs on presentation,
- D-dimer level> 1 μg / mL on presentation,
- High troponin, LDH values,
- High AST, ALT values,
- High inflammatory marker value: Interleukin-6 (IL-6), CRP, Ferritin
- High creatine phosphokinase levels
- Deep lymphopenia

### Who can develop ARDS?

A well-designed study with a small-sample on development of ARDS and death in patients with COVID-19 was published at JAMA (Wu *et al*, 2020).

Accordingly, factors that increase the probability of developing ARDS are;

- advanced age,
- elevated neutrophil count,
- organ failure,
- coagulation dysfunction,
- high LDH
- high D-dimer,
- Fever (T > 39°C).

Notes: Age is associated with both ARDS and death, while fever is associated with the development of ARDS, but it predicts a better outcome.

## COVID 19 Complications are

- Pneumonia
- Acute kidney injury
- Sepsis
- Secondary bacterial infection
- Septic shock
- Thromboembolism
- Left failure / ARDS
- Hospitalization complications
- Cardiomyopathy, arrhythmia, cardiac arrest
- GI bleeding

## ARDS

ARDS developing after acute viral pneumonia is the major cause of morbidity and mortality of COVID-19.

It develops with acute systemic inflammation that develops following direct or indirect injury of the lung. Epithelial and endothelial cell damage in the early exudative stage causes alveolar damage (Fig. **8**).

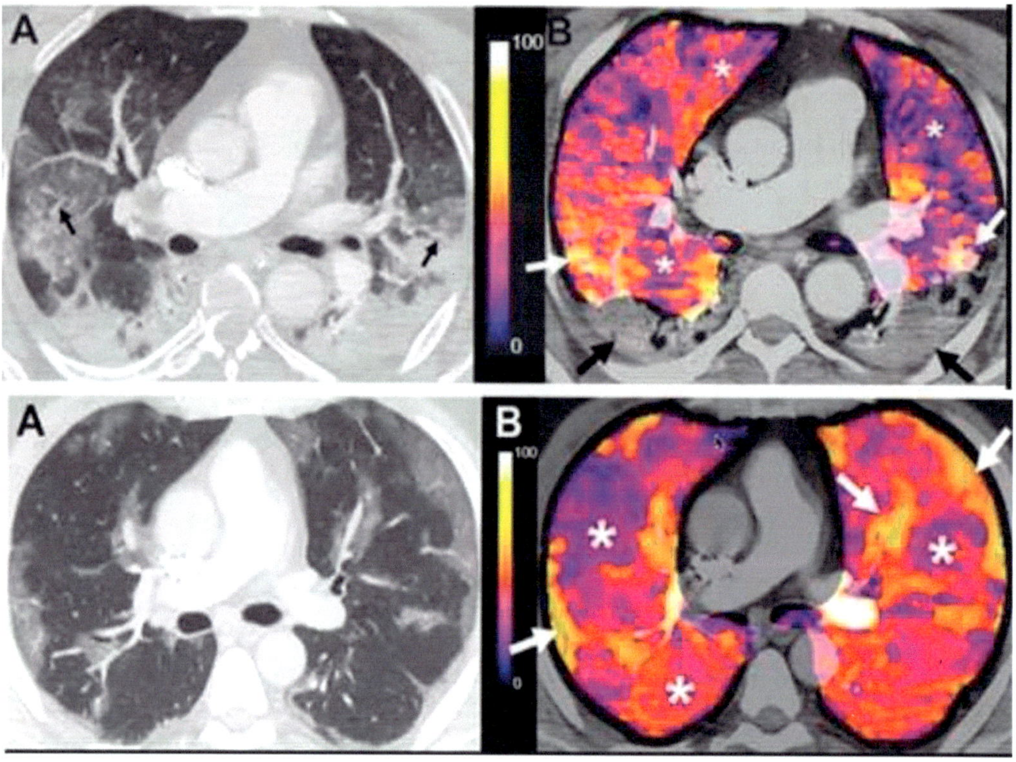


**Fig. (8).** (A/B). In H type ARDS (upper images), there is increased perfusion in GGO areas, mild-t--moderate hypoperfusion in the intact areas of lung, and absence of perfusion in consolidated areas. In L type ARDS (lower images), again, increased perfusion in GGO areas can be noted, and hypoperfused areas in the intact lung.

a. In this patient group, shortness of breath begins approximately 6.5 days after the onset of symptoms.
b. The development of ARDS starts 2.5 days after the onset of shortness of breath.
c. In patients with critical illness, acute hypoxemic respiratory failure due to ARDS is the predominant finding.
d. Hypercapnia is rare.
e. Fever tends to wax and wane during ICU hospitalization.
f. The need for a mechanical ventilator (MV) varies between 30% to 100%.
g. Length of stay in ICU is long; most patients stay intubated for 1 to 2 weeks or longer.

Sepsis, shock, and multi-organ failure occur but appear to be less common compared to ARDS not associated with COVID-19.

The need for vasopressors is variable, but a significant proportion need vasopressor support for hypotension (usually due to sedative agents or cardiac dysfunction).

Data on the risk of secondary bacterial pneumonia are limited, but it does not appear to be an important feature of COVID-19.

- Lung compliance is high compared to other ARDS etiologies, and the barotrauma rate appears to be low, with only 2 percent developing pneumothorax.

Activated vascular endothelial cells become a source of proinflammatory cytokines and reactive oxygen species (ROS) and contribute to the development of coagulopathy, systemic sepsis, a cytokine storm and ARDS. Pulmonary activated platelets are also an important source of proinflammatory cytokines and ROS, as well as exacerbating pulmonary neutrophil-mediated inflammatory responses and contributing to systemic sepsis by binding to neutrophils to form platelet-neutrophil complexes (PNCs). PNC formation increases neutrophil recruitment, activation priming and extraversion of these immune cells into inflamed pulmonary tissue, thereby contributing to ARDS. Sequestered PNCs cause the development of a procoagulant and proinflammatory environment (Morris *et al*, 2020).

## COVID-19 Pneumonia in Pregnancy

CDC reports highlighted that similar rates of pregnant and non-pregnant women of reproductive age are symptomatic when diagnosed with COVID-19 pneumonia ( *Ellington et al*, 2020*)*. A recent report of CDC- MMWR indicated that in women younger than 44 years of age with symptomatic COVID-19, intensive care unit admission, invasive ventilation, ECMO, and death were more likely in pregnant women than in nonpregnant women (Zambrano *et al*, 2020). Therefore, pregnancy is a risk factor for adverse outcome (Table **6**).

**Table 6. The pregnant patient faces the risks of COVID-19 pneumonia together with risks assumed by the pregnancy itself**

| | |
|---|---|
| **Complications of COVID-19 Pneumonia** | Fever<br>Hypoxemia<br>Respiratory Failure/ARDS<br>Sepsis and Shock |
| **Obstetrical Complications** | Preterm Labor<br>Early Rupture of Membranes<br>Increased Risk of Abnormal Fetal Heartbeats |

In a systematic review and meta-analysis published in November 2020, Di Toro *et al.* analyzed 24 articles, including 1100 pregnancies, and reported that the pooled prevalence of pneumonia was 89% (95%CI 70-100), Only 8% had to be admitted to ICU. Three stillbirths and five maternal deaths and three neonatal deaths were reported.

Severe cases of pneumonia requiring supplemental oxygen were reported to be more likely to show bilateral alveolar or interstitial infiltrates on CXR when compared to those with milder course (55·6% *vs.* 0·0%; *P*-value = 0·003) and serum C-reactive protein (CRP) levels >10 mg/dL (33·0% *vs.* 0·0%; *P*-value = 0·05) at admission (San-Juan *et al*, 2020).

The most common laboratory abnormalities are lymphopenia with 47%, and elevated liver enzymes in 17%. ARDS and myocardial injury are the most frequent complications identified so far (Huntley, 2020).

## Definition and Precipitation of ARDS:

According to Berlin criteria; it was defined as new or worsening respiratory distress that occurs within 1 week. However, onset of ARDS associated with COVID-19 was found to be similarly 8 to 12 days in different studies. For early diagnosis and treatment, attention should be paid to the risk of developing ARDS in patients whose disease duration lasts for longer than one week.

ARDS is a condition associated with many disease processes and causes reduced lung compliance and severe hypoxemia. In some COVID-19-associated ARDS patients who meet the ARDS Berlin criteria, lung compliance is relatively good and inconsistent with the severity of hypoxemia (Table 7).

**Table 7. Berlin Criteria in Diagnosis of ARDS.**

| **Berlin Criteria in Diagnosis of ARDS** | |
|---|---|
| Timing | *De novo* or worsening respiratory distress that occurs within 1 week |
| Pulmonary imaging | Bilateral opacity that cannot be explained by effusion, collapse or nodule |
| Causes of edema | Evidence that respiratory distress is not due to heart failure or hypervolemia with objective measures such as echocardiography/ POCUS. |
| Impairment of Oxygenation<br>• Mild<br>• Moderate<br>• Severe | $200\ mmHg \leq PaO_2/FiO_2 < 300mmHg$)<br>$100\ mmHg \leq PaO_2/FiO_2 < 200mmHg$)<br>$PaO_2/FiO_2 \leq 100\ mmHg$)+$PEEP \geq 5cmH_{2O}$ |

Specific characteristics of ARDS related to COVID-19 are somewhat different from ARDS triggered by other causes (Table **8**).

**Table 8. Features of ARDS precipitated by COVID-19 and ARDS triggered by other causes**

| Specific Characteristics of ARDS Related to COVID-19 | Differences from ARDS Precipitated by other Causes |
|---|---|
| **Involvement:** Respiratory system and alveolar epithelial cells | Time of onset; 8-12 days |
| The severity of clinical findings are inconsistent with laboratory and imaging findings and relatively mild. | Lung compliance is relatively normal in some COVID-19-associated ARDS patients. |
| | **Severity classification based on oxygenation index:**<br>When PEEP$\geq$ 5 cmH2O<br>Mild (200 mmHg $\leq PaO_2 / FiO_2 <$300mmHg)<br>Mild to Moderate (150 mmHg$\leq PaO_2 / FiO_2 <$200 mmHg)<br>Moderate to Severe (<150 mmHg) |
| | **Management protocol;**<br>HFNO may be safe even in some moderate to severe cases.<br>The timing of invasive MV can be critical.<br>Corticosteroids: Their effect is not very well established. |

## Treatment of Pneumonia and ARDS

### *Hypoxia Management in Severe and Critical COVID-19 Patient*

#### ***Non-intubated Patient***

#### *Prone Position*

Emerging evidence; shows that pronation is feasible and results in increased oxygenation in patients with COVID-19, regardless of whether they receive supplemental oxygen, HFNO or NIMV support alone. However, it is still unclear whether pronation prevents intubation, accelerates recovery, or reduces mortality.

#### *High-flow Nasal Oxygen Treatment (HFNO)*

HFNO reduces the need for endotracheal intubation in ARDS patients, when compared to standard oxygen therapy. Although HFNO is primarily recommended for patients with mild ARDS in some studies, it ensures that even patients with an oxygenation index of 100 mmHg remain stable for a considerable time window. This situation is somehow inconsistent with the treatment strategies of ARDS caused by other factors.

*Target Levels for Oxygenation*

WHO recommends oxygen saturation to be ≥94% during the first resuscitation and> 90% for maintenance $SpO_2$.

In the patient with critical COVID-19 pneumonia; ideally, $SpO_2$ should be kept between 90-96% at the lowest possible inspired oxygen fraction ($FiO_2$) to meet the oxygenation target. However, this target may differ between patient groups (such as concomitant hypercapnic oxygen deficiency caused by COPD, pregnant patient). Hyperoxia should be avoided.

*Nebulized Treatment*

Nebulizers are associated with aerosolization and potentially increase the risk of SARS-CoV-2 transmission. In suspected or documented COVID-19 patients, nebulized bronchodilator therapy should be reserved for acute bronchospasm ( *e.g.* in case of asthma or exacerbation of COPD). Otherwise, nebulized therapy should generally be avoided, especially for indications without a clear evidence base.

***Intubated Patient***

Most patients who develop ARDS in the course of COVID-19 will need mechanical ventilation. Delaying intubation until the patient is in acute decompensation will harm the patient and healthcare workers and is not recommended. Increased oxygen requirements of the patients should be evaluated with repeated examinations every 1 to 2 hours and blood gas control (Table **9**).

Indications of emergent control of airway (endotracheal intubation) include:

| |
|---|
| Rapid deterioration of the clinical status within hours, |
| No clinical improvement despite high flow oxygen support $FiO_2$> 0.6 and> 50 L / min, |
| Worsening dyspnea, development of hypercapnia, altered mental status, |
| Evidence of hemodynamic instability or multiple organ failure, |

IMV: Because severe COVID-19 patients may deteriorate rapidly, patients receiving HFNO should be closely monitored due to the need for immediate intubation.

Veno-venous extracorporeal oxygenation (V-V ECMO): It is preferred in the patients in extremis, in whom ARDS develops and progresses rapidly.

**Table 9. Oxygen treatment principles and dosages.**

| | | | |
|---|---|---|---|
| ***Oxygen Treatment*** | ***Low-flow $O_2$ systems*** | Up to 6 L / min, with nasal cannula, • Oxygenation up to 10-20 L / min is administered with simple face mask, Venturi face mask, nonrebreather mask | • As the current increases, the risk of aerosolization will increase. |
| | ***HFNO*** | HFNO 14%-63%, NIMV 11%-56% utilization rate • It has been reported that HFNO reduces the need for MV in patients with COVID-19 severe pneumonia • Patients should be followed up clinically and with blood gases every 1-2 hours. • HFNO should be ordered at the lowest possible values. (20 L/min and $FiO_2$ 0.4) • For NIV, a full face mask should be preferred. CPAP should start with a value of 5 to 10 cmH2O. | • There are not enough studies yet on how effective this approach is in avoiding intubation. • In case of a sudden increase in oxygen demand, pulmonary embolism should be ruled out. • New devices have been launched to limit aerosol emission from patients receiving HFNO or NIV; however, its effectiveness on clinical results has not yet been tested. |

## Specific Drug Treatments

Various treatments are being evaluated for COVID-19. Although some of these treatments are clinically available for other indications, their use for COVID-19 continues to be investigated (Table **10**).

**Corticosteroids** (CST) have been recognized as a potential treatment for ARDS because of its role in alleviating inflammation and fibrosis. The agents were found to be associated with increased viral clearance and mortality rate in MERS-CoV and influenza infections.

**Table 10. Some treatment agents and advices for use in COVID-19 pneumonia**

| Drug | Notes- Advices |
|---|---|
| **Plasma** | • Plasma taken from donors fully recovered from COVID-19 is administered to the patient.<br>• FDA approved the agent for investigational use.<br>• Studies have reported that patients with severe COVID-19, who are in mechanical ventilation despite antiviral therapy and have high viral titers, have decreased viral load and disease severity scores 12 days after plasma transfusion (Shen *et al*, 2020).<br>● Based on past experience and available data, efficacy is expected to be best when plasma treatment is given in the early stages of the disease, especially before patients become critically ill. |
| **Empirical Antibiotic Treatment** | Not routinely recommended. Antibiotics are ordered if:<br>• Bacterial pneumonia suspected,<br>• The suspicion of superinfection developing during follow-up (new consolidation or fever in thoracic imaging) (Wang D, 2020). |
| **NSAID** | Acetaminophen and NSAIDS can be considered to relieve pain and other signs of inflammation. The lowest dose of NSAIDs should be given. |
| **IL-6 Inhibitors** | • Tocilizumab is an interleukin-6 (IL-6) receptor inhibitor used for rheumatic diseases and cytokine release syndrome.<br>• High IL-6 levels have been identified in patients with severe COVID-19 and accordingly, case reports have described favorable outcomes with tocilizumab. (Mehta *et al*, 2020; Luo *et al*, 2020)<br>• The treatment guidelines of the Chinese National Health Commission included the agent for patients with severe COVID-19 and high IL-6 levels.<br>● The IDSA guideline panel recommends tocilizumab only in the context of a clinical trial. Additional clinical studies are needed to inform research on the effectiveness of treatment with tocilizumab for patients with COVID-19. |
| **Remdesivir (IV)** | • It is a nucleotide analog that possesses prominent activity against SARS-CoV-2 in both *in vitro* and animal studies. (Sheahan *et al*, 2017).<br>Side effects: nausea, vomiting and elevations in transaminases<br>• Contraindications:<br>- High ALT level (5 times above the normal limits),<br>- Chronic kidney disease (Creatinine clearance <30- 50 mL / min),<br>- pregnancy and breastfeeding<br>• In a case series;<br>Clinical improvement demonstrated in 68% of hypoxic patients<br>- 57% of intubated patients were extubated,<br>- It was reported that 3 of 4 patients who underwent extracorporeal membrane oxygenation (ECMO) were weaned from ECMO (Grein *et al*, 2020)<br>• However; data from, randomized comparison studies are still needed to establish the effect of remdesivir.<br>● IDSA and FDA32; recommends the use of remdesivir in adult and pediatric patients with severe COVID-19 pneumonia. (Conditional recommendation, moderate evidence).<br>● 100 mg IV daily to complete 5 days after 200 mg IV initial dose.<br>● IDSA warns that the benefit of remdesivir is greater in severely ill patients with adequate oxygen support rather than patients under MV or ECMO therapy for emergency and medication shortages. Again, a 5-day treatment is recommended for this patient group instead of 10-day treatment, such as those under MV or ECMO treatment. Remdesivir treatment is stopped if the patient's discharge is planned before the end of the treatment period. |

*(Table 10) cont.....*

| Drug | Notes- Advices |
|---|---|
| **Favipiravir** | It is an RNA polymerase inhibitor used in the treatment of Influenza and produced favorable results in the management of COVID-19.<br>• Although data are limited, SARS-CoV-2 may accelerate RNA clearance.<br>• In a nonrandomized study of patients with non-severe disease in China, favipiravir use had faster viral clearance rates (median 4 *versus* 11 days) and higher rate of radiological improvement (91% *versus* 62% on Day 14) compared to lopinavir-ritonavir. |
| **Lopinavir-ritonavir** | • This combined protease inhibitor used for HIV infection has been found to have in vitro activity against SARS-CoV. (Groneberg *et al*, 2020).<br>In a randomized study; 199 patients with severe COVID-19 were administered lopinavir-ritonavir (400 / 100mg) twice daily for 14 days. There was no improvement in clinical improvement compared to standard treatment. (Cao *et al*, 2020). |
| **Hydroxychloroquine / Chloroquine** | • It is believed to inhibit the progression to ARDS by inhibiting TNF-α and IL-6 production.<br>• *In-vivo* effectiveness has not been clearly established yet.<br>• These agents can prolong the QT interval and should be used in patients with a long QTc interval or with other agents that affect cardiac conduction, with caution and under close monitoring (Simpson *et al*, 2020).<br>• Other side effects include retinopathy or cardiomyopathy (may ensue in prolonged use and in higher doses)<br>Hydroxychloroquine: 400 mg × 2 the first day, then 400 mg, 5 days in total<br>Chloroquine: 500 mg per day (4-7 days) after 1 g on the first day (FDA, 2020)<br>• Antiviral activity of hydroxychloroquine is stronger.<br>● WHO ended the hydroxychloroquine trial of the large SOLIDARITY trial after existing data.<br>● IDSA recommends not to use hydroxychloroquine / chloroquine, hydroxychloroquine / chloroquine + azithromycin in hospitalized patients. (Strong recommendation, moderate level of evidence). https://www.idsociety.org/practice-guideline/covid-19-guidel-ne-treatment-and-management/<br>● In June 2020, FDA; cancelled the authorization for use in severe COVID-19 patients, as the known and potential benefits of these drugs do not outweigh the risks. |
| **Azithromycin plus hydroxychloroquine** | • It is not recommended to routinely use azithromycin in combination with hydroxychloroquine to treat COVID-19.<br>• Both azithromycin and hydroxychloroquine are associated with QTc prolongation, and concomitant use may cause a more severe effect in this context. |
| **Interferon-β** | • There is no direct data evaluating the effect of interferon beta on SARS-CoV-2. However, interferon beta effectively reduces MERS-CoV *in vitro* and has resulted in good results in the animal model of MERS-CoV infection (Hart *et al*, 2020). |
| **Venous Thromboembolism Prophylaxis** | Recommended for all inpatients diagnosed with COVID-19.<br>• There should be no contraindication (active bleeding, severe thrombocytopenia).<br>• Dysregulated coagulation parameters, diffuse intravascular coagulation (DIC) were associated with disease severity and mortality. |

CST use in ARDS patients remains controversial, but this treatment is currently the only pharmacological intervention that can reduce morbidity and mortality (Fig. **9**).

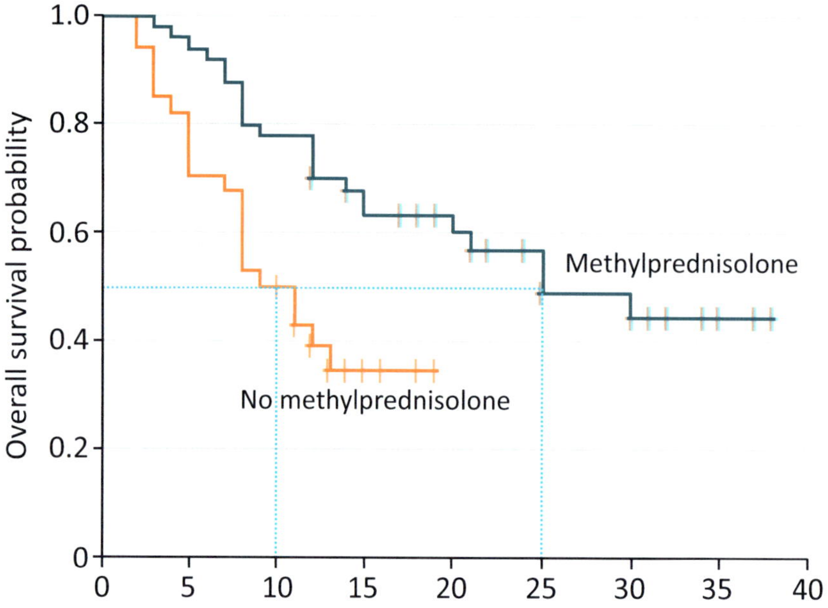


**Fig. (9).** >ARDS development is delayed by the use of methyl prednisolone or it is prevented.

Moreover, methylprednisolone shortened the duration of invasive mechanical ventilation need and reduced mortality in patients with ARDS. However, WHO does not recommend the routine administration of systemic CST to COVID-19 or COVID19-associated ARDS patients.

The IDSA guideline panel recommends glucocorticoid administration in hospitalized patients with critical COVID-19. (Conditional recommendation, Moderate level of evidence).

CST are not recommended for routine treatment (If there are no indications such as COPD attack or refractory septic shock) (CDC, 2020).

**Note:** Dexamethasone 6 mg IV or PO can be substituted for 10 days (or until discharge if earlier) or the equivalent glucocorticoid dose if dexamethasone is not available. The equivalent total daily doses of glucocorticoids alternative to 6 mg dexamethasone per day are 32 mg methylprednisolone and 40 mg prednisone.

## CONCLUSION

Pneumonia is the principal complication to be noticed in a patient who is going to deteriorate in the course of COVID-19. ARDS and respiratory failure are final common pathways leading to death in the patients in extremis. ARDS development is delayed or prevented by the rational use of mechanical ventilation and some agents such as methyl prednisolone. Timely diagnosis and management cannot be overestimated in a patient prone to develop severe pneumonia, ARDS and respiratory failure.

## REFERENCES

Abbasi, B, Akhavan, R & Ghamari Khameneh, A (2020) Evaluation of the relationship between inpatient COVID-19 mortality and chest CT severity score. *Am J Emerg Med,* S0735-6757, 30851-2.

ACR Recommendations for the use of Chest Radiography and Computed Tomography (CT) for Suspected COVID-19 Infection https://www.acr.org/Advocacy-and-Economics/ACR-Position-Statements /Recommendations-for-Chest-Radiography-and-CT-for-Suspected-COVID19-Infection

Ai, T, Yang, Z & Hou, H (2020) Correlation of chest CT and RT-PCR testing in coronavirus disease 2019 (COVID-19) in China. *a report of 1014 cases Radiology,*

Bai, HX, Hsieh, B, Xiong, Z, Halsey, K, Choi, JW, Tran, TML, Pan, I, Shi, LB, Wang, DC, Mei, J, Jiang, XL, Zeng, QH, Egglin, TK, Hu, PF, Agarwal, S, Xie, FF, Li, S, Healey, T, Atalay, MK & Liao, WH (2020) Performance of Radiologists in Differentiating COVID-19 from Non-COVID-19 Viral Pneumonia at Chest CT. *Radiology,* 296, E46-54.
[http://dx.doi.org/10.1148/radiol.2020200823] [PMID: 32155105]

Bajema, KL, Oster, AM, McGovern, OL, Lindstrom, S, Stenger, MR, Anderson, TC, Isenhour, C, Clarke, KR, Evans, ME, Chu, VT, Biggs, HM, Kirking, HL, Gerber, SI, Hall, AJ, Fry, AM & Oliver, SE (2020) Persons evaluated for 2019 novel coronavirus-United States, January 2020. *MMWR Morb Mortal Wkly Rep,* 69, 166-70.
[http://dx.doi.org/10.15585/mmwr.mm6906e1] [PMID: 32053579]

Cao, B, Wang, Y, Wen, D, Liu, W, Wang, J, Fan, G, Ruan, L, Song, B, Cai, Y, Wei, M, Li, X, Xia, J, Chen, N, Xiang, J, Yu, T, Bai, T, Xie, X, Zhang, L, Li, C, Yuan, Y, Chen, H, Li, H, Huang, H, Tu, S, Gong, F, Liu, Y, Wei, Y, Dong, C, Zhou, F, Gu, X, Xu, J, Liu, Z, Zhang, Y, Li, H, Shang, L, Wang, K, Li, K, Zhou, X, Dong, X, Qu, Z, Lu, S, Hu, X, Ruan, S, Luo, S, Wu, J, Peng, L, Cheng, F, Pan, L, Zou, J, Jia, C, Wang, J, Liu, X, Wang, S, Wu, X, Ge, Q, He, J, Zhan, H, Qiu, F, Guo, L, Huang, C, Jaki, T, Hayden, FG, Horby, PW, Zhang, D & Wang, C (2020) A trial of lopinavir-ritonavir in adults hospitalized with severe COVID-19. *N Engl J Med,* 382, 1787-99.
[http://dx.doi.org/10.1056/NEJMoa2001282] [PMID: 32187464]

(2020) https://www.cdc.gov/coronavirus/2019-ncov/hcp/clinical-guidance-management-patients.html

Dai, WC, Zhang, HW, Yu, J, Xu, HJ, Chen, H, Luo, SP, Zhang, H, Liang, LH, Wu, XL, Lei, Y & Lin, F (2020) CT imaging and differential diagnosis of COVID-19. *Can Assoc Radiol J,* 71, 195-200.
[http://dx.doi.org/10.1177/0846537120913033] [PMID: 32129670]

Ellington, S, Strid, P & Tong, VT (2020) Characteristics of Women of Reproductive Age with Laboratory-Confirmed SARS-CoV-2 Infection by Pregnancy Status - United States *Morbidity and Mortality Weekly Report (MMWR) Weekly,* 69, 769-5.
[http://dx.doi.org/] [PMID: ]

Fang, Y, Zhang, H, Xie, J, Lin, M, Ying, L, Pang, P & Ji, W (2020) Sensitivity of Chest CT for COVID-19: Comparison to RT-PCR. *Radiology,* 296, E115-7.
[http://dx.doi.org/10.1148/radiol.2020200432] [PMID: 32073353]

Grein, J, Ohmagari, N & Shin, D (2020) *Compassionate Use of Remdesivir for Patients with Severe COVID-19.*J New England Med.

Groneberg, DA, Poutanen, SM, Low, DE, Lode, H, Welte, T & Zabel, P (2005) Treatment and vaccines for severe acute respiratory syndrome. *Lancet Infect Dis,* 5, 147-55.
[http://dx.doi.org/10.1016/S1473-3099(05)70022-0] [PMID: 15766649]

Guan, WJ, Ni, ZY, Hu, Y, Liang, WH, Ou, CQ, He, JX, Liu, L, Shan, H, Lei, CL, Hui, DSC, Du, B, Li, LJ, Zeng, G, Yuen, KY, Chen, RC, Tang, CL, Wang, T, Chen, PY, Xiang, J, Li, SY, Wang, JL, Liang, ZJ, Peng,

YX, Wei, L, Liu, Y, Hu, YH, Peng, P, Wang, JM, Liu, JY, Chen, Z, Li, G, Zheng, ZJ, Qiu, SQ, Luo, J, Ye, CJ, Zhu, SY & Zhong, NS (2020) Clinical characteristics of coronavirus disease 2019 in China. *N Engl J Med,* 382, 1708-20.
[http://dx.doi.org/10.1056/NEJMoa2002032] [PMID: 32109013]

Hafiz, M, Icksan, AG, Harlivasari, AD, Aulia, R, Susanti, F & Eldinia, L (2020) Clinical, Radiological Features and Outcome of COVID-19 patients in a Secondary Hospital in Jakarta, Indonesia. *J Infect Dev Ctries,* 14, 750-7.
[http://dx.doi.org/10.3855/jidc.12911] [PMID: 32794466]

Hart, BJ, Dyall, J, Postnikova, E, Zhou, H, Kindrachuk, J, Johnson, RF, Olinger, GG, Frieman, MB, Holbrook, MR, Jahrling, PB & Hensley, L (2014) Interferon-β and mycophenolic acid are potent inhibitors of Middle East respiratory syndrome coronavirus in cell-based assays. *J Gen Virol,* 95, 571-7.
[http://dx.doi.org/10.1099/vir.0.061911-0] [PMID: 24323636]

Huang, C, Wang, Y, Li, X, Ren, L, Zhao, J, Hu, Y, Zhang, L, Fan, G, Xu, J, Gu, X, Cheng, Z, Yu, T, Xia, J, Wei, Y, Wu, W, Xie, X, Yin, W, Li, H, Liu, M, Xiao, Y, Gao, H, Guo, L, Xie, J, Wang, G, Jiang, R, Gao, Z, Jin, Q, Wang, J & Cao, B (2020) Clinical features of patients infected with 2019 novel coronavirus in Wuhan, China. *Lancet,* 395, 497-506. [Erratum in: Lancet. 2020 Jan 30; Huntley BJF, Huntley ES, Di Mascio D, Chen T, Berghella V, Chauhan SP. Rates of Maternal and Perinatal Mortality and Vertical Transmission in Pregnancies Complicated by Severe Acute Respiratory Syndrome Coronavirus 2 ]. [SARS-Co-V-2]. [ Infection: A Systematic Review. Obstet Gynecol. 2020 Aug;136]. [2]. [:303-312. doi: 10.1097/AOG.0000000000004010. PMID: 32516273].
[http://dx.doi.org/10.1016/S0140-6736(20)30183-5] [PMID: 31986264]

*Infectious Diseases Society of America Guidelines on the Treatment and Management of Patients with COVID-19.*https://www.idsociety.org/practice-guideline/covid-19-guideline-treatment-and-management/

Kovács, A, Palásti, P, Veréb, D, Bozsik, B, Palkó, A & Kincses, ZT (2020) The sensitivity and specificity of chest CT in the diagnosis of COVID-19. *Eur Radiol,* 1-6.
[http://dx.doi.org/10.1007/s00330-020-07347-x] [PMID: 33051732]

Li, X, Geng, M, Peng, Y, Meng, L & Lu, S (2020) Molecular immune pathogenesis and diagnosis of COVID-19. *J Pharm Anal,* 10, 102-8.
[http://dx.doi.org/10.1016/j.jpha.2020.03.001] [PMID: 32282863]

Liang, T, Cai, H & Chen, Y (2020) *Handbook of COVID-19 prevention and treatment.*Zhejiang University School of Medicine, Zhejiang.

Liu, J, Liu, Y & Xiang, P (2020) Neutrophil-to-lymphocyte ratio predicts severe illness patients with 2019 Novel Coronavirus in the early stage. *J Transl Med,* 18, 206.
[http://dx.doi.org/10.1186/s12967-020-02374-0] [PMID: 32434518]

Luo, P, Liu, Y, Qiu, L, Liu, X, Liu, D & Li, J (2020) Tocilizumab treatment in COVID-19: A single center experience. *J Med Virol,* 92, 814-8.
[http://dx.doi.org/10.1002/jmv.25801] [PMID: 32253759]

Mehta, P, McAuley, DF, Brown, M, Sanchez, E, Tattersall, RS & Manson, JJ (2020) COVID-19: consider cytokine storm syndromes and immunosuppression. *Lancet,* 395, 1033-4.
[http://dx.doi.org/10.1016/S0140-6736(20)30628-0] [PMID: 32192578]

Mizumoto, K, Kagaya, K, Zarebski, A & Chowell, G (2020) Estimating the asymptomatic proportion of coronavirus disease 2019 (COVID-19) cases on board the Diamond Princess cruise ship, Yokohama, Japan, 2020. *Euro Surveill,* 252000180
[http://dx.doi.org/10.2807/1560-7917.ES.2020.25.10.2000180] [PMID: 32183930]

Infectious Diseases Society of America Guidelines on the Treatment and Management of Patients with COVID-19 https://www.who.int/news-room/commentaries/detail/modes-of-transmission-of-virus-c-using-covid-19-implications-for-ipc-precaution-recommendations

Morris, G, Bortolasci, CC, Puri, BK, Olive, L, Marx, W, O'Neil, A, Athan, E, Carvalho, AF, Maes, M, Walder, K & Berk, M (2020) The pathophysiology of SARS-CoV-2: A suggested model and therapeutic

approach. *Life Sci,* 258118166
[http://dx.doi.org/10.1016/j.lfs.2020.118166] [PMID: 32739471]

Ong, CWM, Migliori, GB, Raviglione, M, MacGregor-Skinner, G, Sotgiu, G, Alffenaar, JW, Tiberi, S, Adlhoch, C, Alonzi, T, Archuleta, S, Brusin, S, Cambau, E, Capobianchi, MR, Castilletti, C, Centis, R, Cirillo, DM, D'Ambrosio, L, Delogu, G, Esposito, SMR, Figueroa, J, Friedland, JS, Ho, BCH, Ippolito, G, Jankovic, M, Kim, HY, Rosales Klintz, S, Ködmön, C, Lalle, E, Leo, YS, Leung, CC, Märtson, AG, Melazzini, MG, Najafi Fard, S, Penttinen, P, Petrone, L, Petruccioli, E, Pontali, E, Saderi, L, Santin, M, Spanevello, A, van Crevel, R, van der Werf, MJ, Visca, D, Viveiros, M, Zellweger, JP, Zumla, A & Goletti, D (2020) Epidemic and pandemic viral infections: impact on tuberculosis and the lung. *Eur Respir J,* 562001727
[http://dx.doi.org/10.1183/13993003.01727-2020] [PMID: 32586885]

Ong, SWX, Lee, PH, Tan, YK, Ling, LM, Ho, BCH, Ng, CG, Wang, DL, Tan, BH, Leo, YS, Ng, OT, Wong, MSY & Marimuthu, K (2020) Environmental contamination in a coronavirus disease 2019 (COVID-19) intensive care unit-What is the risk? *Infect Control Hosp Epidemiol,* 1-9.
[http://dx.doi.org/10.1017/ice.2020.1278] [PMID: 33081858]

Pan, F, Ye, T & Sun, P (2020) Time course of lung changes on chest CT during recovery from 2019 novel coronavirus (COVID-19) pneumonia. *Radiology,* 295, 715-21.
[http://dx.doi.org/10.1148/radiol.2020200370] [PMID: 32053470]

Revel, MP, Parkar, AP, Prosch, H, Silva, M, Sverzellati, N, Gleeson, F & Brady, A (2020) COVID-19 patients and the radiology department - advice from the European Society of Radiology (ESR) and the European Society of Thoracic Imaging (ESTI). *Eur Radiol,* 30, 4903-9.
[http://dx.doi.org/10.1007/s00330-020-06865-y] [PMID: 32314058]

Rubin, GD, Ryerson, CJ, Haramati, LB, Sverzellati, N, Kanne, JP, Raoof, S, Schluger, NW, Volpi, A, Yim, JJ, Martin, IBK, Anderson, DJ, Kong, C, Altes, T, Bush, A, Desai, SR, Goldin, O, Goo, JM, Humbert, M, Inoue, Y, Kauczor, HU, Luo, F, Mazzone, PJ, Prokop, M, Remy-Jardin, M, Richeldi, L, Schaefer-Prokop, CM, Tomiyama, N, Wells, AU & Leung, AN (2020) The Role of Chest Imaging in Patient Management during the COVID-19 Pandemic: A Multinational Consensus Statement from the Fleischner Society. *Radiology,* 296, 172-80.
[http://dx.doi.org/10.1148/radiol.2020201365] [PMID: 32255413]

San-Juan, R, Barbero, P, Fernández-Ruiz, M, López-Medrano, F, Lizasoáin, M, Hernández-Jiménez, P, Silva, JT, Ruiz-Ruigómez, M, Corbella, L, Rodríguez-Goncer, I, Folgueira, MD, Lalueza, A, Batllori, E, Mejía, I, Forcén, L, Lumbreras, C, García-Burguillo, A, Galindo, A & Aguado, JM (2020) Incidence and clinical profiles of COVID-19 pneumonia in pregnant women: A single-centre cohort study from Spain. *EClinicalMedicine,* 23100407
[http://dx.doi.org/10.1016/j.eclinm.2020.100407] [PMID: 32632417]

Sheahan, TP, Sims, AC, Graham, RL, Menachery, VD, Gralinski, LE, Case, JB, Leist, SR, Pyrc, K, Feng, JY, Trantcheva, I, Bannister, R, Park, Y, Babusis, D, Clarke, MO, Mackman, RL, Spahn, JE, Palmiotti, CA, Siegel, D, Ray, AS, Cihlar, T, Jordan, R, Denison, MR & Baric, RS (2017) Broad-spectrum antiviral GS-5734 inhibits both epidemic and zoonotic coronaviruses. *Sci Transl Med,* 9eaal3653
[http://dx.doi.org/10.1126/scitranslmed.aal3653] [PMID: 28659436]

Shen, C, Wang, Z, Zhao, F, Yang, Y, Li, J, Yuan, J, Wang, F, Li, D, Yang, M, Xing, L, Wei, J, Xiao, H, Yang, Y, Qu, J, Qing, L, Chen, L, Xu, Z, Peng, L, Li, Y, Zheng, H, Chen, F, Huang, K, Jiang, Y, Liu, D, Zhang, Z, Liu, Y & Liu, L (2020) Treatment of 5 critically ill patients with COVID-19 with convalescent plasma. *JAMA,* 323, 1582-9.
[http://dx.doi.org/10.1001/jama.2020.4783] [PMID: 32219428]

Shi, H, Han, X, Jiang, N, Cao, Y, Alwalid, O, Gu, J, Fan, Y & Zheng, C (2020) Radiological findings from 81 patients with COVID-19 pneumonia in Wuhan, China: a descriptive study. *Lancet Infect Dis,* 20, 425-34.
[http://dx.doi.org/10.1016/S1473-3099(20)30086-4] [PMID: 32105637]

Simpson, S, Kay, FU, Abbara, S, Bhalla, S, Chung, JH, Chung, M, Henry, TS, Kanne, JP, Kligerman, S, Ko, JP & Litt, H (2020) Radiological Society of North America Expert Consensus Statement on Reporting Chest

CT Findings Related to COVID-19. Endorsed by the Society of Thoracic Radiology, the American College of Radiology, and RSNA - Secondary Publication. *J Thorac Imaging,* 35, 219-27. [http://dx.doi.org/10.1097/RTI.0000000000000524] [PMID: 32324653]

(2020) https://www.fda.gov/media/136534/download

Wang, D, Hu, B, Hu, C, Zhu, F, Liu, X, Zhang, J, Wang, B, Xiang, H, Cheng, Z, Xiong, Y, Zhao, Y, Li, Y, Wang, X & Peng, Z (2020) Clinical characteristics of 138 hospitalized patients with 2019 novel coronavirus–infected pneumonia in Wuhan, China. *JAMA,* 323, 1061-9. [http://dx.doi.org/10.1001/jama.2020.1585] [PMID: 32031570]

Wei, WE, Li, Z, Chiew, CJ, Yong, SE, Toh, MP & Lee, VJ (2020) Presymptomatic Transmission of SARS-CoV-2 - Singapore, January 23-March 16, 2020. *MMWR Morb Mortal Wkly Rep,* 69, 411-5. [http://dx.doi.org/10.15585/mmwr.mm6914e1] [PMID: 32271722]

WHO. Novel Coronavirus (2019-nCoV) technical guidance: Patient management (2020) https://www.who.int/publications/i/item/clinical-management-of-covid-19

Wu, C, Chen, X, Cai, Y, Xia, J, Zhou, X, Xu, S, Huang, H, Zhang, L, Zhou, X, Du, C, Zhang, Y, Song, J, Wang, S, Chao, Y, Yang, Z, Xu, J, Zhou, X, Chen, D, Xiong, W, Xu, L, Zhou, F, Jiang, J, Bai, C, Zheng, J & Song, Y (2020) Risk factors associated with acute respiratory distress syndrome and death in patients with coronavirus disease 2019 pneumonia in Wuhan, China. *JAMA Intern Med,* 180, 934-43. [http://dx.doi.org/10.1001/jamainternmed.2020.0994] [PMID: 32167524]

Yang, R, Li, X & Liu, H (2020) Chest CT Severity Score: An Imaging Tool for Assessing Severe COVID-19. *Radiol Cardiothorac Imaging,* 2e200047 [http://dx.doi.org/10.1148/ryct.2020200047]

Zambrano, LD, Ellington, S, Strid, P, Galang, RR, Oduyebo, T, Tong, VT, Woodworth, KR, Nahabedian, JF, III, Azziz-Baumgartner, E, Gilboa, SM & Meaney-Delman, D (2020) Update: Characteristics of Symptomatic Women of Reproductive Age with Laboratory-Confirmed SARS-CoV-2 Infection by Pregnancy Status - United States, January 22-October 3, 2020. *MMWR Morb Mortal Wkly Rep,* 69, 1641-7. [http://dx.doi.org/10.15585/mmwr.mm6944e3] [PMID: 33151921]

Zhou, F, Yu, T, Du, R, Fan, G, Liu, Y, Liu, Z, Xiang, J, Wang, Y, Song, B, Gu, X, Guan, L, Wei, Y, Li, H, Wu, X, Xu, J, Tu, S, Zhang, Y, Chen, H & Cao, B (2020) Clinical course and risk factors for mortality of adult inpatients with COVID-19 in Wuhan, China: a retrospective cohort study. *Lancet,* 395, 1054-62. [http://dx.doi.org/10.1016/S0140-6736(20)30566-3] [PMID: 32171076]

# CHAPTER 12

# Pregnancy, COVID-19, and Children: Dangerous Trio?

**Abstract:** It has not been proven that the infection is transmitted to the baby in the uterus. It is currently known that pregnant women with COVID-19 are mostly infected in the last period of pregnancy. In general, the clinical course of the disease is similar to non-pregnant ones. Most drugs can be given to these women in the treatment of COVID-19 and its complications, while some are dangerous. In addition, women with COVID-19 can and should breastfeed their babies with adherence to universal precautions and hygiene. Tomography can be elicited in pregnant women due to this vital requirement. When pregnant women are suspected of having COVID-19, they have priority for treatment and hospitalization.

Compared to adults, children have less tendency to be infected with the disease, and they recover from the disease with milder symptoms. Stronger immunity in children fed with breast milk and other vaccines is also a supportive assumption. Fever and respiratory complaints are common in children. Increased inflammatory markers and low lymphocyte count (and percentage) in complete blood count (lymphopenia) are less common in children.

**Keywords:** COVID-19, Children, Diagnosis, Mother, Newborn, Pandemic, Pregnancy, Treatment.

Infections and especially pneumonia during pregnancy can be one of the common causes of death. In 1957-58 Asian flu, 10% of deaths were recorded in pregnant women, and death rates were more common than non-pregnant women. In general, respiratory diseases in pregnant women are a more serious problem than the other population.

In the 2002-2003 SARS disease epidemic, a clinical course in pregnant women is worse than non-pregnant women. It has also been reported that preterm birth and miscarriage rates increase. 4 out of 7 pregnant women who were admitted in the first 3 months (trimester) resulted in miscarriage/abortion, and 4 out of 5 pregnant women who were referred after 24 weeks resulted in premature birth (Wong, 2004).

**Ozgur KARCIOGLU, Selman YENIOCAK and Mandana HOSSEINZADEH**

It has been reported that immunity based on T-helper 2 cells, which is dominant in pregnant women, is a system that protects the fetus and exposes pregnant women to infection (Dashraath *et al.*, 2020). Therefore, the need for different principles of care in COVID-19 pandemics in pregnant women has been underlined.

Only five of the 1308 cases registered in the MERS epidemic in Saudi Arabia between 2012-2016 were pregnant women and all of them resulted badly (Assiri, 2016). All of the cases were between the ages of 27-34, and all required admission to ICU. Two women died, and two infant deaths (perinatal death) were recorded.

## WHAT ARE THE CHARACTERISTICS OF PREGNANT WOMEN WITH COVID-19?

Pregnant women with COVID-19 are younger than pregnant women with SARS and MERS, between the ages of 23-40. Shortness of breath is seen in up to 18% (Guan, 2020). Fever was reported as 84%, and cough was 28% (Dashraath, 2020). Similar to non-pregnant women, the main complaints are fever, cough, shortness of breath, and the most common finding is lymphopenia. The main finding in radiology is peripherally distributed shadowing on CXR, while bilateral diffuse ground glass opacities (GGO) are typical in tomography (Kong 2020, Shi 2020).

### Should there be a Different Warning for Pregnant Healthcare Workers?

Yes, there is. In well-designed clinical studies, it has been reported that high-protection masks such as N95 result in insufficient oxygen intake after 1 hour of physical activity in the late pregnancy (second and third trimester) (Tong 2015, Roberge 2014).

### Could the Pregnant Women with Covid-19 Transmit the Disease to the Baby?

No. That is, such a possibility is negligible. During pregnancy, there is an increased risk of all kinds of respiratory infections such as influenza (flu). It has not been proven that the infection is transmitted to the baby in the uterus. When it comes to COVID-19, it is known that pregnant women are mostly infected in the last period of pregnancy. In general, the clinical course of the disease is similar to non-pregnant ones.

Few cases have been reported that represent the transmission of COVID-19 from mother to baby before or during delivery (Rasmussen 2020). The COVID test was found positive in a newborn 30 hours after its birth on February 5, 2020 in Wuhan.

COVID-19 pneumonia requiring mechanical ventilation has been reported in a 30-week pregnant woman (Wang, 2020). Pregnancy was terminated by cesarean section (C/S) and she recovered.

Of note, placenta and amniotic fluid swabs in pregnant women infected with COVID-19 were completely negative for COVID-19. Likewise, no relationship has been established between early termination of pregnancy (abortion) and COVID-19, SARS, and MERS infections.

## How is Protection from Covid-19 during Pregnancy?

Individual isolation and social solidarity provide protection for pregnant women. It is also important not to visit hospital unless it is mandatory.

## What are the General Treatment Methods in Pregnant Women?

Pregnant women with suspected or diagnosed CoVID-19 infection should receive supportive therapy (oxygenation, hydration, antibiotic therapy, and others) like other patients. In addition, fetus should be followed up, and uterine contractions should be closely monitored. Be aware of preterm birth and birth control should be individualized.

The indication of emergency C / S and delivery in pregnant with CoVID-19 infection is a difficult decision. Obstetrics, ICU, and infection specialists should have a consensus on a joint decision and individualized treatment plan.

Attention should be paid to pregnancy warnings in drug use. Personal risk-benefit balance should be taken into account on every step. Consultation should be sought from obstetrics and gynecology whenever necessary.

### Fever Treatment:

Taking plenty of fluids and warm showers every few hours, along with cooling the ambient temperature is more effective than many agents in reducing fever.

### Medications:

Paracetamol is the safest choice of agents. Although the NSAID group "profen"s (ketoprofen / dexketoprofen / ibuprofen / flurbiprofen) are effective agents against fever, care should be taken as they may hide the signs and symptoms of COVID-19 infection. Nonetheless, alleviating fever appears to be an important goal of the symptomatic treatment, thus antipyretic medications are mainstays of treatment in many instances.

## Are the Drugs used in the Treatment of Covid-19 Harmful during Pregnancy?

**Tocilizumab,** which is safely recommended as an anti-inflammatory in COVID-19 cases, cannot be used in pregnancy, since there are not enough studies. It has even been reported that the drug should be discontinued before pregnancy.

The use of chloroquine and its metabolites generally appears to be safe and effective. Since the volume of distribution (Vd) is high, it requires higher doses (at least 500 mg chloroquine) during pregnancy (Gao, 2020). These high doses can be associated with systolic hypotension which is aggravated by compression of the enlarged uterus on the inferior vena cava in the supine pregnant woman. Therefore, left lateral decubitus position should be emphasized to assume.

**Azithromycin** is one of the drugs that should be avoided during pregnancy. It can cause developmental disorders (malformations) in the newborn.

**Lopinavir / ritonavir** treatment, which has been used for a long time in the treatment of AIDS, is among the useful strategies for pregnant women. There are no suggestions for changes in pregnancy, including dose reduction, for these agents.

**Remdesivir,** one of the broad-acting anti-nucleotide antiviral agents, seems safe in pregnancy. Phase 3 studies are carried out for effectiveness. Favipiravir, another polymerase inhibitor, cannot be used in pregnant women.

Although the use of corticosteroids is not recommended routinely, it can be used within an individualized plan in selected cases such as ARDS.

## Can the Woman with COVID-19 Breastfeed her Baby?

Yes. Transmission of COVID-19 to a child through breast milk has not been demonstrated by breastfeeding. On the contrary, the benefits of breastfeeding are immense, and the child should not be deprived of it with a diagnosis or suspicion of COVID-19. This should be taken into account only if the mother is using antiviral and other drugs. Even if the mother is very sick, it is tried to be given to the child by expressing the milk or by another suitable method.

## Is there Anything to Pay Attention to After Birth?

When the baby is given to the mother, the infection in the mother can be transmitted to the baby *via* breathing and droplets. Washing hands before touching the baby and using a mask will be protective.

## COVID-19 in Newborns and Children:

There are more than 27 million of registered COVID-19 cases worldwide, while very few cases of newborns and children are recorded, which means that the children's immune system protects them.

Since the beginning of the COVID-19 pandemics, until March 22, 2020, there were no deaths between the ages of 0 and 9. There is a 0.2% mortality rate between the ages of 10 and 19. 96% of the children have mild disease (Dong, 2020). Analyzing the whole situation, the clinical status is milder in children when compared to the adults. However, it should be remembered that they can be severe in selected cases.

There is hardly any transmission from mother to child through the placenta. Deaths from children are also very exceptional. In newborns born to COVID-19 infected mothers, the tests were mostly negative.

A multicenter cohort study was conducted among newborns born to mothers with COVID-19 in 34 neonatal intensive care units (NICUs) in Turkey (Oncel MY, 2020). Eight of 125 mothers (6.4%) were admitted to an ICU for MV, among whom six died (4.8%). Four of 120 newborns (3.3%) had a positive RT-PCR test result. Although samples taken on the first day were negative, one neonate became positive on the second day and the other two on the fifth day.

In cases such as neonatal jaundice, systems are to be developed in which parents can take care of the baby bedside at home against the dangers of leaving the house.

## Can Children Take COVID-19 Medications Used by Adults?

The safety of lopinavir / ritonavir in the neonatal period and premature infants has not been established. Apart from that, other drugs including oseltamivir and chloroquine can be used.

In summary, COVID-19 infection during pregnancy may increase the need for admission into ICU in pregnant women and the risk of maternal death. The rate of spontaneous miscarriage and premature birth are also likely to be high.

In the baby, the risks of growth retardation, perinatal death, and respiratory distress syndrome increase.

Can tomography be obtained for the diagnosis of COVID-19 in pregnant women?

Clinical deterioration in patients with COVID-19 occurs as a result of respiratory failure due to multiple organ failure, especially pneumonia. For this reason, identification of disease effects in the lung is the most important tool in enlightening the extent and severity of the disease. Tomography can be elicited in pregnant women due to this vital requirement.

Important note: When pregnant women are suspected of having COVID-19, they have priority for treatment and hospitalization (Algorithm **1**).

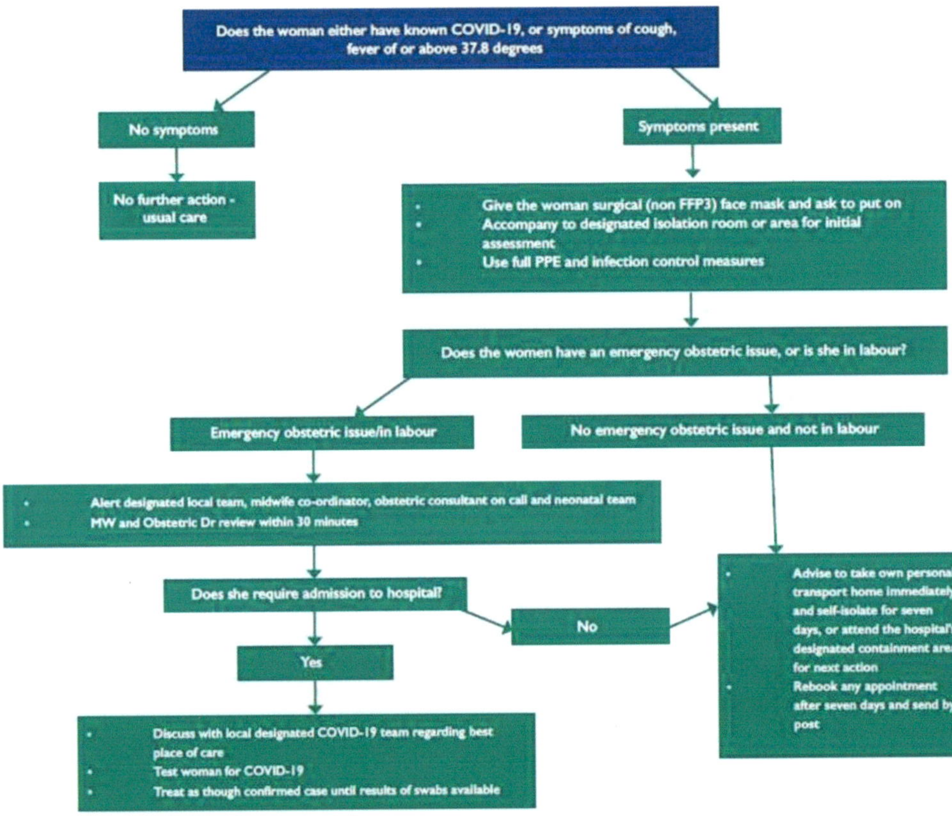


**Algorithm 1.** The algorithm below is the most recent recommendation for pregnant women.

## COVID-19 IN CHILDREN: IT IS NOT A FAIRY TALE, IT IS A REALITY

Children account for 1% to 5% of COVID-19 cases in the large total. In a study involving 44,672 confirmed COVID-19 cases by February 11, 2020, 965 people (2.2%) died, only one of them was under 19 years old (Epidemiology Working Group for NCIP Epidemic Response, Chinese Center for Disease Control and

Prevention, 2020). Those under 10 years of age at the time of diagnosis are reported at a rate of 0.9%. Among 22,000 cases in Italy, the rate of children is 1.2% and there is no death (Livingston, 2020). 2% in China and 5% in the USA were the share of children among all cases, respectively (CDC, 2020). Guan *et al.* stated that 0.9% of those affected in a large series in China were under the age of 15 (Guan, 2020).

Compared to adults, children have less tendency to be infected with the disease, and they recover from the disease with milder symptoms. Although there is no difference in terms of encountering the virus, their findings are much less common. Deaths are very rare in childhood. Ludvigsson *et al.* combined the findings of 45 studies in their systematic review (Ludvigsson, 2020). They reported that children showed a better clinical course than adults and deaths were very rare.

What could be the reason why COVID-19 is rare in children? This is most likely due to the relatively low availability of ACE-2 receptors in children. Stronger immunity in children fed with breast milk and other vaccines is also a supportive assumption.

## Are the Children "Carriers of COVID-19"?

Both yes and no. There are scarce literature data on this issue. In Switzerland, the researchers found that in only 8% of households did a child develop symptoms before any other household contacts (Posfay-Barbe, 2020). The finding is in accord with similar studies which cited that children are index cases in less than one-tenth of familial clusters with COVID-19.

## Are the Signs and Symptoms in Children Different from Adults?

It is basically no different. Fever and respiratory complaints are common. In fact, the fever response is sharper and more common than adults. Up to 98% of the patients have fever at some point in the disease course. However, severe pneumonia is much less common in children. Although nasal discharge is not expected in adults, it can be seen in some children. Clinical manifestations and laboratory findings somewhat differ from those of adults (Figs. **1 & 2**).

Pearl: Children present into the hospitals without any symptoms more commonly than adults, or have milder symptoms than all others.

Although rare, pediatric multisystem inflammatory syndrome temporally associated with COVID-19 infection is a severe disease.

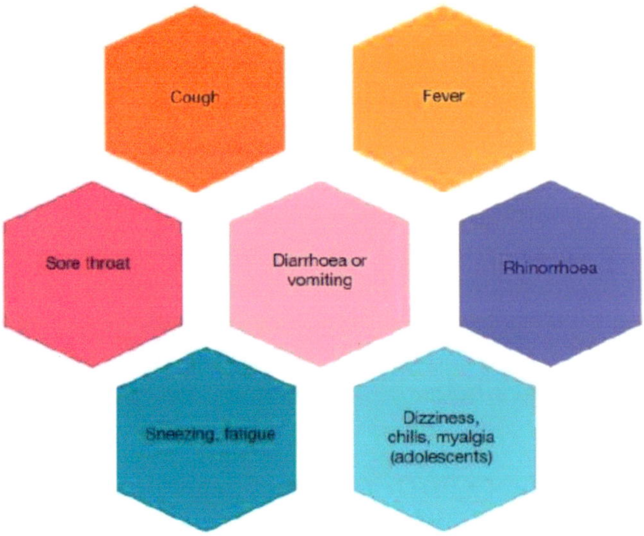


**Fig. (1).** Common clinical manifestations of symptomatic COVID-19 infection in children (Adapted from Naja, 2020).

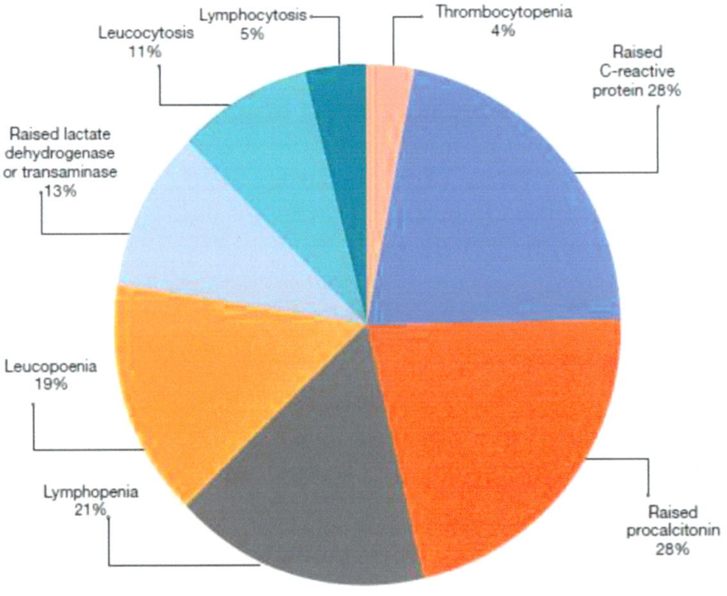


**Fig. (2).** Common laboratory findings to be expected in symptomatic COVID-19 infection in children (Adapted from Naja, 2020).

The table below can be used to distinguish COVID-19 from diseases such as cold, flu, and common cold. It should be kept in mind that the rate of correct diagnosis is not 100% even by the most experienced physician, and it is necessary to refer to the family health center or hospital in case of doubt (Table **1**).

**Table 1. Characteristics of symptomatology seen in the courses of three common diseases to take into account in the differential diagnosis**

| Symptoms | COVID-19 | Cold | Flu |
|---|---|---|---|
| **Evolution** | Symptoms range from mild to severe | Gradual onset of symptoms | Abrupt onset of symptoms |
| **Fever** | Common | Rare/Mild | Common |
| **Fatigue** | Sometimes | Sometimes | Common |
| **Cough** | Common (dry) | Rare/Mild | Common (dry) |
| **Sneezing** | - | Common | - |
| **Aches and pains** | Sometimes | Common | Common |
| **Runny or stuffy nose** | Rare/Mild | Common | Sometimes |
| **Sore throat** | Sometimes | Common | Sometimes |
| **Diarrhea** | Rare/Mild | - | Sometimes |
| **Headaches** | Sometimes | Rare/Mild | Common |
| **Shortness of breath, dyspnea** | Sometimes | - | - |

Of note, 'pediatric multisystem inflammatory syndrome' which can be encountered in the course of COVID-19 deserves special attention (Table **2**).

## Is COVID-19 more Risky for Children with Asthma or Allergies? What are the Risks?

For the physician, asthma is not a single or monotonous disease. Mild and severe asthma are not put together. A patient who has to use the inhaler medicine in his bag infrequently, can walk comfortably at hospital admission, can speak in long sentences, and whose respiratory rate is within normal limits for age is no different from a patient without asthma in terms of risks. In addition, patients who have to use their inhaler at high doses continuously, who have a history of intubation / mechanical ventilation, and who use steroids are at high risk for poor prognosis. Similar points can be highlighted for allergy. A history of anaphylaxis is particularly important because the risk of developing allergies or even anaphylaxis to the treatments that will be given will be much higher than that of other people. If the child is taken to the hospital with suspected COVID-19, a history of allergy, asthma and anaphylaxis must be recorded.

**Table 2. Clinical features in children with pediatric multisystem inflammatory syndrome temporally associated with COVID-19.**

| Frequency Seen | Clinical Feature |
|---|---|
| All | Persistent fever >38.5°C |
| Most | Hypotension |
| | Oxygen requirement |
| Some | Conjunctivitis |
| | Rash |
| | Mucous membrane changes |
| | Swollen or hard hands and feet |
| | Lymphadenopathy |
| | Neck swelling |
| | Sore throat |
| | Abdominal pain, diarrhea or vomiting |
| | Headache, confusion, or syncope |
| | Cough or respiratory symptoms |

## Are the Laboratory Findings Different in Children?

No, they are not. The leukocyte count (WBC) in children with COVID-19 is normal or low as in adults. Increased inflammatory markers and low lymphocyte count (and percentage) in complete blood count (lymphopenia) are less common in children. It has been reported that lymphopenia is seen in only 3 to 3.5% of the afflicted children (Lu, 2020). There are studies that associate high procalcitonin levels with severity of disease (Henry, 2020). Studies on IL-6 are also being conducted.

## Which Children get COVID-19?

Similar to adults, the presence of comorbid diseases is the most significant risk factor. 1391 children, who had contact with adults with COVID-19 diagnosed in China, were screened, whether symptomatic or not (Lu *et al.* 2020). 171 children (3/5 are boys) were diagnosed and hospitalized. The median age of the children in this study was 6.7 years. The most common findings were fever, cough, and redness in the throat. The median duration of fever is 3 days (range: 1 to 16 days). Diarrhea was detected in 8.8%, while tachypnea and tachycardia were found in 28% and 42%, respectively. Although the tests are positive, there are neither radiological findings nor symptoms in 27 children (15.8%). There were radiological findings in 12 children without any symptoms. All 3 children requiring admission to ICU and mechanical ventilation have comorbid diseases (hydronephrosis, leukemia, intussusception). Lymphopenia was detected in 3.5% of cases. Radiological findings are mostly ground glass opacities (1/3 cases), local patchy opacity (18%) and bilateral patchy shadowing (12%).

**Newborns:** An analysis by the WHO examined 149 pregnant women and revealed that pregnancy does not pose a risk factor for COVID-19 per se (WHO, 2020). Nevertheless, it has been reported that COVID-19 infection while pregnant can lead to fetal distress, premature birth, and respiratory distress (Zhu, 2020). It is accepted that there is no transmission from the mother to the child through the placenta.

39 newborns delivered by 38 pregnant women with COVID-19 were examined in detail (Schwartz, 2020). Thirty of 39 children have been tested for COVID-19 and all are negative.

## How is the Covid-19 Virus Transmitted to Children?

It is not different with adults. Children are more active than adults in putting their hands to their mouths and faces. It will be very easy for the child to encounter the virus if the adult brings a virus-infected item to the house from outside, or does not comply with hygiene practices. For example, if there is a toddler at home, it would be appropriate to put the shoes at home in a bag or leave them completely outside the door.

## Should Masks and Gloves be used for Children who are Going Out Necessarily?

This precaution, which applies to other people, is of course valid for children, too. Masks with high protection, such as N95 or N99 are absolutely not suitable for children. Since the oxygen consumption per kilogram of children is much higher than adults, these masks, which can prevent easy breathing, can cause hypoxia and syncope.

## Since The Mortality Rate in Children is Close to Zero, Covid-19 has Nothing to do with Children, Right?

Not that much. Children are carriers. Asymptomatic children with the virus can walk around freely and infect adults and the elderly.

## Should Children be Locked up at Home?

School closures and children staying at home have been examined in some important studies and it has been suggested that it has negative consequences (Wang, 2020). These undesirable effects can be prolonged "screen time", irregular sleep due to lack of exercise, diet problems, weight gain and loss of respiratory-circulatory health status. Sprang *et al.* reported that the risk of post-traumatic stress disorder is higher in children after prolonged home closure (Sprang, 2013).

**Disease severity in children:** In one of the largest series published, only 5.2% of children had severe disease and 0.6% had critical illness (Dong, 2020). Here, severe illness was defined as shortness of breath, central cyanosis, and a decrease in O2 saturation below 92%. Critical illness is the development of respiratory failure, shock, and symptoms of multiple organ failure. In this series, the rate of severe and critical illness in children under 1 year of age is the highest in all childhood periods with 10.6%.

The rate of children among COVID-19 patients hospitalized in the USA was reported as 1.6% to 2.5%, and no intensive care was required in any case (CDC, 2020). In Lu's series of 171 cases, the only death occurred in a 10-month-old child with intussusception with multiorgan failure (Lu, 2020).

## Does the Baby's Breastfeeding Affect the Covid-19 Clinical Course?

Yes. With the high secretory IgA and some other substances contained in breast milk, passive natural immunity is provided in every child. During the COVID-19 pandemic, maintaining and supporting breastfeeding is essential to prevent infection. In case of suspected contact or clinically supported infection, it is recommended that the mother donate breast milk by wearing a mask and providing the necessary hygiene rules to breastfeeding or milking (Gokcay, 2020). Maintenance and sustaining breastfeeding during pandemics is very important because breast milk has immunological, anti-infective and immunomodulatory effects as well as unique nutritional properties (Lawrence, 2016).

**Intact immunity** plays an important role in overcoming the disease with mild course. Disease transmission *via* breast milk has not been reported in children.

Cellular components found in breast milk that directly affect immunity;

- Leukocytes
- Macrophages
- Polymorphonuclear leukocytes
- Lymphocyte

• Stem cells

## How is the Diagnosis Made?

The diagnosis is established by searching for the nucleic acid of the virus in samples taken from the respiratory tract in most countries around the world, that is, RT-PCR study. In some countries such as China, it has been found more appropriate to diagnose it with the clinical focus. In this system, at least two of the clinical findings are expected to accompany laboratory and radiological findings (Fig. **3**).

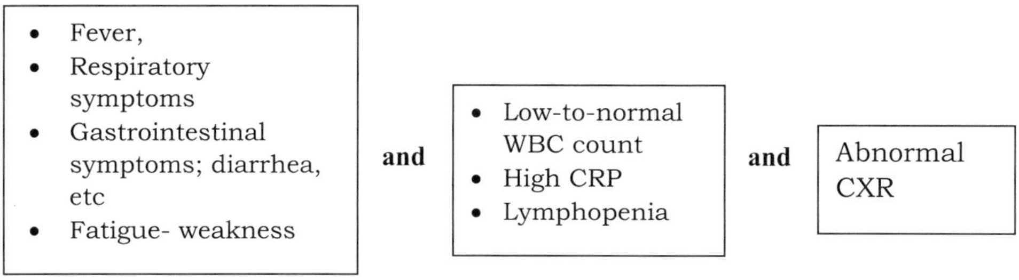


**Fig. (3).** At least two of the clinical findings are expected to accompany laboratory and radiological findings to establish the diagnosis of COVID-19. Some researchers stated that some other viral pneumonias such as influenza and H1N1 infection should be ruled out for diagnosis (Dong, 2020).

## Imaging Principles for Pediatric COVID-19 Suspected Cases

First of all, high-radiation imaging (*e.g.* CT) is not recommended as a screening test for children with suspected COVID-19. This is also true for children with mild clinical symptoms. However, imaging is recommended when there are risk factors for disease progression or worsening.

Chinese researchers emphasized that it is appropriate to scan children with x-ray and tomography if necessary for diagnostic examination (Shen, 2020). Differential diagnosis includes influenza virus, parainfluenza virus, adenovirus, respiratory syncytial virus, rhinovirus, human metapneumovirus and other viral agents. It has been reported that bacterial pneumonia agents, Mycoplasma pneumonia and Chlamydia pneumonia should also be differentiated from COVID-19.

It is more appropriate to start with CXR in children with mild to severe symptoms and signs. CT should only be requested if the results are thought to affect the clinical course (accompanying pneumothorax, bacterial co-infection). In certain situations, magnetic resonance imaging (MRI) may also be considered for early diagnosis of COVID-19 pneumonia because it contains little radiation. The first RT-PCR test may be ordered if there are mild to severe findings in children who are negative for COVID-19 if the radiology is compatible with COVID-19. In cases where testing and other facilities are limited, CXR may be requested within the initial assessment tools (Fig. **4**).

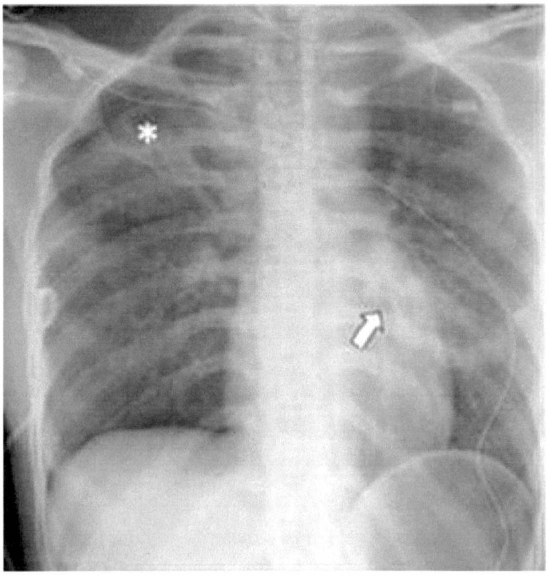

**Fig. (4).** A 15-year-old girl with a history of asthma and a positive COVID-19 RT-PCR test. She was admitted with fever and respiratory distress. Ground-glass opacities are observed in both peripheral (asterisk) and central regions (arrow) on chest radiography. These are vague findings for pediatric COVID-19 infection. At the same time, right apical pneumothorax is seen.

## Can Sequential Cxr be Requested?

Yes, but may be ordered in assessing treatment efficacy, in case of clinical deterioration, and in determining the situations of life support devices ( *e.g.* tracheal intubation).

## Can CXR be Ordered After Recovery?

No, unless there are symptoms. It can be used in the investigation of long-term lung damage if there is clinical suspicion and in cases with severe clinical course.

The main principles in treatment are the management of hypoxia, inhalation therapies, nutritional support, and restoration of fluid and electrolyte balance.

Even in children diagnosed with COVID-19 by PCR, CT findings were mostly reported as negative (77%) (Steinberger, 2020). Among the findings seen are GGO, peripheral distribution, crazy paving pattern, halo, and reversed halo sign. Lesions are predominantly in the lower lobes.

As children get older, the possibility of more severe disease increases. Nevertheless, there have not been great changes in children who have a CT scan and are checked again. Therefore, it is recommended that CT scans should be avoided as much as possible, not to be exposed to unnecessary radiation (Table **3**, Fig. **5**).

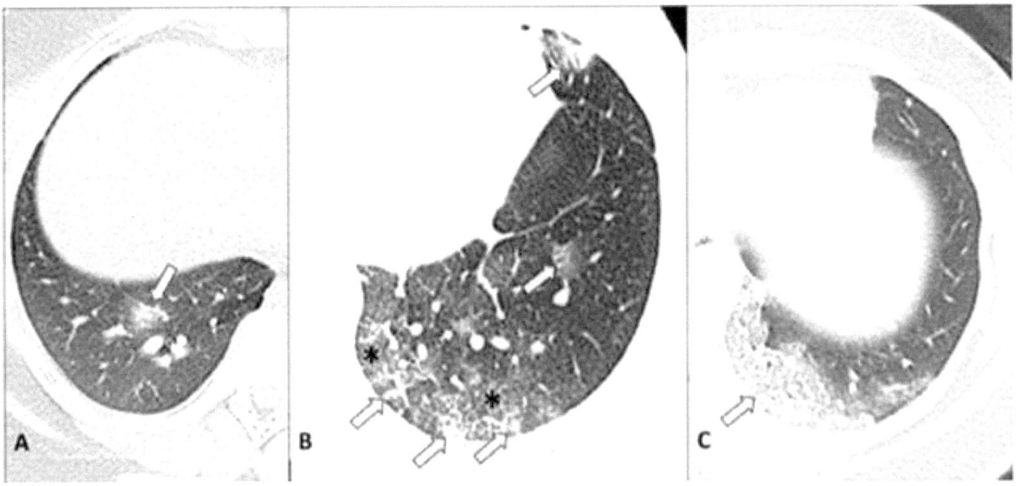


**Fig. (5).** Computed tomography images in 3 different patients in 3 different stages of COVID-19 pneumonia (early, progressive, and advanced). (A) Findings of early phase COVID-19 pneumonia in a 14-year-old girl with Hodgkin lymphoma diagnosed with PCR (+). The patient presented with fever and cough. In the axial section, GGO (arrow) and ill-defined central consolidation are compatible with the "halo" sign. (B) In the progressive phase, a 15-year-old PCR (+) girl has a travel history to Europe. She presented with an increasing cough and shortness of breath. In the axial section, there are GGOs (arrow) and central consolidation areas. Among these areas, GGO (asterisks) started to fill the lung parenchyma. (C) A 16-year-old PCR (+) girl was brought with severe shortness of breath. In the axial section there are areas of confluent consolidation in the lower left posterior lobe (arrow). Findings are consistent with advanced stage COVID-19 pneumonia.

## Discharge Criteria

The Chinese consensus group recommended discharge with the following criteria:

-Fever that does not ensue for three days,

- improvement in respiratory symptoms,
- Negative SARS-CoV-2 test.

Management recommendations are generally same with the adults. However, there are unique features to be individualized in each patient (Fig. **6**).

**Table 3. Findings on X-ray and tomography for pediatric COVID-19 classification.**

| Classification | CXR | CT |
|---|---|---|
| **Typical** | Bilaterally distributed peripheral and / or subpleural "ground glass opacities" (GGO) and / or consolidation | Bilateral, peripheral and / or subpleural GGO and / or predominant consolidation pattern in the lower lobe<br>"Halo" sign (early finding) |
| **Indeterminate** | Unilateral peripheral or central GGO and / or consolidation<br>Bilateral peribronchial thickening and / or peribronchial opacities<br>Multifocal or diffuse GGO and / or consolidation (no specific distribution pattern) | Unilateral peripheral or central GGO and / or consolidation<br>Bilateral peribronchial thickening and / or peribronchial opacities<br>Multifocal or diffuse GGO and / or consolidation (no specific distribution pattern)<br>"Crazy paving" sign |
| **Atypical** | Unilateral segmental or lobar consolidation<br>Central unilateral / bilateral GGO and / or consolidation<br>Single round shape consolidation ± air bronchogram<br>Pleural effusion<br>Lymphadenopathy | Unilateral segmental or lobar consolidation<br>Central unilateral / bilateral GGO and / or consolidation<br>discrete small nodules (centrilobular, tree-i--bud)<br>Lung cavitation<br>Pleural effusion<br>Lymphadenopathy |
| **Negative** | No finding indicative of pneumonia | No finding indicative of pneumonia |

## How Can we Tell Kids About COVID-19?

Charts or tables devised to train healthcare workers, and other adults on the signs and symptoms of the disease will be perceived as hard to understand and boring for kids. Instead, we should prepare fun and playful tools mostly based on visual elements to tell them about anything.

We should always bear in mind that it is very difficult and almost impossible to teach kids anything without amusing and attracting interest and excitement. Different age and developmental groups will require different approaches, images, and tools among children.

A training tool such that as follows will attract kids and in turn, will render them open to get the essential message in the teaching element (Fig. 7).

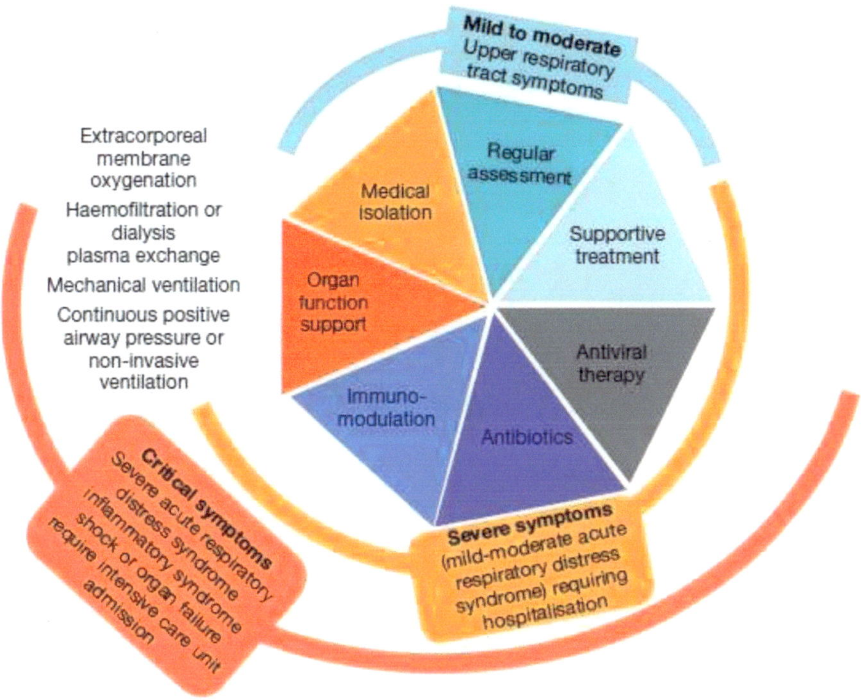


**Fig. (6).** Management recommendations for COVID-19 infection in children and adolescents (Adapted from Mustafa *et al*, 2020).

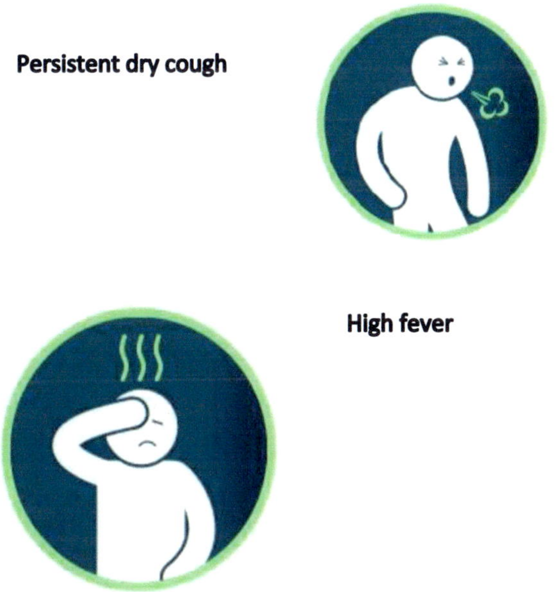


*(Fig. 7) contd.....*

**To stop the spread:**

**Wash your hands at least for 20 to 30 seconds**

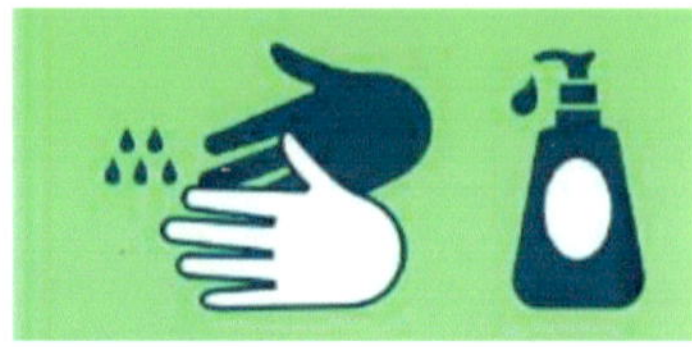

**Cover your face with a napkin or handkerchief while coughing. If these are unavailable, use your inner elbow for this purpose. Never take your barehands to your mouth or face.**

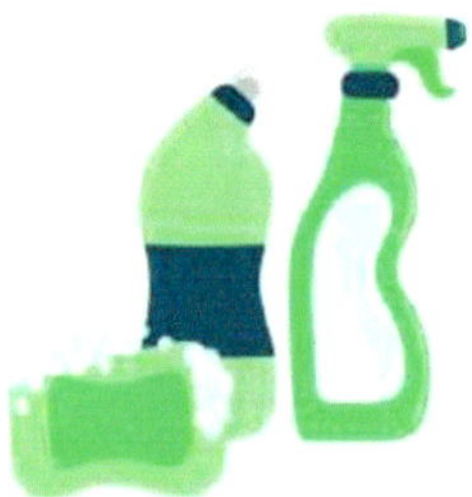

**Your parents can clean the house very frequently. You can help them, but you should stay away from the chemicals they use for this activity. These are very dangerous for you.**

1. 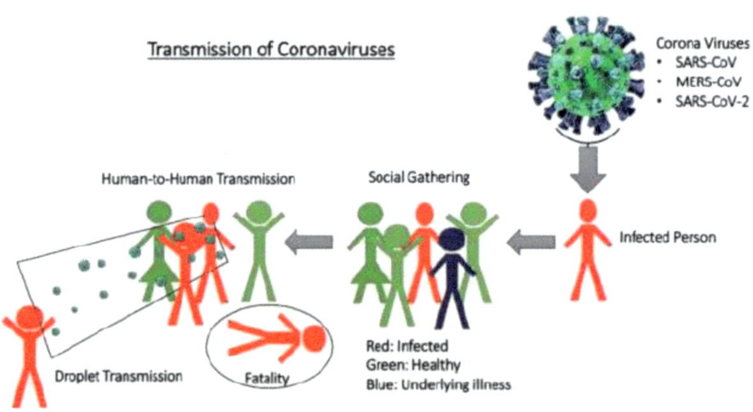

**Stay home should you develop a complaint such as fever or cough. Do not get in close contact with others. Tell your teacher or principals if you feel unwell at school.**

*(Fig. 7) contd.....*

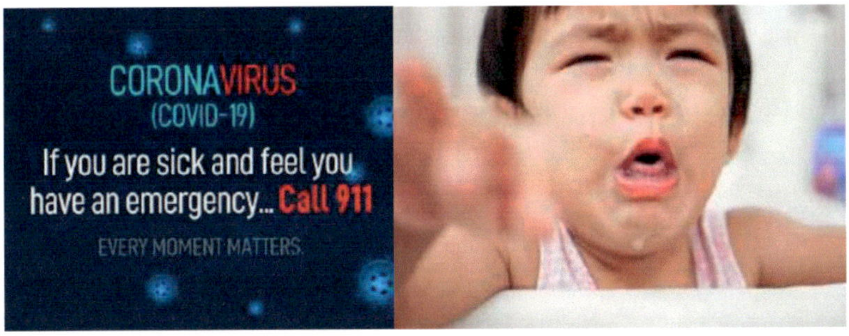


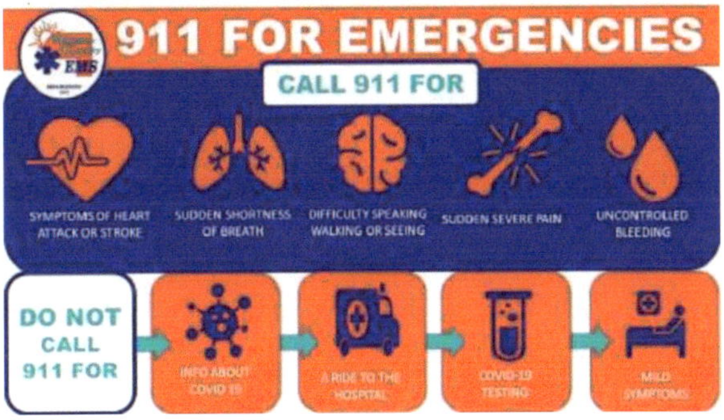


**Dial 911 /112 if you do not get well rapidly and concerned about yourself. Tell the paramedics or other officers about your condition without panic or excitement. Tell your parents also in a calm manner.**

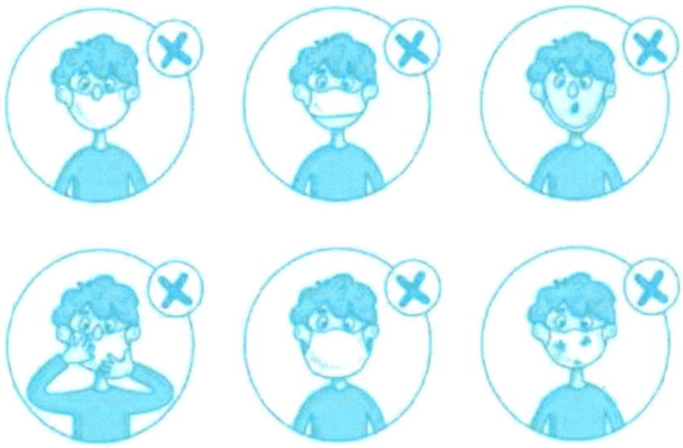

**How to talk about wearing mask properly to your child? (Adapted from Unicef;** https://www.unicef.org/coronavirus/covid-19-and-masks-tips-families

Left upper to right lower:

- Don't pull below the nose
- Don't leave the chin exposed
- Don't pull below the chin
- Don't touch the mask while wearing it
- Don't wear a loose mask
- Don't wear a dirtv. damaged or

**Fig. (7).** How can I realize I am getting sick?.

## CONCLUSION

In pregnant women, the main complaints are fever, cough, shortness of breath and most common finding is lymphopenia, similar to non-pregnant women. The main finding in radiology is peripherally distributed shadowing on CXR, while bilateral diffuse ground glass opacities are typical in tomography.

Children of all age groups may be prone to be infected with COVID-19. There is also no clear gender choice. Although the clinical course is considered to be milder in general compared to adults, it should be known that it may be severe especially in young children and those with comorbid diseases. For example, the fever response is sharper and more common than adults. Most drugs including oseltamivir and chloroquine can be used in children.

## REFERENCES

Assiri, A, Abedi, GR, Al Masri, M, Bin Saeed, A, Gerber, SI & Watson, JT (2016) Middle East Respiratory Syndrome Coronavirus Infection During Pregnancy: A Report of 5 Cases From Saudi Arabia. *Clin Infect Dis,* 63, 951-3.
[http://dx.doi.org/10.1093/cid/ciw412] [PMID: 27358348]

(2020) Severe Outcomes Among Patients with Coronavirus Disease 2019 (COVID-19) — United States, February 12–March 16, 2020. (CDC COVID-19 Response Team). *Morbidity and Mortality Weekly Report,* 2020, 69.

Y, Dong, X, Mo & Y, Hu (2020) Pediatrics 2020;16:16. Epidemiological Characteristics of 2143 Pediatric Patients With 2019 Coronavirus Disease in China. *Pediatrics,* 16, 16.

Dashraath, P (2020) Coronavirus Disease 2019 (COVID-19) Pandemic and Pregnancy. *Am J Obstet Gynecol,* S0002-9378, 30343-4.
[http://dx.doi.org/10.1016/j.ajog.2020.03.021]

Dong, Y, Mo, X & Hu, Y (2020) Epidemiological Characteristics of 2143 Pediatric Patients With 2019 Coronavirus Disease in China. *Pediatrics,* 16, 16.
[http://dx.doi.org/10.1542/peds.2020-0702]

*Epidemiology Working Group for NCIP Epidemic Response, Chinese Center for Disease Control and Prevention.*
[http://dx.doi.org/10.3760/cma.j.issn.0254-6450.2020.02.003] [PMID: 32064853]

Gao, J, Tian, Z & Yang, X (2020) Breakthrough: Chloroquine phosphate has shown apparent efficacy in treatment of COVID-19 associated pneumonia in clinical studies. *Biosci Trends,* 14, 72-3.
[http://dx.doi.org/10.5582/bst.2020.01047] [PMID: 32074550]

Gokcay, G & Keskindermirci, G (2020) Breastmilk and Covid-19 *J Ist Faculty Med.*
[http://dx.doi.org/10.26650/IUITFD.2020.0025]

Guan, WJ, Ni, ZY, Hu, Y, Liang, WH, Ou, CQ, He, JX, Liu, L, Shan, H, Lei, CL, Hui, DSC, Du, B, Li, LJ, Zeng, G, Yuen, KY, Chen, RC, Tang, CL, Wang, T, Chen, PY, Xiang, J, Li, SY, Wang, JL, Liang, ZJ, Peng, YX, Wei, L, Liu, Y, Hu, YH, Peng, P, Wang, JM, Liu, JY, Chen, Z, Li, G, Zheng, ZJ, Qiu, SQ, Luo, J, Ye, CJ, Zhu, SY & Zhong, NS (2020) Clinical Characteristics of Coronavirus Disease 2019 in China. *N Engl J Med,* 382, 1708-20.
[http://dx.doi.org/10.1056/NEJMoa2002032] [PMID: 32109013]

Henry, BM, Lippi, G & Plebani, M (2020) Laboratory abnormalities in children with novel coronavirus disease 2019. *Clin Chem Lab Med,* 58, 1135-8.
[http://dx.doi.org/10.1515/cclm-2020-0272] [PMID: 32172227]

Kong, W & Agarwal, PP (2020) Chest Imaging Appearance of COVID-19 Infection. *Radiol Cardiothorac Imaging,* 2e200028
[http://dx.doi.org/10.1148/ryct.2020200028]

Lawrence, RA & Lawrence, RM (2016) *Breastfeeding: A Guide for the Medical Profession.*Elsevier Philadelphia.

Livingston, E & Bucher, K (2020) Coronavirus Disease 2019 (COVID-19) in Italy. *JAMA,* 323, 1335. [published Online First: 2020/03/18].

[http://dx.doi.org/10.1001/jama.2020.4344] [PMID: 32181795]

Lu, X, Zhang, L, Du, H, Zhang, J, Li, YY, Qu, J, Zhang, W, Wang, Y, Bao, S, Li, Y, Wu, C, Liu, H, Liu, D, Shao, J, Peng, X, Yang, Y, Liu, Z, Xiang, Y, Zhang, F, Silva, RM, Pinkerton, KE, Shen, K, Xiao, H, Xu, S & Wong, GWK (2020) SARS-CoV-2 Infection in Children. *N Engl J Med,* 382, 1663-5. [http://dx.doi.org/10.1056/NEJMc2005073] [PMID: 32187458]

Ludvigsson, JF (2020) Systematic review of COVID-19 in children shows milder cases and a better prognosis than adults. *Acta Paediatr,* 109, 1088-95. [http://dx.doi.org/10.1111/apa.15270] [PMID: 32202343]

Mustafa, NM & A Selim, L (2020) Characterisation of COVID-19 pandemic in paediatric age group: a systematic review and meta-analysis. *J Clin Virol,* 128104395 [http://dx.doi.org/10.1016/j.jcv.2020.104395] [PMID: 32417675]

Naja, M, Wedderburn, L & Ciurtin, C (2020) COVID-19 infection in children and adolescents. *Br J Hosp Med (Lond),* 81, 1-10. [http://dx.doi.org/10.12968/hmed.2020.0321] [PMID: 32845750]

Oncel, MY, Akın, IM & Kanburoglu, MK (2020) A multicenter study on epidemiological and clinical characteristics of 125 newborns born to women infected with COVID-19 by Turkish Neonatal Society. *Eur J Pediatr,* 1-10. [published online ahead of print, 2020 Aug 10]. [published correction appears in Eur J Pediatr. 2020 Aug 22;]. [http://dx.doi.org/10.1007/s00431-020-03767-5] [PMID: 32776309]

Posfay-Barbe, KM, Wagner, N, Gauthey, M, Moussaoui, D, Loevy, N, Diana, A & L'Huillier, AG (2020) COVID-19 in Children and the Dynamics of Infection in Families. *Pediatrics,* 146e20201576 [http://dx.doi.org/10.1542/peds.2020-1576] [PMID: 32457213]

Rasmussen, SA, Smulian, JC, Lednicky, JA, Wen, TS & Jamieson, DJ (2020) Coronavirus Disease 2019 (COVID-19) and pregnancy: what obstetricians need to know. *Am J Obstet Gynecol,* 222, 415-26. [http://dx.doi.org/10.1016/j.ajog.2020.02.017] [PMID: 32105680]

Roberge, RJ, Kim, JH & Powell, JB (2014) N95 respirator use during advanced pregnancy. *Am J Infect Control,* 42, 1097-100. [http://dx.doi.org/10.1016/j.ajic.2014.06.025] [PMID: 25278401]

Schwartz, DA (2020) An Analysis of 38 Pregnant Women with COVID-19, Their Newborn Infants, and Maternal-Fetal Transmission of SARS-CoV-2: Maternal Coronavirus Infections and Pregnancy Outcomes. *Arch Pathol Lab Med* Epub ahead of print [http://dx.doi.org/10.5858/arpa.2020-0901-SA] [PMID: 32180426]

Shen, K, Yang, Y & Wang, T (2020) National Center for Children's Health, Beijing, China; Group of Respirology, Chinese Pediatric Society, Chinese Medical Association; Chinese Medical Doctor Association Committee on Respirology Pediatrics; China Medicine Education Association Committee on Pediatrics; Chinese Research Hospital Association Committee on Pediatrics; Chinese Non-government Medical Institutions Association Committee on Pediatrics; China Association of Traditional Chinese Medicine, Committee on Children's Health and Medicine Research; China News of Drug Information Association, Committee on Children's Safety Medication; Global Pediatric Pulmonology Alliance. Diagnosis, treatment, and prevention of 2019 novel coronavirus infection in children: experts' consensus statement. *World J Pediatr,* 16, 223-31. [http://dx.doi.org/10.1007/s12519-020-00343-7] [PMID: 32034659]

Shi, H, Han, X & Jiang, N (2020) Radiological findings from 81 patients with COVID-19 pneumonia in Wuhan, China: a descriptive study. *Lancet Infect Dis.* [http://dx.doi.org/10.1016/S1473-3099(20)30086-4]

Sprang, G & Silman, M (2013) Posttraumatic stress disorder in parents and youth after health-related disasters. *Disaster Med Public Health Prep,* 7, 105-10. [http://dx.doi.org/10.1017/dmp.2013.22] [PMID: 24618142]

Steinberger, S, Lin, B, Bernheim, A, Chung, M, Gao, Y, Xie, Z, Zhao, T, Xia, J, Mei, X & Little, BP (2020)

CT Features of Coronavirus Disease (COVID-19) in 30 Pediatric Patients. *AJR Am J Roentgenol,* 215, 1303-11.
[http://dx.doi.org/10.2214/AJR.20.23145] [PMID: 32442030]

Tong, PS, Kale, AS, Ng, K, Loke, AP, Choolani, MA, Lim, CL, Chan, YH, Chong, YS, Tambyah, PA & Yong, EL (2015) Respiratory consequences of N95-type Mask usage in pregnant healthcare workers-a controlled clinical study. *Antimicrob Resist Infect Control,* 4, 48-57.
[http://dx.doi.org/10.1186/s13756-015-0086-z] [PMID: 26579222]

Wang, G, Zhang, Y & Zhao, J (2020) *Mitigate the effects of home confinement on children during the COVID-19 outbreak*
[http://dx.doi.org/10.1016/S0140-6736(20)30547-X]

WHO. Report of the WHO-China Joint Mission on Coronavirus Disease 2019 (COVID-19) https://www.who.int/docs/default-source/coronaviruse/who-china-joint-mission-on-covid-19-final-report.pdf

Wong, SF, Chow, KM, Leung, TN, Ng, WF, Ng, TK, Shek, CC, Ng, PC, Lam, PW, Ho, LC, To, WW, Lai, ST, Yan, WW & Tan, PY (2004) Pregnancy and perinatal outcomes of women with severe acute respiratory syndrome. *Am J Obstet Gynecol,* 191, 292-7.
[http://dx.doi.org/10.1016/j.ajog.2003.11.019] [PMID: 15295381]

Zhu, H, Wang, L, Fang, C, Peng, S, Zhang, L, Chang, G, Xia, S & Zhou, W (2020) Clinical analysis of 10 neonates born to mothers with 2019-nCoV pneumonia. *Transl Pediatr,* 9, 51-60.
[http://dx.doi.org/10.21037/tp.2020.02.06] [PMID: 32154135]

# CHAPTER 13

# COVID-19 and The Elderly: Is It Different From The Young?

**Abstract:** There are some differences in the way the symptoms are perceived and expressed by the elderly. Senses and perception can be blunted due to difficulties and impairments in the structure and function of the nerves. For example, the perception of pain, which is sharper and more severe in young people, can be felt milder, more uncertain, or ill-defined in the elderly.

In the elderly, too, the main complaints can be listed as fever, dry cough, and shortness of breath. There may be mild to severe sore throat, loss of sense of smell, weakness, muscle and joint pain, headache, diarrhea, rarely runny nose, and cough with phlegm. They are more prone to have a more severe disease course. Researchers reported that the fatality rate in all cases in China was 1.4%, while it was 22% in cases over 80 years old. This chapter aims to delineate specific difficulties the elderly face when they were infected with COVID-19 and to discuss possible solutions for this vulnerable group in the pandemic period.

**Keywords:** COVID-19, Diagnosis, Elderly, Geriatric care, Pandemic, Treatment.

Case example

The daughter of the 84-year-old nursing home patient from Izmir calls 911 (112 in Turkey). The patient has pre-diabetes, chronic lung disease, and a history of deep vein thrombosis. He complained of cough, runny nose, and mild fever in the past week. His fever has not been recorded today. His cough has gradually increased recently. The patient did not travel, but relatives from Europe visited him three weeks ago. They did not tell about any complaints. Her fingerstick blood sugar has been found slightly elevated, and her daughter says she looks worse than usual.

Advancing age is not just something in the calendar; instead, it is impaired cellular repair mechanisms, progressive senescence of every part of the body, and finally, suffering from depletion of physiological reserves of the bodily systems for homeostasis.

Ozgur KARCIOGLU, Selman YENIOCAK and Mandana HOSSEINZADEH

## WHAT KIND OF SYMPTOMS SHOULD RAISE SUSPICION OF COVID-19 IN THE ELDERLY?

In fact, the complaints and symptoms of young and middle-aged people are not very different. Nevertheless, there will be some differences in the way the symptoms are perceived, and expressed. Senses and perception can be blunted due to difficulties and impairments in the structure and function of the nerves. For example, the perception of pain, which is sharper and more severe in young people, can be felt milder, more uncertain, or ill-defined in the elderly.

To give an extreme example, elderly people can even have a heart attack without chest pain. Fever does not increase sharply in the elderly as in young people. Similarly, we can think that all symptoms related to COVID-19 can be felt lighter, so the risk of being unrecognized will be substantial.

Pearl: In the elderly, too, the main complaints can be listed as fever, dry cough, and shortness of breath. There may be mild to severe sore throat, loss of sense of smell, weakness, muscle and joint pain, diarrhea, rarely runny nose, and cough with phlegm.

The important point here is that each patient will experience the disease with a different combination of symptoms and symptoms. For example, one patient will be referred as shortness of breath and sore throat, fever and cough in the other patient, diarrhea, and muscle pain in the other.

## IS THERE ANY DIFFERENCE BETWEEN OTHER EPIDEMICS AND COVID-19 IN THIS REGARD?

Yes. SARS in 2002, H1N1 (swine flu) in 2009, and MERS in 2012 also had a severe impact on the society, but there was no different involvement according to age within the short time periods they reigned. Their case fatality rate was higher than COVID-19, at 35% and 10%, yet the effect size was significantly smaller.

## IS COVID-19 DIFFERENT IN THE ELDERLY?

Yes. Not only COVID-19, but almost all diseases, from heart attack to brain infarction, have a different presentation and clinical course in older individuals. For example, while the time from the onset of symptoms to death is 11.5 days in the elderly with COVID-19, it is 14 days in young people (Wang *et al*, 2020).

Difficulties in history taking, signs and symptoms are often subtler, recovery takes longer time, and differences in the effects of drugs are the main points that draw attention. Beyond these, comorbidities directly affect the mortality rate.

The elderly is more susceptible to infections, including COVID-19, due to weak immunity. They are also slower in recovery. The complications of the disease and adverse effects of the drugs and other treatment complications can be more frequent and severe.

If there is smoking, vitamin deficiency, diabetes mellitus, protracted course and difficulty in recovery will be more pronounced.

In the report published by the WHO in the first months of the pandemics, the fatality rate in all cases in China was 1.4%, while it was 22% in cases over 80 years old.

23% of the population in Italy is 65 years old and above. Close to 90% of COVID-19 deaths have been recorded in individuals aged 70 and over (WSJ). Those over the age of 80 constituted 58% of deaths. It is also known that these rates vary according to geography and countries. For example, the percentage of inflicted elderly people in Europe is much higher than those in the Middle East or Africa, directly reflecting the characteristics in the age distribution of the population besides the age predilections of the virus.

On March 16, 2020, CDC stated that the test (PCR) should be done first for the elderly, and those with chronic comorbid diseases, and immunosuppression. In practice, it has been reported that elderly patients with fever and respiratory symptoms who have negative influenza tests should undergo COVID test immediately. It was also noted that testing the elderly with mild symptoms and complaints by taking them in other environments, not immediately to ED, may prevent excessive crowdedness in EDs (Malone *et al*, 2020) (Fig. **1**).

## IS THERE A DIFFERENCE IN COMPLAINTS AND FINDINGS IN ELDERLY PEOPLE WITH COVID-19 COMPARED TO YOUNG PEOPLE?

Yes. For example:

**Fever** is one of the main complaints. Due to the compromised immune system and other problems of the elderly, they cannot generate the fever response like young people. It has been reported that the fever response is suppressed in elderly patients diagnosed with COVID-19 (High, 2020). In a study, fever was found in only 1/3 of the elderly at the first admission (Lam, 2016). The temperature limit is considered as 37.8C in a single measurement or 37.3C in consecutive measurements.

**Cough:** The elderly may experience chronic cough problems due to different reasons such as long-term smoking and chronic lung diseases. Therefore, it may be difficult for them to notice cough triggered by COVID-19.

**Shortness of breath:** For reasons similar to cough, many chronic problems may cause shortness of breath in the elderly. There is difficulty in distinguishing this from newly developed shortness of breath due to COVID-19. Furthermore, the development of shortness of breath in the elderly may cause rapid deterioration due to the decrease in other organ reserves.

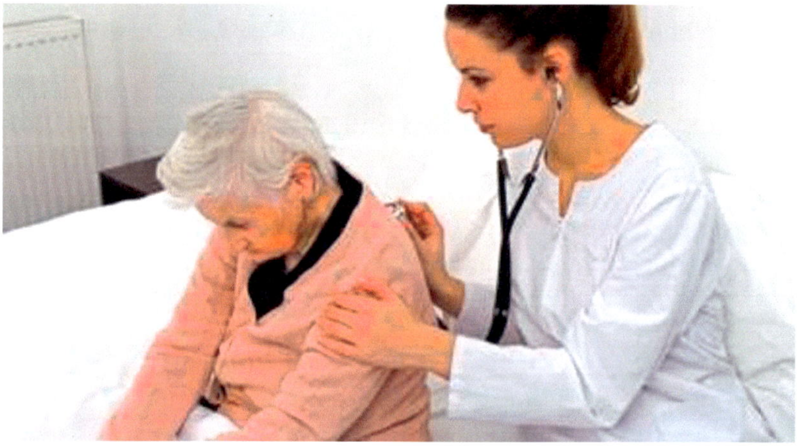

**Fig. (1).** Evaluation of the elderly patient may necessitate a suitable environment in or outside the emergency department to elicit a thorough history and elaborate examination.

**Tachycardia**: An expected finding in severe COVID-19 cases. Under normal conditions, a pulse rate above 100 is tachycardia and often indicates that something is wrong in the body. This finding can be hidden, as the elderly use many medications due to heart disease and high blood pressure. Beta-blockers and calcium channel blockers typically diminish the tachycardia response. This issue should be asked while evaluating the heart rate of any given patient.

**Consciousness and cognitive functions:** It is the most difficult issue to evaluate in the elderly. Even with language barriers and speech difficulties aside, the elderly may have numerous impairments inflicting mental status and cognition in disease processes, such that circulatory deficiencies and respiratory distress causing hypotension and hypoxia.

**Anosmia:** It has been accepted to be one of the most specific findings. In other words, in the event that sudden loss of smell is accompanied by one or more of the other complaints and findings, it should prompt one think of COVID-19 unless proven otherwise. Due to the deterioration of nerve functions in the elderly, this will not be as sharp as in young people.

**Muscle and joint aches:** It may be difficult to differentiate de novo ones in the elderly from those reasons such as chronic rheumatic diseases.

**Loss of appetite, nausea:** The elderly is mostly already lacking appetite. The effects of various medications used, liver failure or pancreatitis and coronary ischemia or CVA may also cause nausea. The physician should perform a complete examination to rule out differential diagnoses.

**Diarrhea:** Due to the slow functioning of the immune system, the impairment of antibody production and gastric acid release, resistance to microbial agents from the digestive system decreases, as a result, gastroenteritis and diarrhea are more common. This can cause the diarrhea in COVID-19 to be mixed with diarrhea precipitated by other causes.

**Fatigue:** There are many elderly people who have long been suffering from weakness due to malnutrition and other chronic conditions.

With all these difficulties, there may be delays in the recognition and treatment of COVID-19 as in almost any disease in the elderly, and even this can lead to sudden deterioration and death.

## THERE ARE SPECIAL DIFFICULTIES FOR THE ELDERLY IN THE TREATMENT AND FOLLOW-UP PROCESS.

1. The isolation period will pose special difficulties for the elderly than the young, because they have some essential requirements in the medium to long term. They are dependent on others for many issues ranging from walking aid to food and needs for self-care and may have difficulties with their travel restrictions.
2. Due to cognitive problems, there may be difficulties in administering the treatment as necessary, for example taking medications on time.
3. During the follow-up process at home, it will be more difficult to recognize new problems and take action, *e.g.,* it will be difficult for them to notice that their fever rises again, a sore throat, *etc.* appears.
4. The already fragile psychology of the elderly can be destroyed by reduced social support and depression may occur more frequently or become more severe. This may lead to failure of treatment and malnutrition. It has also been revealed that in such cases the rate of suicide also increases.

Medications given to young people in treatments may not be suitable for elderly people due to organ failure. For example, if there is kidney failure, it may not be appropriate to administer a drug that is excreted from the kidney through the urine, or a dose reduction may be required. Likewise, drug interactions may have grave consequences in the elderly. The treatment regimen should not be regulated without taking previous medications into account. Differences in the metabolism of the elderly should also be taken into account.

Since the elderly cannot express their feelings and complaints sufficiently, such as thirst, they easily become dehydrated, which can lead to impaired cognitive functions, altered level of consciousness, coma, and even delirium.

## WHAT CAN BE DONE?

- Due to the difficulties in the diagnostic processes of COVID-19, the issue of atypical presentations should be emphasized in the training of triage and emergency healthcare workers. Experience will be needed in interpreting fever, pulse rate, and shortness of breath.
- The elderly who receive home treatment, in isolation or in quarantine should be called regularly from the administrative (or observatory) center, and technological tools such as visual protection and follow up should be put into use when appropriate.
- Interactions of drug doses in the elderly, problems in elimination, and differences in metabolism should be considered in treatment decisions.
- Knowing that their psychology is fragile, one should be alert to issues such as depression and suicidal thoughts, and if necessary, support from a clinical psychologist or psychiatrist should be obtained.

## CONCLUSION

It is known that the elderly is more susceptible to infections, including COVID-19, due to weak immunity. They are also slower in recovery. The complications of the disease and adverse effects of the drugs and other treatment complications can be more frequent and severe. Difficulties in history taking, signs and symptoms are often subtler, recovery takes longer time, and differences in the effects of drugs are the main points that draw attention. Beyond these, comorbidities directly affect the mortality rate. Physicians should be alert for rapid deterioration and need for aggressive management in the elderly with COVID-19.

## REFERENCES

High, KP, Bradley, SF, Gravenstein, S, Mehr, DR, Quagliarello, VJ, Richards, C & Yoshikawa, TT (2009) Clinical practice guideline for the evaluation of fever and infection in older adult residents of long-term care facilities: 2008 update by the Infectious Diseases Society of America. *Clin Infect Dis,* 48, 149-71. [http://dx.doi.org/10.1086/595683] [PMID: 19072244]

With Aging Population, Has World's Highest Daily Deaths from Virus *Wall Street Journal Italy.*https://www.wsj.com/articles/italy-with-elderly-population-has-worlds-highest-death--ate-from-virus-11583785086

Lam, PP, Coleman, BL & Green, K (2016) Predictors of influenza among older adults in the ED. *BMC Infect Dis,* 16, 615.
[http://dx.doi.org/10.1186/s12879-016-1966-4] [PMID: 27793117]

Malone, ML, Hogan, TM & Perry, A (2020) COVID-19 in Older Adults: Key Points for Emergency Department Providers. *J Geriatr Emerg Med,* 1, 1-11.

Wang, G, Wu, C, Zhang, Q, Yu, B, Lü, J, Zhang, S, Wu, G, Wu, Y & Zhong, Y (2020) Clinical characteristics and the risk factors for severe events of elderly coronavirus disease 2019 patients. *Zhong Nan Da Xue Xue Bao Yi Xue Ban,* 45, 542-8.
[http://dx.doi.org/10.11817/j.issn.1672-7347.2020.200292] [PMID: 32879104]

# CHAPTER 14

# Principles of Treatment

**Abstract:** It is well established that there is no 'standard' protocol for the treatment of COVID-19. The use of certain antiviral agents and antibiotics such as azithromycin has been concluded to be beneficial, and therefore, their use has been recommended. Namely, remdesivir and favipiravir may be the best potential antiviral drugs for the treatment of COVID-19. However, treatments should be tailored for every given patient in regard to the signs and symptoms, the severity of the disease, age and comorbid diseases, organ failures, phase of the disease, pregnancy status, and possible drug interactions.

The use of NSAIDs as an antipyretic, analgesic, and anti-inflammatory agents appears to be indicated in viral infections such as COVID-19, also during pandemic periods. There is no evidence to support NSAIDs not to be used in COVID-19 infections due to their side effects. NSAIDs are used after paracetamol, if necessary, to manage the symptoms of COVID-19.

Although it has been postulated that deficiencies of certain vitamins and minerals (*e.g.*, vitamins C and D), multi-center, community-based, well-designed studies are necessary to clarify their relationship with COVID-19, especially before recommending them for treatment.

In brief, treatments should be individualized, and evidence-based principles must be followed.

**Keywords:** Antibiotics, Antivirals, COVID-19, NSAID, Pandemic, Treatment, Vitamin C, Vitamin D.

## ANTIVIRALS

The sooner antiviral agents are started in the treatment of COVID-19, the more effective the treatment of the disease can be anticipated. Delayed antiviral therapy has previously been declared as an independent risk factor for long-term viral spread and detection of viruses and is also associated with grave outcomes (Wang *et al*, , 2018).

There is no established 'standard' protocol for the treatment of COVID-19. The use of certain antiviral agents has been concluded to be beneficial , and therefore,

**Ozgur KARCIOGLU, Selman YENIOCAK and Mandana HOSSEINZADEH**

their use has been recommended (Fig. **1**). However, it is not recommended to use three or more antiviral drugs simultaneously (Diagnosis and Treatment Protocol for Novel Coronavirus Pneumonia. Trial Version 7).

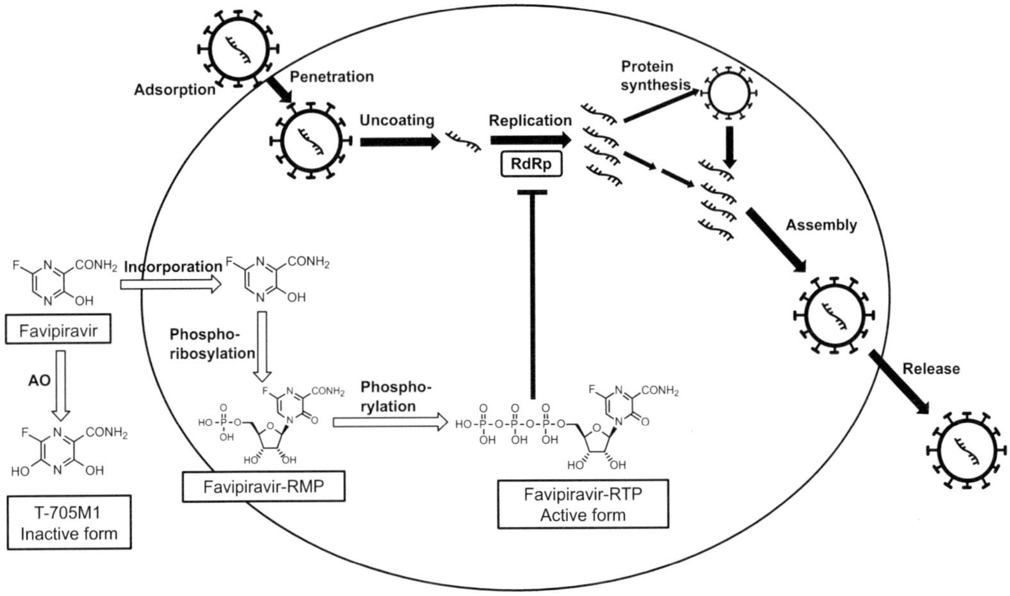


**Fig. (1).** The mechanism of action of favipiravir (T-705) against the virus. Favipiravir is incorporated into cells and transformed by host cells into favipiravir ibofuranosyl - 5 ′ - triphosphate (favipiravir - RTP). The triphosphate form, favipiravir-RTP, inhibits the activity of RNA-dependent RNA polymerase (RdRp) of RNA viruses. AO: Aldehyde oxidase; RMP: Ribosyl monophosphate

Antiviral agents that can be used in the management of COVID-19 were listed in Table **1**.

**Table 1. Antiviral Agents That Can Be Used in The Management of Covid-19.**

| **I. Nucleotide Analogues** |
|---|
| Favipiravir |
| Ribavirin |
| Remdesivir |
| Nafamostat |
| Nitazoxanide |
| Valipiravir |
| **II. Neuraminidase inhibitors** |
| Oseltamivir |
| Zanamivir |

*(Table 1) cont.....*

| **I. Nucleotide Analogues** |
|---|
| Peramivir |
| **III. Lopinavir/ Ritonavir** (Kaletra ®) |
| **IV. Umifenovir** (Arbidol ®) |

## Nucleotide Analogues (NA)

NA have different mechanisms of action, including lethal mutagenesis, specific or non-specific chain termination, and inhibition of nucleotide biosynthesis (Arabi *et al*, , 2018). Although some treatment options awaiting validation have been reported in the treatment of COVID-19, including various broad-spectrum antivirals such as valipiravir and remdesivir, there are currently no specific antiviral drugs that have been identified (Beigel *et al*, 2019; Li *et al*, 2020).

### *1. Favipiravir*

Favipiravir (FPV) is an antiviral agent derived from pyrazine carboxamide 6-Fluoro-3-hydroxy-pyrazine-2-carboxamide. It acts by transforming favipiravir into ibofuranosyl-5′-triphosphate (T - 705 - RTP), which is its active metabolite by being ribosylated and phosphorylated in the cell (Furuta *et al*, 2017). T - 705 - RTP competes with purine nucleosides and interferes with viral replication by being incorporated into the viral RNA. Thus potentially inhibiting RNA-dependent RNA polymerase (RdRp) of RNA viruses (Fig. **1**, Furuta *et al*, , 2005).

It is administered in COVID-19 with the thought that it shortens the time for relief of symptoms. It stops viral replication by inhibiting RNA polymerase on CoV (Mifsud *et al*, 2019; Wang *et al*, 2020). In a study conducted in China on its effectiveness in COVID-19 treatment, it was concluded that FPV is useful. FPV is administered 1600 mg twice a day on the first day and 600 mg in 2nd-14$^{th}$ day. LPV / RTV was orally at 400/100 mg twice a day. Additionally, all participants received standard care. In this study, patients treated with FPV were reported to have faster viral clearance and better radiological recovery than patients treated with LPV / RTV. Diarrhea (5.71%) and liver-kidney damage (2.86%) were seen as side effects (Cai *et al*, 2020).

FPV is 54% bound to plasma proteins. The elimination half-life is about 2 to 5.5 hours, and the bioavailability rate is 97.6%. The mean Cmax is 51.5 μg / mL, the main volume of distribution is 15-20 L, and its metabolites are excreted by the kidneys. Use of FPV in patients with moderate renal impairment (GFR 30-60 ml / min) causes a 1.5-fold increase in Cmin compared to patients with normal renal function; however, there is no data regarding its use in patients with GFR <30 mL / min (Joshi *et al*, 2020).

## Posology

### a) Treatment Dose:

1800 mg twice daily on day 1, followed by 600-800 mg twice daily for up to 14 days in mild to moderate COVID-19.

**b) Prophylaxis:** 1600 mg orally twice a day on day 1, then 2-25. 600-800 mg twice a day (NCT04448119) every day.

In order to determine the potential use and reliability of FPV and other antivirals in COVID-19, literature data evaluating the use of FPV in various databases were searched (Pilkington *et al*, 2020). Within the scope of this study, the data of 29 studies and 4299 patients and the side effects were examined The incidence of the compared side effects is shown in Table **2** below.

**Table 2. Incidences of side effects (SE) attributed to oseltamivir, umifenovir, lopinavir / ritonavir and FPV.**

| - | FPV SE | Oseltamivir, Umifenovir, Lopinavir/Ritonavir SE |
|---|---|---|
| Grade 1-4 SE | 28,2% | 28,4% |
| SE that necessitates discontinuation of the drug | 1,1% | 1,2% |
| Serious SE | 0,4% | 0,4% |
| Gastrointestinal SE | 8,7% | 11,5% |
| Hyperuricemia | 5,8% | 1,3% |

According to this study, it was concluded that FPV shows a favorable safety profile for total and serious side effects, and is safe and tolerable in short-term use.

In a study where 1798 articles were compiled to analyze the efficacy and safety of FPV in the treatment of COVID-19, the group who received FPV + standard care treatment, the control group who received other antivirals + standard care + supportive care (respiratory support, antibiotics, immunomodulators, and some herbal medicines) compared (Shrestha *et al*, , 2020). In this study, clinical recovery following treatment with FVP in COVID-19 patients, the time when RT-PCR turned negative after treatment, side effects during treatment, $O_2$ and mechanical ventilation requirements were searched for. Controlled clinical trials, prospective and retrospective studies using FPV in the management of COVID-19 patients were included in qualitative analysis, studies with treatment and control groups were included in quantitative analysis. As a result of this study, the following data were obtained:

1. There was no significant difference in risk ratios between both groups (day 7: RR 1.13, 95% CI 0.55 to 2.33; day 14: RR 1.06, 95% CI 0.84 to 1.33)
2. It was concluded that there was no significant risk difference (RD) for viral clearance between both groups (day 7: RD 0.06, 95% CI - 0.34 to 0.45; day 14: RD 0.03, 95% CI - 0.17 to 0.24)
3. Treatment group overall risk ratios (RR) compared with the control group showed a significant improvement in clinical improvement and improvement of CT findings on days 7 and 14 of treatment (Day 7: RR 1.25, 95% CI, 1.01 to 1.53 Day 14: RR 1.29, 95% CI, 1.08 to 1.54).
4. Lack of improvement in clinical symptoms and signs and lack of improvement in CT findings were reported to be lower in the treatment group than in the control group albeit not statistically significant (OR 0.59, 95% CI, 0.30 to 1.14; participants: 376; studies: 3; I2: %) 39).
5. The need for $O_2$ support in the treatment group was reduced, but it was not statistically significant (OR 0.76).
6. It was concluded that there was a statistically insignificant decrease in tolerable side effects such as increased transaminases, nausea, vomiting, and diarrhea observed in the treatment group (OR 0.69). There were no serious life-threatening adverse effects following FPV therapy.

In this study, it was concluded that although there was no significant difference in viral clearance, $O_2$ supplementation requirement and side effect profile, patients achieved remarkable clinical and radiological improvements following FPV treatment compared to the control group.

**Side Effects:** The most common side effects are hyperuricemia (15.5%) and AST-ALT increase (7.4%), while neutropenia, triglyceride increase, mild-moderate diarrhea, decrease in body weight, vomiting and decrease in locomotor activity, psychiatric symptoms are other known side effects (Joshi *et al*, 2020).

**Contraindications:** It is contraindicated in pregnancy and lactating women, hypersensitivity, severe hepatic, and renal failure. It is also avoided in pregnant and suspected pregnant women due to its teratogenic potential observed in animal studies. It is recommended to use effective contraceptive methods during treatment and up to 7 days after treatment. It should be administered with caution in hyperuricemia patients with gout or a history of gout. (Nagata *et al*, 2015; Delang *et al*, 2018).

In conclusion, FPV appears to be a reasonable option among the best antiviral drugs that can be used in the treatment of COVID-19.

## *2. Ribavirin*

Ribavirin (RBV) is the most commonly used synthetic agent with broad spectrum antiviral activity against many DNA and RNA viruses. It inhibits RNA replication by blocking the viral replicase protein (Chu *et al*, 2004). RBV was used in combination with cortisone in the Hong Kong SARS 2003 epidemic, oseltamivir + cortisone in some centers, and in another study conducted in Canada in the same epidemic, it was used in combination with antibiotics + oseltamivir (Poutanen *et al*, 2003). It was used in empirical therapy shortly after the onset of the COVID-19 outbreak, with the greatest benefit being reported in early treatment of pneumonia before development of sepsis or organ failure (Peiris *et al*, 2003; Lee *et al*, 2003; Habib *et al*, 2019).

RBV causes hypocalcemia and hypomagnesemia and decreases hemoglobin concentrations. This feature impairs its antiviral efficacy against COVID-19 (Beigel *et al*, 2019).

Ribavirin is recommended to be used in combination with ifn-alpha or lpv / rtv. studies have shown that the risk of developing ards and death is lower in patients treated with combined drugs.

It is used by 500 mg IV injection in adults, for a maximum of 10 days (Diagnosis and Treatment Protocol for Novel Coronavirus Pneumonia. Trial Version 7).

## *3. Remdesivir (GS-5734)*

Remdesivir (RDV) is a phosphoramidate prodrug, an adenosine nucleotide analogue with broad-spectrum antiviral activity against filoviruses, paramyxoviruses, pneumoviruses, pathogenic CoVs such as SARS-CoV and MERS-CoV (Sheahan *et al*, 2017).

It acts by inhibiting SARS-CoV and MERS-CoV replication in animal model tissue cultures. It has shown antiviral activity in the treatment of MERS and SARS in animal models caused by CoVs (Sheahan *et al*, 2017; Agostini *et al*, 2018). RDV has broad spectrum anti-CoV activity. It has been suggested that RDV may also be an option for the treatment of COVID-19 patients (Brown *et al*, 2019; Liu *et al*, 2020).

RDV + INF-β was shown to have superior antiviral activity than LPV / RTV in both *in vitro* and MERS-CoV mouse model (Sheahan *et al*, 2017). It has been reported that the prophylactic LPV / RTV + INF-β combination reduces virus titers without affecting other disease parameters, while the therapeutic LPV / RTV + INF-β combination improves lung function, but does not reduce virus replication or severe lung pathology. Therefore, it has been postulated that RDV may be the best potential antiviral drug for the treatment of COVID-19. Today, there are some unfinished studies that have been initiated to evaluate the efficacy and safety of RDV in patients hospitalized with COVID-19 infection (Tian *et al*, 2020).

A randomized, double-blind, placebo-controlled, multicenter study of RDV was conducted in China between February and March, 2020 (Wang *et al*, 2020). A total of 237 patients hospitalized with pneumonia caused by SARS-CoV-2 were included in the study. The first group received a 200 mg IV RDV loading dose on day 1, followed by a 100 mg / day IV RDV maintenance dose on days 2 to 10, and placebo for 10 days in the second group. RDV treatment did not result in a significant change in clinical recovery times (hazard ratio 1 · 23 [95% CI 0 · 87-1 · 75]). Side effects were reported in 102 (66%) patients in the first group receiving RDV treatment, and in 50 (64%) patients in the second group receiving placebo treatment. These side effects are cited in the Table **3**. As a result of this study, it has been reported that there is no benefit of RDV treatment in the clinical improvement of COVID-19.

The largest-ever study on RDV against COVID-19 is an international multi-center, double-blind, randomized, placebo-controlled study conducted between February and April, 2020 (Beigel *et al*, 2020). A total of 1063 patients with COVID-19 pneumonia were randomly divided into two groups to receive IV RDV and placebo in addition to supportive care. Median time to recovery was reported as 11 (95% CI, 9 to 12) days for group 1 receiving RDV treatment, and 15 (95% CI, 12 to 19) days for the other group receiving placebo treatment. In addition, the 14-day mortality rates were 7.1% in the RDV group and 11.9% in the placebo group (hazard ratio for death, 0.70; 95% CI, 0.47 to 1.04). Serious side effects were reported in 114 patients (21.1%) of the first group of patients receiving RDV treatment and in 141 (27.0%) of the second group patients who received placebo treatment. Side effects in the RDV group were noted as anemia in 47 (9.0%) patients, acute kidney injury, increased serum creatinine or reduced creatinine clearance in 38 (7.3%) patients, fever in 17 (3.3%) patients, hyperglycemia or increased blood glucose level was observed in 17 (3.3%) patients, and liver enzyme elevation in 31 (5.9%) patients. Main findings from the study of Beigel *et al*, are shown in the Table **4**.

In critical COVID-19 cases, RDV is given by 200 mg IV in 30 minutes; then 100 mg is given for 2 to 10 days. If RDV cannot be used or is contraindicated, the same dose of crushed hydroxychloroquine (HCQ) or chloroquine phosphate (CQ) can be given via NG (Interim Clinical Guidance for Patients Suspected of / Confirmed with COVID-19 in Belgium.16 Mars 2020; Version 3). It can be used in patients with confirmed COVID-19 disease who are treated with mechanical ventilation in the ICU. However, it is not used in patients with multiorgan failure, those with creatinine clearance <30 ml / min, high transaminases and concomitant use of LPV / RTV drug; those treated with dialysis or hemofiltration, and receiving inotropic agents. These criteria mean that most patients will not be eligible for RDV use.

**Table 3. The side effects and their rates in group members who received RDV and placebo treatment (Adapted from Wang *et al*, 2020).**

| - | **RDV Group** | **Placebo Group** |
|---|---|---|
| - | **N=158**<br>**%/n** | **N=79**<br>**%/n** |
| **Side/ Adverse Effects** | 66 / 102 | 64 / 50 |
| Constipation | 14 / 21 | 15 / 12 |
| Hypoalbuminemia | 13 / 20 | 15 / 12 |
| Hypokalemia | 12 / 18 | 14 / 11 |
| Anemia | 12 / 18 | 15 / 12 |
| Rash | 12 / 18 | 3 / 2 |
| Thrombocytopenia | 10 / 16 | 6 / 5 |
| Elevated bilirubin levels | 10 / 15 | 9 / 7 |
| Leukocytosis | 7 / 11 | 8 / 6 |
| Hyperglycemia | 7 / 11 | 8 / 6 |
| Increased neutrophils | 6 / 10 | 5 / 4 |
| Blood urea nitrogen (BUN) increased | 6 / 10 | 6 / 5 |
| Hyperlipidemia | 6 / 10 | 10 / 8 |
| Nausea | 5 /8 | 3 / 2 |
| Elevated liver function tests | 5 / 7 | 12 / 9 |
| Diarrhea | 3 / 5 | 3 / 2 |
| Vomiting | 3 /4 | 3 / 2 |
| Hyponatremia | 3 /4 | 3 / 2 |
| Hyperkalemia | 3 / 4 | 1 / 1 |

**Table 4. Important data from the study of Beigel *et al*, (Beigel *et al*, 2020).**

| **Variable / Characteristic** | **RDV Group** | **Placebo Group** |
|---|---|---|
| **Number of patients** | 541 | 522 |
| **Median Recovery Time** | 11 | 15 |
| **Mortality Rates (14 days) (%)** | 7,1 | 11,9 |

*(Table 4) cont.....*

| Variable / Characteristic | RDV Group | Placebo Group |
|---|---|---|
| **Incidences of Serious Side Effects (% / n)** | 21,1 / 114 | 27,0 / 141 |
| -Anemia | 9,0 / 47 | 7,9 / 43 |
| - Renal complications | 7,3 / 38 | 7,4 / 40 |
| - Fever | 3,3 / 17 | 5,0 / 27 |
| - Hyperglycemia | 3,3 / 17 | 4,1 / 22 |
| - Elevated liver function tests | 5,9 / 31 | 4,1 / 22 |

## *4. Nafamostat Mesylate*

This antiviral drug, which is a synthetic serine protease inhibitor, provides anti-infective effect by reducing cathepsin B release and preventing membrane fusion. It is used in influenza, MERS, and Ebola virus diseases. The treatment of COVID-19 infection is still under investigation (Hsieh *et al*, 2007; Nishimura *et al*, 2015). It has been reported to block cell entry of SARS-CoV-2 (McKee *et al*, 2020).

## *5. Nitazoxanide*

This antiprotozoal drug regulates growth, reproduction, and survival of a number of extracellular and intracellular protozoans, helminths, anaerobic and microaerophilic bacteria, and viruses. It has been reported to be effective against a wide variety of viruses, including animal or human CoVs (Rossignol *et al*, 2016).

It is a broad spectrum antiviral agent that is being developed for the treatment of influenza and other respiratory viral infections. Phase 3 clinical research is currently underway for acute uncomplicated influenza treatment. In *in vitro* studies, tizoxanide, an active circulating metabolite of nitazoxanide, inhibits the growth of a wide variety of influenza A and B strains, including influenza A subtypes H1N1, H3N2, H3N2v, H3N8, H5N9, H7N1 and oseltamivir resistant strains. Tizoxanide inhibits the replication of a wide variety of other RNA and DNA viruses, including RSV, parainfluenza, coronavirus, rotavirus, norovirus, hepatitis B, hepatitis C, dengue, yellow fever, Japanese encephalitis, HIV (Rossignol, 2014).

In a study accessed as a preprint, it was reported that Nitazoxanide was effective in the treatment and prophylaxis of SARS-CoV-2, but clinical studies should be conducted in order to determine the optimal dose to achieve this effect (Rajoli*et al*, 2020).

## Neuraminidase Inhibitors (NAI) (Oseltamivir, Zanamivir, Peramivir)

Oral oseltamivir is the most widely available agent among the neuraminidase inhibitors (NAI). In patients with influenza A (H1N1) infection, a reduction in mortality was observed with treatments using NAI, mostly oral oseltamivir. Early NAI treatment, which is initiated within 2 days of symptom onset, has been associated with a reduction in mortality compared to delayed treatment (Muthuri *et al*, 2014). In addition, it has been shown that there is a decrease mortality from influenza A (H5N1) with expedient treatment with oseltamivir before the onset of respiratory failure (Adisasmito *et al*, 2010). The Clinical Practice Guidelines of the Infectious Diseases Association of America (IDSA) recommend oseltamivir for all patients hospitalized with influenza. The treatment period is 5 days and is usually extended to 10 days for patients with ARDS, pneumonia or immunodeficiency (Uyeki *et al*, 2019).

Nebulized zanamivir solution has been administered to patients on mechanical ventilation, but the commercial formulation contains lactose and should not be used for nebulization. Peramivir is the only influenza antiviral agent approved by the FDA that can be used IV. The IV form of Zanamivir was recently approved by the European Medicines Agency (EMA). These agents were found to have comparable activity with oseltamivir in hospitalized influenza patients. In a study comparing high-dose of IV zanamivir with oral oseltamivir, some of the ED patients given high-dose of IV zanamivir had a shorter duration of the viral disease (Marty *et al*, 2017). NAI has been shown to be effective as an empirical treatment in MERS-CoV infection. Although there is no definitive evidence of the efficacy of Oseltamivir in the treatment of COVID-19; its oral form is widely used in Chinese hospitals for suspected or confirmed COVID-19 cases. It is recommended to be ordered as soon as possible (Lu, 2020; Bleibtreu *et al*, 2018).

## Lopinavir / Ritonavir (Kaletra)

Lopinavir (LPV) and ritonavir (RTV) are protease inhibitors that block viral replication. LPV has been reported to demonstrate antiviral activity against SARS *in vitro* at a concentration of 4 µg / ml (Chu *et al*, 2004). However, when combined with ribavirin, LPV is much more effective, showing antiviral activity even at a concentration of 1 mcg / mL. RTV is used together to pharmacokinetically increase the half-life of LPV through cytochrome P450 inhibition. LPV / RTV combination has been shown to be effective against SARS-CoV and MERS-CoV in patients and tissue culture (Chu *et al*, 2004; Arabi *et al*, 2018). LPV is a type of protease inhibitor used in the treatment of human immunodeficiency virus 1 (HIV-1) infection together with RTV. LPV / RTV combination, which is also used in the treatment of HIV infection, can help antiviral therapy by using it together with ribavirin in the early stages of the disease. It has been concluded that LPV / RTV can be beneficial, although it does not appear to be very effective in COVID-19 patients (Chu *et al*, 2004; Lindsey *et al*, 2020).

LPV / RTV has been recommended to high-risk groups of patients with COVID-19 pneumonia (elderly patients or patients with underlying diseases) (Lim *et al*, 2020). LPV / RTV combination shows synergistic effect when used together with ribavirin (Young *et al*, 2020).

In a study conducted in Hong Kong, some of the patients received only ribavirin and LPV / RTV + ribavirin combination was administered to some patients in the treatment of SARS. It has been reported that the risk of death caused by ARDS or SARS-CoV is lower in patients who received combination therapy than those receiving only ribavirin (2.4% *vs* 28.8%, p = 0.001) (Chu *et al*, 2004). In another study, more effective treatment results were reported in terms of shortening of virus transmission time and recovery after LPV / RTV treatment than with other treatments. Randomized clinical trials for LPV / RTV and IV remdesivir in the treatment of COVID-19 are still ongoing (Zhou *et al*, 2020). However, in a study by Gautret *et al*, one group of COVID-19 patients (n=21) received LPV / RTV, the second group (n=16) Umifenovir (Arbidol), and the third group (n=7) was treated without antiviral drugs. No statistically significant difference was found between these patient groups in regard to the rates of improvement or deterioration in clinical condition after treatment (Gautret *et al*, 2020).

In a randomized clinical study conducted with 199 patients with severe COVID-19, it was concluded that the group with LPV / RTV added to the treatment did not have a reduction in the clinical recovery time compared to the standard care group, so LPV / RTV treatment did not provide any benefit (Cao *et al*, 2020).

In an experimental study comparing the efficacy of prophylactic and therapeutic Remdesivir (RDV) versus prophylactic and therapeutic LPV / RTV-INFb, RDV improved lung functions, reduced viral loads and severe lung damage, in contrast, prophylactic LPV / RTV-IFNb has been reported to reduce viral loads slightly, without affecting other disease markers in mice (Sheahan *et al*, 2020).

It is difficult to assess whether LPV / RTV has a role in COVID-19 as monotherapy or as an element of combination therapy with available data. On the other hand, if the patient has HIV, LPV / RTV should be used as part of a standard antiretroviral regimen combination (Chu *et al*, 2004). Whether LPV / RTV treatment provides clinical benefit requires a larger data-based studies. The adult dosage of LPV / RTV combined therapy, its side effects, the conditions that should not be used with some drugs and the situations to be considered in its use are summarized in the Table **5** (Chan *et al*, 2003).

**Table 5. Adult dosage of LPV / RTV combined therapy, side effects, conditions that should not be used with certain drugs and conditions to be considered during treatment.**

| **Therapeutic Doses** | 200 / 50 mg orally twice a day, 5-10 days |
|---|---|
| **Side / adverse effects** | Allergic / Dermatologic: Hypersensitivity reactions, angioedema, Stevens-Johnson syndrome, toxic epidermal necrolysis, erythema multiforme<br>Cardiac: QT prolongation and Torsades de Pointes, AV block, PR prolongation<br>Metabolic: Hyperglycemia, hypertriglyceridemia<br>Organ systems: renal failure, pancreatitis, hepatotoxicity<br>Hematological: Anemia, leukopenia, neutropenia<br>GI: Nausea, vomiting, diarrhea<br>Psychological: Sleep disorders, anxiety. |
| **Contraindications Of Use With Coexisting Disorders.** | Avoid use of LPV / RTV in the presence of ischemic heart disease, cardiomyopathy, structural heart disease, QT prolongation, liver disease. |
| **Warnings- Notes** | • Daily follow-up of ECG, blood glucose, triglyceride, BUN, creatinine, electrolyte, CBC.<br>• If the tablets are crushed and administered by gastric catheter, its absorption may be reduced by approximately 50%. |

## Umifenovir (Arbidol)

It is a broad-spectrum antiviral agent with activity against a range of enveloped and non-enveloped viruses, produced in Russia. The antiviral mechanism is the inhibition of virus-mediated fusion with the target envelope and resultant blockage of virus entry into target cells (Boriskin *et al*, 2008). *In vitro*, it has been shown to inhibit many viral infections, including hepatitis B virus, Ebola virus, Lassa virus, human herpes virus 8, poliovirus and vesicular stomatitis virus (Pécheur *et al*, 2016; Hulseberg *et al*, 2019).

In some tests conducted in Russia, it has been shown that the drug is effective in COVID-19, and it has similar efficacy in direct clinical and *in vitro* comparisons with oseltamivir (Leneva *et al*, 2005; 2016). In February 2020, the Chinese National Health Commission recommended its use as a potential treatment during the COVID-19 pandemic (Lu *et al*, 2020; Zheng *et al*, 2020). **Umifenovir** is used orally at a dose of 3x200 mg / day in adults and for a maximum of 10 days (Diagnosis and Treatment Protocol for Novel Coronavirus Pneumonia. Trial Version 7).

In a study, some of the COVID-19 patients were given LPV / RTV together with Umifenovir (Arbidol) as a combined treatment, and LPV / RTV was administered orally to the other part as monotherapy. It was stated that the clinical improvement of the group receiving combined therapy was more favorable than the group receiving monotherapy (Deng *et al*, 2020). In a study conducted in Wuhan in January 2020, patients were given 400 mg of umifenovir three times a day for 9 days. In the group treated with umifenovir relative to the control group, it was shown to reduce viral load identified by (RT-PCR) and decrease mortality (0% and 16%) (Wang *et al*, 2020).

## Chloroquine

**Chloroquine Phosphate:** Chloroquine phosphate (CQ) has *in vitro* activity against COVID-19 and reduces the virus transmission time. This drug has been used in the treatment of malaria for years. Its therapeutic range is very narrow. Therefore, it is recommended that its use in suspected or confirmed COVID-19 should be limited to hospitalized patients (Interim Clinical Guidance for Patients Suspected of Confirmed with COVID-19 in Belgium. 16 Mar 2020, Version 3; Gao *et al*, 2020). Several randomized controlled trials have been conducted to test the effect of CQ in treating COVID-19. Therapeutic effects were observed in terms of treatment of fever, improvement in thoracic CT findings and delayed disease progression. CQ has been declared as a medical antiviral agent for the treatment of COVID-19 infection in the sixth edition of the new COVID-19 Pneumonia Diagnosis and Treatment Plan published by the Chinese National Health and Care Commission on February 19, 2020 (Wang M *et al*, 2020).

In a study conducted on 22 COVID-19 patients, members of a group of 10 patients received 500 mg oral CQ twice a day for 10 days, and the other 12 patients received 400/100 mg oral LPV / RTV twice a day for 10 days. It has been concluded that treatment with CQ has a slight advantage over LPV / RTV in terms of improvement in clinical symptoms and laboratory tests (Huang *et al*, 2020).

CQ has been reported to inhibit the *in vitro* replication of several CoV strains. Recent publications support the hypothesis that CQ can improve clinical outcomes of patients infected with SARS-CoV-2. CQ prevents the binding of SARS-CoV-2 to target cells by interfering with the receptor glycosylation of ACE2, which SARS-CoV-2 uses as a cell surface receptor in the lung, heart, kidney and intestine. Effects of CQ on CoV by different mechanisms are shown in Table **6**.

The recommended dose for adults is 2x500 mg / day orally, for a minimum of 5 and a maximum of 10 days. If severe GI reactions occur, the dose is reduced in half (1x500 mg / day). Dose adjustment may be required in kidney or liver dysfunction.

**Table 6. Effects of CQ on CoV by different mechanisms. (Wang PH *et al*, 2020; Savarino *et al*, 2003).**

| |
|---|
| 1. It prevents the binding of SARS-CoV-2 to target cells by interfering with the receptor glycosylation of ACE2.<br>2. It may also limit the biosynthesis of sialic acids that may be required for the binding of SARS-CoV-2 to the cell surface.<br>3. If some viral particles bind to the cell surface, it can prevent the formation of autophagosomes by increasing the endosomal pH.<br>4. It changes the pH of lysosomes and inhibits cathepsins; this leads to the formation of an autophagosome that cleaves the SARS-CoV-2 spike protein.<br>5. It can inhibit virus replication by decreasing cellular mitogen-activated protein (MAP) kinase activation.<br>6. CoV can alter maturation by disrupting the proteolytic processing of the M protein; It can alter the virion assembly and budding.<br>7. It can act indirectly by reducing the production of pro-inflammatory cytokines and / or by activating anti-SARS-CoV-2 CD8 + T-cells. |

**Severe adverse effects** include QT prolongation, Torsades de Pointes, decreased seizure threshold, anaphylaxis or anaphylactoid reaction, neuromuscular disorder, neuropsychiatric disorders (may trigger delirium), pancytopenia, neutropenia, thrombocytopenia, aplastic anemia, hepatitis.

**There are also common side effects** such as nausea, vomiting, diarrhea, abdominal pain, headache, and extrapyramidal symptoms. During the treatment, the QT interval is monitored in the serial complete blood count and ECG controls. Side effects and incidence rates of Chloroquine are noted in Table 7.

**Table 7. Some of the side effects and incidence rates of Chloroquine (Chloroquine Side Effects, 2020).**

| | **Incidence Rates of Side Effects** | | | |
|---|---|---|---|---|
| | **>10%** | **1%-10%** | **0,1%-1%** | **0,01%-0,1%** |
| **Ocular/ ophthalmological** | - | Temporary blurred vision | - | Retinopathy, irreversible retinal damage |
| **Dermatological** | Itching | Rashes and urticaria | Alopesia and pigmentation disorders | exacerbation of psoriatic lesions, erythema multiforme, toxic epidermal necrolysis, Stevens-Johnson syndrome |
| **Gastrointestinal** | Nausea, vomiting, diarrhea | - | - | abdominal pain, liver dysfunction, and hepatitis |
| **Neurological** | Headache | - | neuropathy, ototoxicity | convulsions and polyneuropathy |

*(Table 7) cont.....*

| | Incidence Rates of Side Effects | | | |
|---|---|---|---|---|
| | **>10%** | **1%-10%** | **0,1%-1%** | **0,01%-0,1%** |
| **Psychiatric** | Sleep disorders | depression | - | hallucinations, psychiatric disorders |
| **Cardiovascular** | - | - | Cardiomyopathy | Life-threatening arrhythmias (including QT prolongation, Torsades de Pointes, ventricular tachycardia, and fibrillation) |
| **Hematological** | - | - | - | Bone marrow depression; aplastic anemia, agranulocytosis, pancytopenia, thrombocytopenia, neutropenia |
| **Musculoskeletal** | - | - | Myopathy | - |

**It is contraindicated in patients** under 18 or over 65 years of age, pregnancy, previously diagnosed porphyria, G6PD deficiency, end-stage liver and kidney diseases, arrhythmia, heart failure and myocardial infarction, retinal disease, hearing loss mental illnesses, skin diseases and epilepsy. In addition, it should not be used with drugs such as digitalis glycosides, heparin, penicillamine, amiodarone, bepridil, domperidone, droperidol, haloperidol, macrolides astemizole, methadone, procainamide, hydrochlorothiazide, quinolones, cisapride, indapamide, chlorpromazine, streptomycin, octreotide, and monoamine oxidase inhibitors (Multicenter collaboration group, 2020).

## Hydroxychloroquine (HCQ) (Plaquenil®)

HCQ is one of the disease modifying antirheumatic drugs, a powerful immunomodulator that prevents inflammation flare-ups (cytokine storm) and organ damage (Ruiz-Irastorza *et al*, 2010). The chemical structure of HCQ is very similar to CQ; It is exactly the same except for an additional hydroxyl molecule at the terminal. The hydroxyl molecule makes HCQ less permeable to the blood-retinal barrier and provides faster clearance in the retinal pigment cell. Thus, it reduces the risk of retinal toxicity with HCQ compared to CQ. Additionally, the narrow therapeutic and safety index margin of CQ makes HCQ a safer option than CQ (Marmor *et al*, 2016).

It has recently been reported that HCQ is stronger than CQ *in vitro*, so it can be used at lower doses (Yao *et al*, 2020). In particular, HCQ can increase intracellular pH and inhibit lysosomal activity in antigen presenting cells, including plasmacytoid dendritic cells and B cells. Thus, antigen processing and major histocompatibility complex (MHC) prevent class II-mediated autoantigen presentation (Lotteau *et al*, 1990). This process reduces T cell activation, differentiation, and expression of co-stimulatory proteins and cytokines (*e.g.* IL-1, IL-6) produced by T and B cells (Wu *et al*, 2017; van den Borne *et al*, 1997).

Like CQ, HCQ also inhibits receptor binding and membrane fusion, which are two essential steps required for cell entry by CoVs. Impaired terminal glycosylation of ACE2 can reduce the binding efficiency between ACE2 and the SARS-CoV spike-protein in host cells. After HCQ and CQ enter a cell, both are concentrated in low pH organelles such as endosomes, Golgi vesicles, and lysosomes. As the virus uses endosomes as its cellular entry mechanism, increasing the pH of the endosomes with CQ therapy has a negative effect on the fusion process of the virus and endosome. Inhibition of SARS-CoV spread has been observed in cells treated with CQ before or after infection, suggesting both the prophylactic and therapeutic advantages of CQ in combating SARS viruses (Vincent *et al*, 2005).

Vomiting and diarrhea are the most common side effects of CQ and HCQ. Long-term exposure to CQ can cause serious side effects such as retinopathy, cardiovascular disorders, and cardiomyopathy (Schrezenmeier *et al*, 2020). While CQ has a number of serious adverse effects on fetal development, HCQ is highly recommended for pregnant patients with autoimmune disease as it prevents the development of congenital heart block due to its potential inhibitory effect of type I interferon (IFN) production. Considering its safety profile during pregnancy, HCQ rather than CQ is a potential therapeutic solution for these patients (Izmirly *et al*, 2012; Lisney *et al*, 2017).

In summary, HCQ is thought to be a better therapeutic approach than CQ in the treatment of COVID-19 infection. There are three main reasons for this:

- HCQ attenuates the severity of COVID-19 by inhibiting cytokine storm by reducing CD154 expression in T cells.
- HCQ can provide a similar antiviral effect in pre and post infection stages found with CQ.
- HCQ has fewer side effects; it is safe during pregnancy.

In order to evaluate the efficacy of HCQ at Wuhan University Hospital in China, a study was conducted including 62 adult patients who were confirmed to be COVID-19 by RT-PCR, had pneumonia in thoracic CT, $SaO_2$ / $SpO_2$ ratio> 93% or $PaO_2$ / $FiO_2$ ratio> 300 mmHg. In addition to standard maintenance therapy, the first group of 31 patients was given 200 mg of HCQ twice a day for 5 days. Again, only standard care treatment was administered to the control group (n= 31). It was reported that patients with COVID-19 treated with HCQ had a significantly shortened course of pneumonia, cough and fever, compared to the control group (Chen *et al*, 2020).

In a systematic review and meta-analysis of 53 randomized trials, Chen *et al*, concluded that CQ is associated with a high total risk of adverse effects compared with the placebo or no intervention in the overall population (Chen, 2020). Given the small number of COVID-19 participants included, we should be cautious regarding the conclusion stating that HCQ is linked with an increased incidence of adverse effects in patients with COVID-19.

In a study coordinated by the University of Méditerranée in Marseille, COVID-19 patients older than 12 years of age were divided into two groups, 24 as the HCQ treatment group and 24 as the control group. The treatment group received 200 mg HCQ, three times a day for 10 days, while additional azithromycin (AZT) were used if necessary. Significant increase in the clearance of the viral nasopharyngeal carrier measured by RT-PCR within just 3 to 6 days of COVID-19 in the treatment group compared to the control group. A faster SARS-CoV-2 clearance was noted after six days of treatment with either HCQ alone or HCQ + AZT (70% versus 12%; P <0.001). AZT added to HCQ has also been reported to be significantly more effective for virus elimination. In addition, the combination of HCQ and AZT showed a synergistic effect. On the other hand, addition of AZT to HCQ may increase the risk of QTc prolongation (Gautret *et al*, 2020).

***Does HCQ Have any Benefit in Prophylaxis?***

In a randomized controlled study examining the use of HCQ after contact with an infected individual without a mask and / or a shield, for at least 10 minutes, at a distance of less than 1.5 meters (post-exposure), the agent was administered at a dose of 600 mg for 5 days. After 2 weeks of follow-up, the risk of developing infection was found to be no different from the placebo group (Boulware *et al*, 2020). In a similar study, HCQ was administered for 8 weeks at a dose of 600 mg / day for prophylactic purposes in comparison with placebo in asymptomatic, PCR-negative and non-infected healthcare workers working in COVID-19-related units for at least 20 hours a week (pre-exposure). Again, the risk of developing infections was similar in the two groups (Abella *et al*, 2020). With these findings, it was concluded that there is no benefit of HCQ prophylactic use in pre- or post-exposure periods.

It is administered orally for 5 to 10 days at the time of diagnosis or suspicion, 400 mg after 12 hours, 2x200 mg in the following 5 days. If HCQ is unavailable, CQ 600 mg (10 mg / kg) in case of diagnosis or suspicion, 300 mg (5 mg / kg) after 12 hours, then 300 mg (5 mg / kg) BID for up to 5 days or 1000 mg at diagnosis and 12 hours then 500mg, then 300mg per day (2x300 mg in severe cases) orally for up to 5 days. It is contraindicated in cases with QTc> 500 msec, myasthenia gravis, porphyria, retinal pathology and epilepsy (Interim Clinical Guidance for Patients Suspected of / Confirmed with COVID-19 in Belgium.16 Mars 2020; Version 3).

### *The Dark Side of The Moon: Doubts about HCQ Effectiveness*

The Turkish Thoracic Society (TTD) Respiratory System Infections Working Group evaluated 12 clinical studies conducted with HCQ / CQ in terms of clinical efficacy and prepared an opinion statement (TTD, 2020). In 8 of these studies, HCQ was not found to be effective or worse results were obtained in those who used this drug. In one study, it was not found to be effective; however, a definite judgment could not be made due to the fact that the patient group using HCQ had more severe and higher concomitant chronic diseases at presentation. In another study, patients using HCQ had better clinical outcomes, but it could not be concluded because patients using HCQ use a higher rate of systemic CSD. In two studies, it was observed that mortality was lower in HCQ users. In all three published meta-analyzes, there was no evidence that HCQ is effective. Similarly, there was no difference in clinical efficacy between early or late initiation of treatment, and HCQ was found to be ineffective in patients with mild-moderate COVID-19 (Cavalcanti *et al*, 2020; Tang *et al*, 2020). Based on the results of these studies, TTD stated that it is useful to review the recommendation for the use of HCQ in the treatment of COVID-19. After this view, no clinical benefit was observed in any evaluation parameter of HCQ use in a randomized controlled study conducted by NIH (Self *et al*, 2020).

## PRINCIPLES OF ANTIBIOTIC TREATMENT IN COVID-19

### Co-infections in COVID-19

The association of SARS-CoV-2 with other respiratory pathogens is a common and potentially important condition. Along with COVID-19, these co-infections have the potential to affect the diagnosis, clinical course, treatment, hospital stay, discharge time and mortality rates of the patients. It is not known how it affects the clinical course or blood laboratory and radiological findings to assess the prognosis of COVID-19 in the presence of co-infection. The number of studies on this subject is small, and while most studies focus only on SARS-CoV-2, co-infection studies have been somewhat neglected.

Co-infection in COVID-19 patients resembles the spectrum of bacterial superinfection in Influenza A / B, the first co-infection in hospitalized patients is usually 11-35%, more frequent bacterial pneumonias caused by streptococcus pneumonia and staphylococcus aureus (Klein *et al*, 2016).

**Viral co-infections (VCI):** COVID-19 can also occur with other viral infections. Influenza and SARS-CoV-2 can occur in patients as VCI and present with similar symptoms. Flu usually occurs during the winter months and is determined by various factors such as the burden of the disease, the availability and effectiveness of the vaccine in that season, the characteristics of the circulating viruses, and the duration of the winter season.

According to the Centers for Disease Control and Prevention (CDCP) data in the USA, it was reported that approximately 36 million patients had symptomatic flu in the 2018-2019 season, resulting in approximately 17 million hospital visits, 490,000 hospitalizations and 34,000 deaths(CDCP, 2020).

The rate of co-infection in patients exhibit pandemic and seasonal variations (Joseph *et al*, 2013). Considering the seasonal increase in the incidence of influenza A and B as a viral agent with COVID-19 and VCI, especially in winter months, the necessity and importance of getting the flu vaccine comes to the fore. In a study to evaluate whether seasonal influenza vaccine or pneumococcal vaccines could help reduce COVID-19 mortality, it was reported that these vaccines could decrease mortality (Thindwa *et al*, 2020).

**Bacterial co-infections (BCI):** In a prospective study of co-infection screening in 257 patients with COVID-19 in China Influenza A / B, human respiratory syncytial virus, parainfluenza type 1/2/3/4, human metapneumovirus, coronaviruses 229E, OC43, NL63 and HKU1, human bocavirus, human adenovirus, human rhinovirus, herpes simplex virus, cytomegalovirus, Epstein Barr virus, Mycoplasma pneumonia, Chlamydia pneumonia, Legionella pneumoniae, Haemophilus influenzae, Moraxella catarrhalis, Klebsiella pneumoniae, Streptococcus pneumoniae, Staphycoccus pneumoniae, Mycobacteria, *Pneumocystis* carinii, Bordetella pertussis and fungi such as aspergillus, Cryptococcus neoformans A / B, mucor, candida, Histoplasma capsulatum; it was reported that viral, bacterial and fungal co-infections were detected in 243 (94.2%) patients (Zhu *et al*, 2020). Of the 243 patients with co-infection, 236 (91.8%) were bacterial, 81 (31.5%) were viral and 60 (23.3%) were fungal agents.

**Fungal co-infections:** In a study where current literature reviews were conducted to investigate the bacterial / fungal co-infection rate in patients with COVID-19, it was reported that bacterial / fungal co-infection was detected in 62 (8%) of 806 patients who were hospitalized (Rawson *et al*, 2020). In the literature review of Lansbury *et al.*, it was reported that co-infection with fungal pathogens was detected in only 3 patients among 30 articles and 3834 patients. (Lansbury L *et al*,

2020).

**Parasitic co-infections:** There is some evidence that helminth infections can alleviate the viral pneumonia process. Although some studies have suggested that helminth infection may impair responses to viral immunization and viral infection, there is no clear clinical evidence that it worsens results (Hartmann *et al*, , 2019; Osborne *et al*, 2014; Schwartz *et al*, 2018).

## Use of Antibiotics in the Treatment of COVID-19

### Why are Antibiotics Used?

Along with its pathogenesis, co-infections play an important role in the exacerbation of infection and in death rate by increasing the difficulties in the diagnosis, treatment and prognosis of COVID-19 disease and even the disease symptoms (Bengoechea *et al*, 2020). Since BCI cannot be ruled out, antibiotic treatment should be considered in critically ill patients with COVID-19 (Bassetti *et al*, 2020).

In a comprehensive, multi-center study conducted in China, it was reported that 58% of the patients who received COVID-19 treatment in hospital received IV antibiotic treatment (Guan *et al*, 2020). In a study conducted in Wuhan, China, the rate of antibiotic use was reported to be 95%. Again, in another study conducted in Jiangsu city of China, it was reported that a single antibiotic, especially moxifloxacin, was added to the treatment of all patients empirically (Wu *et al*, 2020).

Studies on empirical antibiotic use and applications in COVID-19 patients all over the world, except China, are limited. To investigate this issue, an international web-based survey was conducted with 166 participants from 23 countries and 82 different hospitals, 50.3% infectious diseases, 28.5% intensive care and 11.5% internal medicine specialists, dealing with the care and treatment of COVID-19 patients (Beović *et al*, 2020). According to this study, 61.8% (n: 102/166) of the participants reported that antibiotic use in COVID-19 patients was not different from local guidelines and 82.9% (n: 136/166) from local community-acquired pneumonia guidelines.

### How Do We Decide On Antibiotic Treatment?

It was accepted that the most important reason for starting antibiotics was clinical presentation, followed by laboratory inflammation markers and radiological findings. Among the laboratory markers, the most important parameters were listed as procalcitonin, followed by neutrophil count, WBC count and C-reactive protein (Beović *et al*, 2020).

In conclusion, we recommend to stop inappropriate antibiotic use in the empirical treatment of co-infection and / or superinfections concurrent with COVID-19, to choose the most appropriate antibacterial agent according to local guidelines, and to start as soon as possible based on microbiological results. Empirical antibiotherapy should be initiated in accordance with local and current guidelines in patients where microbiological tests are not possible or who are not considered for hospitalization.

Antibiotics in the macrolide group (erythromycin, clarithromycin and azithromycin) have not only antibacterial activity, but also immunomodulatory effects, including anti-inflammatory effects. Recently, the antiviral effects of macrolides have attracted much attention. Erythromycin is the first macrolide with proven efficacy in the treatment of rhinovirus and influenza viruses. Later, clarithromycin and azithromycin have also proven effective for rhinovirus, RSV and influenza virus (Lee *et al*, 2017; Lendermon *et al*, 2017). In addition to the respiratory viruses mentioned above, Zika and Ebola viruses have been reported to be inhibited by azithromycin (Madrid *et al*, 2015; Bosseboeuf *et al*, 2018). Influenza virus has been shown to be significantly inhibited by treatment with azithromycin prior to infection. In the early stage of influenza virus infection, azithromycin prevented influenza virus uptake into host cells. In addition, azithromycin targeted the newly formed virus as a result of growth from host cells and inactivated its endocytic activities. These findings show the potential of azithromycin treatment before and after influenza virus infection (Bosseboeuf *et al*, 2018).

It has been reported that azithromycin therapy in combination with HCQ may be an effective antiviral therapy for COVID-19 (Gautret *et al*, 2020).

**Angiotensin 1 Receptor Blockers (AT1RBs) (-sartans: Losartan, telmisartan, olmesartan)**

Angiotensinogen is broken down by renin, an enzyme released by the kidney, and is converted to inactive angiotensin (AT) I. On the other hand, carboxypeptidase ACE converts AT I to AT II in octapeptide structure, which is the active molecule of the renin angiotensin system (RAS). AT II hormone plays an important role in the development of hypertension by regulating vascular tone, fluid volume and electrolyte balance. AT II acts by binding to two types of receptors called AT1 and AT2. Its physiological effects are mostly achieved through AT1 receptors. These effects include vasoconstriction, aldosterone release, antidiuretic hormone (ADH) synthesis, sympathetic activation, and salt absorption from renal tubules.

All these effects predispose the organism to the development of hypertension (Unger, 2000). Since AT1RBs prevent AT II from binding to the AT1 receptor, this molecule has affinity to AT2 receptors causing the opposite effects (Fig. **2**). As a result, stimulation of AT2 receptors will cause increased vasodilation. AT1RBs also cause an increase in serum AT peptides such as AT 1-7, AII, AIII and AIV. These peptides affect vasoconstriction, renal blood flow and vascular hypertrophy in accordance with the receptors to which they bind (Shibasaki *et al*, 1999).

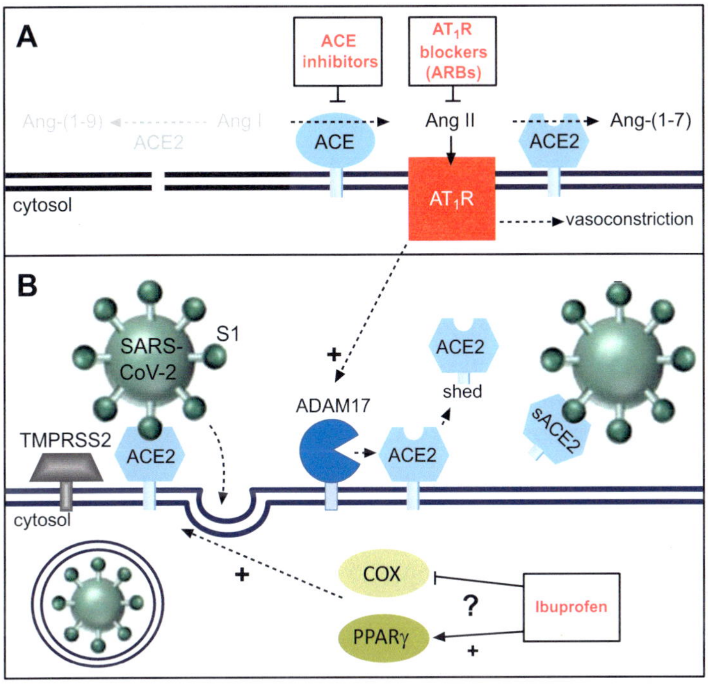


**Fig. (2).** Angiotensin (AT) -converting enzyme-2 (ACE2) converts AT-I to AT- (1-9) and AT-II to AT- (1-7) (Panel A). If ACE inhibitors (ACEI) exist in the tissue, the conversion of AT-I to AT-II is inhibited (Panel B). ACE2 is also bound to SARS-Cov-2 after treatment with "serine protease transmembrane protease, serine 2" (TMPRSS2). If disintegrin and metalloprotease 17 (ADAM17) and membrane-bound ACE2 are cleaved, soluble (s) ACE2 appears and they cannot facilitate SARS-Cov-2 entry, they keep the virus in the solution. With AT-II type-1 receptors (AT1R), they increase ADAM17 activity, and AT1R blockers (ARB) inhibit this. Ibuprofen increases the synthesis of ACE2, possibly via cyclooxygenase (COX) inhibition and Peroxisome Proliferator-Activated Receptor gamma (PPAR-γ) activation.

COVID-19 uses the ACE2 receptor binding motif (RBM) similar to SARS-CoV. In other words, the COVID-19 spike-protein and the SARS-CoV spike-protein share almost the same structure in the RBM domain, and the ACE2 receptor site is the gateway the virus uses to enter the type II alveolar cell. ACE2 receptors are mainly found in type II alveolar cells in the lungs. It is not yet known whether susceptibility to COVID-19 infection is due to individual differences in this region where the virus attaches as it enters the cell (Jin *et al*, 2020; Wan *et al*, 2020; Xu *et al*, 2020). The expression of ACE2 on the cell surface is not related to sex but increases with age (Cao *et al*, 2020).

ACE2 is the shared binding site of both the 2002-2003 pandemic SARS-CoV and possibly the strain precipitating the current COVID-19 pandemic. Therefore, the recommendation to treat AT1RBs to increase the expression of ACE2 in SARS patients seems hypothetical. However, for COVID-19, most likely, observations made in studies on SARS-CoV suggest otherwise. ACE2 receptors are mainly found in type II alveolar cells in the lungs. COVID-19, spike-protein binding to ACE2 receptors, leads to ACE2 down-regulation; As a result, it has been reported that ACE causes excessive angiotensin production, which in turn, contributes to lung damage. Because AT1R stimulated by angiotensin causes an increase in pulmonary vascular permeability and thus mediates the increase of lung injury (Imai *et al*, 2005; Kuba *et al*, 2005).

It should be noted that approximately half of SARS-CoV patients developed hypotension during their hospitalization (Yu *et al*, 2006). There is no comprehensive information available on hypotension rates in COVID-19 patients hospitalized in this epidemic. Now it is early to estimate what percentage of SARS patients of the ongoing epidemic can be safely treated with AT1RBs without the risk of severe hypotension. A provisional recommendation for the administration of AT1RBs such as losartan and telmisartan as COVID-19 therapeutics for the treatment of patients prior to the development of SARS has not yet been proven. In the general population, the percentage of people chronically using AT1RB can be compared between the percentage of hospital admissions of patients with COVID-19 infected with severe symptoms.

AT1RBs have been widely used in clinical practice for the control of hypertension and kidney disorders since the 1990s (Deppe *et al*, 2010). It uses ACE2 as the receptor binding site for the spike-protein of COVID-19 (Wan *et al*, 2020; Lu *et al*, 2020). There are some publications reporting that AT1RBs may be beneficial for patients with COVID-19 pneumonia (Sun *et al*, 2020). It has been shown that losartan and olmesartan, which are AT1RB, which are widely administered to lower blood pressure in hypertensive patients, increase cardiac ACE2 expression in rats after myocardial infarction induced by coronary artery ligation (Ishiyama *et al*, 2004). Losartan has also been shown to upregulate renal ACE2 expression in chronically treated rats (Klimas *et al*, 2015). Consistent with these observations, higher urinary tract ACE2 levels were observed in hypertensive patients treated with olmesartan (Furuhashi *et al*, 2015). Taken together, these observations suggested that chronic AT1R blockade resulted in ACE2 upregulation in both rats and humans.

## Corticosteroids

So far, no definitive conclusions have been found regarding the effects of immunosuppressants in severe influenza virus infections and thus, their therapeutic use is controversial (Beigel *et al*, 2019). Corticosteroids, which are known as an option for immunomodulatory treatment in the treatment of SARS-CoV, affect the whole body and have a very strong effect and have anti-inflammatory and immunosuppressive effects, provide early recovery of fever and less harmful radiographic leaks (Chu *et al*, 2004). The use of corticosteroids to treat influenza virus has been associated with a higher risk of superinfection, long-term viral replication, and an increased risk of death (Rodrigo *et al*, 2016). On the other hand, it has been reported that corticosteroid treatment for MERS-CoV infections was not significantly associated with mortality, but a delay in MERS-CoV RNA clearance was observed (Arabi *et al*, 2018).

In case of progressive deterioration of oxygenation indicators and rapid progression of imaging (CT) findings, glucocorticoids / CSD can be used for a short time (3-5 days) for patients in whom overactivation of the body's inflammatory response is suspected.

It is recommended that the dose not exceed the equivalent of 1-2 mg / kg / day methylprednisolone. It has been reported that a larger glucocorticoid dose will delay the elimination of CoV due to immunosuppressive effects (Diagnosis and Treatment Protocol for Novel Coronavirus Pneumonia. Trial Version 7). Care should be taken when using glucocorticoids, as they can suppress the body's immune system and slow the clearance of the virus (The 3/4/2020 Chinese Health and Public Health Ministry Guideline on Novel Coronavirus Disease (COVID-19) Diagnosis and Treatment (Revision # 6). Low-dose corticosteroids have been used to treat those with severe COVID-19 infection for possible benefit by attenuating inflammatory lung damage, as cytokine storm was observed. However, corticosteroids did not reduce mortality in SARS-CoV and MERS-CoV infections according to the WHO guideline (WHO). Clinical management of severe acute respiratory infection. Novel coronavirus (nCoV) infection is 2020. Arabi *et al*, 2018). It has been reported in some publications that corticosteroids should not be used in CoV infection, did not provide benefit in previous SARS or MERS outbreaks and could increase viral spread (Lee *et al*, 2004).

Some publications reported supporting evidence for the use of CSD in COVID-19. In a study, the use of low-dose CSD decreased mortality in patients with ARDS (Sun *et al*, 2019).

## Effectiveness of IV Pulse CSD in the Treatment of COVID-19

Some investigations have been conducted to evaluate the effectiveness of pulse CSD treatment in COVID-19. In a randomized controlled study investigating the effectiveness of pulse methylprednisolone (PMP) administration in treatment of COVID-19 patients, 34 out of 68 patients were administered 250 mg / day methylprednisolone IV for 3 days in addition to standard therapy and their data were compared with 34 patients who received only standard therapy (Edalatifad *et al*, 2020). It was concluded that patients who received PMP for their treatment had significantly reduced mortality rate, recovery time and discharge time compared to patients who received standard therapy ($p < 0.001$; p: 0.006; p: 0.003, respectively). In a study conducted in Spain, 1 mg / kg / day methylprednisolone was added to the treatment of 396 COVID-19 patients 10 days after the onset of symptoms as a median time and compared with 67 patients who received standard treatment. It was observed that in-hospital mortality of patients who received CSD was lower than those who did not, and it reduced mortality by 41.8% ($p = 0.044$; $p = 0.710$) (Fernandez-Cruz *et al*, 2020). In addition, CSD pulse dose was administered to 86 patients of the group given CSD in the treatment. Patients who received PMP and those who received 1 mg / kg / day methylprednisolone were compared and no statistically significant difference was found between in-hospital mortality rates.

It is unclear whether the use of CSD in ARDS is effective. Three cohort studies evaluated in a meta-analysis reported increased mortality from CSD use in people with influenza-related ARDS (Ruan *et al*, 2014).

In the guidelines, it has been reported that systemic corticosteroids are not routinely recommended and should not be given as an adjunctive therapy in the treatment of COVID-19 (WHO). Clinical management of severe acute respiratory infection when novel coronavirus (nCoV) infection is. 2020. Clark *et al*, 2020; Russell *et al*, 2020).

In the review published in JAMA in July 2020, it was stated that new information and evidence revealed that dexamethasone reduced mortality, but the beneficial effect was limited to those who need supplementary oxygen and / or MV and severe patients with a protracted clinical course (Wiersinga WJ, 2020). In the randomized Evaluation of COVID-19 Therapy (RECOVERY) study, 2104 patients were randomized to receive 6 mg dexamethasone + other treatments for 10 days, and 4321 patients to receive only other treatments without steroids (Horby P, 2020). 28-day mortality is lower in the dexamethasone group. (21.6% *vs* 24.6%; age adjusted rate ratio, 0.83 [95% CI, 0.74-0.92]; $P < .001$). In a smaller retrospective cohort study reported from Wuhan, a lower mortality rate was observed among 201 patients who received methylprednisolone (hazard ratio, 0.38 [95% CI, 0.20-0.72]) (Wu, 2020).

Although it has been reported that treatment with methylprednisolone may be beneficial for patients with ARDS following COVID-19, the effect of CST in such patients is still to be elucidated (Wu, 2020).

On 2 September 2020, WHO published a guide for physicians on the use of CST in patients with COVID-19 (WHO, JAMA, 2020). These most recent guidelines advocated use of systemic CST for the treatment of patients with severe and critical COVID-19, while the agents are not recommended for those with non-severe COVID-19, as the treatment was not associated with any benefits.

This issue was also evaluated thoroughly by Lamontagne *et al*, A living WHO guideline in September 2020, who made a strong recommendation for use of CST in severe and critical COVID-19 because there is a lower risk of death among people treated with systemic CST (moderate certainty evidence) (Lamontagne, 2020). The panel collected data from eight randomized trials (7184 participants) and found that systemic CST probably reduce 28 day mortality in patients with critical covid-19 (moderate certainty evidence; 87 fewer deaths per 1000 patients (95% CI; 124 fewer to 41 fewer)), and also in those with severe disease (moderate certainty evidence; 67 fewer deaths per 1000 patients (100 fewer to 27 fewer)). They have also advocated that all or almost all fully informed patients with severe and critical COVID-19 would choose this treatment. In contrast, the panel concluded that patients with non-severe COVID-19 would decline this treatment because they would be unlikely to benefit and may be harmed.

Summary: In case of deterioration of oxygenation and rapid progression of imaging (CT) findings, CST- glucocorticoids can be used for a short time (3-5 days) for patients in whom overactivation of the body's inflammatory response (cytokine storm) is suspected. Considering the side effects in general, CSDs can be tried after other alternative therapeutic agents have been tried in the treatment of COVID-19 patients. In the treatment of COVID-19, systemic CSDs are not routinely recommended as an adjunct therapy and should not be given, but it can be used with severe or critically ill patients who need additional $O_2$ or MV and whose symptoms persist for a long time.

## N-acetyl-cysteine (NAC)

Severe COVID-19 infection leads to a cytokine storm syndrome associated with acute respiratory distress syndrome (ARDS), multiple organ failure, and increased mortality. This syndrome is characterized by increased secretion of interleukin (IL)-2, IL-7, granulocyte colony stimulating factor, interferon-inducible protein

10, monocyte chemoattractant protein 1, macrophage inflammatory protein 1-α, and tumor necrosis factor (TNF)-α (Mehta *et al*, 2020). Reactive oxygen species and oxidative stress activate important redox sensitive transcription factors such as NF-κB and activator protein-1, leading to the coordinate expression of the proinflammatory genes of IL-6, IL-8 and TNF-a (Conner *et al*, 1996).

N-Acetylcysteine (NAC), a well-known mucolytic agent used in respiratory tract infections, is a thiol containing free radical scavenger and a precursor to glutathione (Sanguinetti, 2015). Glutathione is an endogenous antioxidant that is often depleted in patients with oxidative stress or systemic inflammation, including those with chronic obstructive pulmonary disease (COPD) and ARDS. After systemic administration, NAC is rapidly converted to cysteine, the precursor to glutathione (Sadowska *et al*, 2007).

The beneficial effect of 1200 mg / day oral NAC in the management of COPD exacerbations has been previously demonstrated (Sanguinetti, 2015). Adding this dose of NAC to conventional therapy improves oxidative stress and inflammatory response in patients with community-acquired pneumonia (Zhang *et al*, 2018). The positive effects of NAC have been associated with inhibition of IL-8, IL-6, and TNF-a expression, and release of respiratory syncytial virus (RSV) in alveolar type II cells infected with influenza virus A and B (Mata *et al*, 2011). Therefore, it is beneficial to add 1200 mg / day oral NAC to the treatment protocol in order to potentially prevent the development of cytokine storm syndrome and ARDS in patients with COVID-19 (Andreou *et al*, 2020).

Some agents used in the treatment of COVID-19 and their key characteristics are shown in Table **8**.

**Table 8. Some agents used in the treatment of COVID-19 and their key characteristics.**

| Agent | Mechanisms of Effect | Indications | Recommended Dose | Contraindications |
|---|---|---|---|---|
| **1.Antivirals** | | | | |
| **1.Lopinavir/ Ritonavir** | Protease inhibition | SARS-CoV, MERS-CoV, HIV-1 | 2x200 / 50 mg / day, oral, no more than 10 days | Heart and liver disease |
| **2.Nucleotide Analogues** | | | | |
| a) Ribavirin | Blockage of viral replicase polyprotein | RSV,HCV | 500 mg, IV, no more than 10 days | Heart diseases, pregnancy, hemoglobinopathies |
| b) Remdesivir | Interferes with viral polymerase | SARS-CoV, MERS-CoV, Ebola | 200 mg / 30 min IV inf. then 100 mg 2-10 days. | Liver and kidney failure |

*(Table 8) cont.....*

| Agent | Mechanisms of Effect | Indications | Recommended Dose | Contraindications |
|---|---|---|---|---|
| c) Favipiravir | Viral replication inhibition | İnfluenza | 2x1600 mg / day; then 2x600 mg / day, 5 days. | Pregnancy |
| d) Nafamostat | Protease inhibition | MERS-CoV, Ebola | - | Hypersensitivity reaction |
| e) Nitazoxanide | Antiprotease | CoV | - | Hypersensitivity reaction |
| **3. Neuraminidase inhibitors (NAI)** | | | | |
| a. Oseltamivir | NAI | Influenza A,B, Avian flu (H5N1), MERS-CoV | 2x75 mg / day, oral, 5 days | Hypersensitivity reaction |
| b. Zanamivir | NAI | Influenza A,B, Avian flu (H5N1), MERS-CoV | 2x10mg / day, via inhalation and IV, 5 days. | Hypersensitivity reaction |
| c. Peramivir | NAI | Influenza A,B, Avian flu (H5N1), MERS-CoV | 800 mg / day, oral, 5 days; 300 mg / day, single dose IM; 800 mg single dose IV | Hypersensitivity reaction |
| d. Umifenovir (Arbidol) | Blockage of viral entry to target cells | Influenza A,B, HCV | 3x200 mg / day, oral, 5-10 days. | Hypersensitivity reaction |
| **4. Chloroquines** | | | | |
| a. CQ | Blockage of receptor binding and membrane fusion used for viral entry to target cells of CoV | Malaria, Rheumatic diseases | 2x500mg / day, oral, 5-10 days | End stage liver and / or kidney disease, Heart and Retinal disease, Epilepsy |
| b. HCQ | Blockage of receptor binding and membrane fusion used for viral entry to target cells of CoV | Malaria, Rheumatic diseases | Two doses of 400 mg 12 hours apart, followed by 2x200 mg / day, oral, 5-10 days | QTc> 500 ms, Myasthenia gravis, Porphyria, Retinal disease, Epilepsy |
| **Tocilizumab** | Monoclonal antibodies | Liver disease, Rheumatic arthritis | Initial dose is 4-8 mg / kg. IV injection in 100 ml saline. Repeat dose after 12 hours | Tbc, active infection, Hypersensitivity reaction |

## CAN WE USE PAINKILLERS AND ANTI-INFLAMMATORY AGENTS IN COVID-19?

As of September 2020, COVID-19 afflicted more than 27.000.000 people in the world and caused nearly 900.000 deaths. The increase observed in the total number of cases in several months has sparked a concern that COVID-19 has threatened the world's well-being as never before and it is going to maintain its dreadful status in the next years.

The use of antipyretic, analgesic and NSAIDs has been extensively discussed in the pandemic period. Before the outbreak, the utilization of antipyretic, analgesic and NSAIDs has been widespread in the treatment of pain and fever. These signs and symptoms are precipitated mainly by cytokine storm, major pathophysiologic pathway inflicting these patients. It is well established that cytokine storm , which is a hyperactive inflammatory response, triggers COVID-19 symptoms such as fever, muscle pain, sore throat . This has also been suggested to represent the link to the severity of the disease. Treatments recommended to support a non-hospitalized patient with a confirmed or suspected COVID infection are shown in Table **9**.

**Table 9. Treatments recommended to support a non-hospitalized patient with a confirmed or suspected COVID infection.**

| Intervention | Description |
|---|---|
| **Fever** | Having plenty of fluids and a warm shower at intervals of several hours will be most effective means to alleviate fever. Also ventilate the house / environment, dress thin or not at all, keep the ambient temperature low (18-22$^{0}$C). |
| **Antipyretic-pain medications:** | Paracetamol can be the first choice. Caution should be taken since the NSAID group "profens" (*i.e.,* ibuprofen / ketoprofen / dexketoprofen / flurbiprofen) are active antipyretic and NSAID agents, as they can disguise / increase the signs and symptoms of COVID-19 infection (Micallef, 2020). However, this opinion was not supported on the basis of evidence and does not appear to be a real threat in the management. Instead, recent reports pointed out that NSAIDs can in fact alleviate the manifestations of cytokine storm. |
| **Tocilizumab (anti-interleukin-6 receptor antibody)** | The agent can be used as an immunomodulator, to suppress inflammation and to alleviate fever. Its beneficial efficacy is remarkable during the cytokine storm period. |
| **Corticosteroids** | Methylprednisolone is useful in patients with ARDS with its anti-inflammatory effects, it may be effective on inflammatory muscle pain. It is recommended only in the treatment of ARDS (Wu, 2020). Mostly not recommended if there are not any other indications. |
| **Vitamin supplements** | The beneficial efficacy of vitamins C and D have not been proven yet in routine treatment. Thus it appears to be useful only in people with deficiency, malnutrition and debility. |

There is a data scarcity to determine which agents can be safely used in patients with a definitive or presumptive diagnosis of COVID-19. Therefore, both public and the medical community had a concern that NSAIDs can exert detrimental effects on patients with COVID-19 in this pandemic era.

The severity of the course of the disease is associated with an exaggerated immune response. It is postulated that overt activation of neutrophil leukocytes is one of the main causes (Barnes, 2020). Elevated levels of CRP and other inflammatory markers indicate that the pro-inflammatory response plays a crucial role in COVID-19 infection (Martinez, 2020). In the pathophysiology of moderate-to severe COVID-19, pneumonia and ARDS triggered by increased pulmonary inflammation lead to thickened lung secretions, widespread lung damage and obstruction of the airways, and entry into the fatal path begins with this mechanism. Increased proinflammatory cytokines (cytokine storm) in serum and microthrombi also play a critical role in this mechanism.

## How to Decide for Treatment of Pain in The Pandemic Period?

The American College of Surgeons recommend that not only medical factors, but also logistical circumstances be considered when making treatment decisions (ACS, 2020). For pain management, factors that should be taken into consideration when deciding whether to see a patient in person, change the appointment to telemedicine, postpone the visit, and perform a procedure include:

- Acuity
- Co-morbid psychiatric (*e.g.* severe pain-related depression) and social (*e.g.* single mother of young children with limited resources) considerations
- Pain level and accompanying functional impairment
- Likelihood of the visit/ procedure providing meaningful benefit
- Likelihood of the patient to seek scarce emergency services, or be started on opioids
- Need for physical examination
- Risk association with in-person visit or procedure
- Work status (*e.g.* is the patient currently working or likely to return to work with

## Adequate Pain Treatment?

## Paracetamol and NSAIDs

NSAIDs, especially "profen group" is commonly used as an anti-inflammatory agent globally, have been pointed out to facilitate the adhesion of the virus to the cell by up-regulation of ACE2 receptors in patients with COVID-19, but it has not been supported by concrete evidence. There are no clear data to support that NSAIDs should not be used specifically in patients diagnosed with or suspected to have COVID-19 (Pergolizzi, 2020).

The deadliest complication of COVID-19 infection is sepsis, along with cardiovascular and / or respiratory complications. This situation is predominantly seen in elderly and patients with comorbidities (Zhou, 2020). It should be kept in mind that long-term use of NSAIDs such as ibuprofen, naproxen and diclofenac are associated with higher rates of CVD, such as myocardial infarction, heart failure and stroke (Bhala, 2013).

Acute respiratory infections are associated with an already increased risk of stroke and myocardial infarction, and short-term use of NSAIDs during illness is associated with an increased risk (Wen, 2018). For example, the use of NSAIDs in acute respiratory infections has been reported to increase the propensity for AMI (OR: 3.41), but it is thought that there may be no significant increase of the risk with NSAIDs since the OR value for AMI is considered to be 2.65, even if NSAIDs are not used at all (Wen, 2017). It is not known whether any of these proposed factors apply to the COVID-19 pandemic. Evidence to date is not strong enough to support the full refusal of the use of NSAIDs.

NSAIDs are used if paracetamol's analgesic effect is insufficient, or for conditions such as severe musculoskeletal pain or resistant fever.

### How About Aspirin?

People taking low-dose aspirin should continue their treatment for secondary prevention of cardiovascular disease (Little, 2020).

### Should Pregnant Women Take NSAIDS?

It is evident that treatment and prophylaxis with aspirin and NSAIDs should not be interrupted in pregnant women (Kwiatkowski, 2020). It was also concluded that there is no suggestion that NSAIDs should be withheld in pregnant patients with suspected or diagnosed COVID-19. Kakodkar *et al*, also reported in their article published in April 2020 that WHO also stated that it had not issued a negative interpretation for ibuprofen and/or other NSAIDs and that it was appropriate to continue the medication (Kakodkar, 2020).

### Renin-Angiotensin System (RAS) Inhibitors

The idea that RAS inhibitors and ibuprofen increase ACE2 receptors is based on the results of a study by giving high doses of ibuprofen in diabetic rats, such as 40 mg / kg (Qiao, 2015). This dose is deliberately an overdose such as 3 g in a 70 kg person. This does not mean that these findings can be extrapolated to an outcome associated with the usual dose of ibuprofen in man.

## Specific Pain Syndromes and COVID-19

### - *Headache*

Headache has been reported in 11% to 34% of cases with COVID-19 in different series (Borges do Nascimento. 2020, Zhang 2020, Chen 2020, Xu 2020). In addition, around 6% to 10% of the symptomatic patients with COVID-19 reported headache as a presenting symptom (Bolay, 2020). Headache is one of the principal indications in which NSAIDS are preferred as the first-line agent. In the article published in April 2020, It was reported that no evidence-based data prevents the use of **RAS** inhibitors and NSAIDS such as ibuprofen in suspected patients with COVID-19 with headache (Maassen VanDenBrink, 2020).

**- Musculoskeletal pain and NSAIDS:** Orthopedists from Italy, De Girolamo *et al*, stated that the warnings for not using ibuprofen in May 2020 lead to a point that reduces the quality of life of orthopedic patients (De Girolamo, 2020).

## Safety and NSAIDs

In the last IDSA report, the issue regarding the use of NSAID agents in COVID-19 cases was also examined and it was stated that there is no warning that NSAIDs should not specifically used in patients with COVID-19, however, possible adverse effects need to be taken into consideration (Bhimraj, 2020). It has been mentioned that any cause-effect relationship regarding the use of NSAID has not been established in patients with deterioration. GI hemorrhage is the best known widespread adverse effect of NSAIDS. Nonetheless, profen group has been shown to cause fewer GI hemorrhages when compared to other NSAIDs (British National Formulary, 2014).

In the UK, **"The Expert Working Group on the Commission of Human Medicines"** stated that no link could be proven between ibuprofen and severe course or exacerbation of COVID-19 (Gov.UK.). Again, the UK health authority NHS emphasized that paracetamol may be the first choice and there is no clear data preventing the use of ibuprofen in the treatment of acute pain and fever (NHS England, 2020). Previously, it is reported that there is no definite data on NSAIDs increasing the complications of community-acquired pneumonia (Basille 2017).

Another critical issue regarding safety is that the feared side effects of NSAIDs are **dose-related** consequences of the agents. In other words, a comparison of short-term oral NSAID and IV continuous infusion in a severely symptomatic patient will certainly yield different results. For example, IV administered NSAID significantly increases the risk of stroke / CVA in patients with critical condition and/or respiratory distress, but there is no such risk in oral administration (Voiriot, 2018). In a new article, Zolk *et al*, also suggested that NSAIDs should be used in the COVID-19 pandemic period at the lowest effective dose and for a short time and reported that no untoward effects are expected (Zolk, 2020).

More recently, a population-based Danish cohort study was conducted by Lund *et al*, (Lund, 2020). The median age of the sample was 50 years, and 58% were female. They reported that treatment with NSAIDs was not linked with 30-day mortality, hospital admission, ICU admission, mechanical ventilation, or renal replacement therapy in Danish patients with COVID-19. The Danish researchers had previously demonstrated that NSAIDs were not associated with 30-day intensive care unit admission or death in adjusted analyses in patients with influenza.

## The Differences Between the Agents

Diclofenac, one of the most commonly used NSAIDs, has been accused of marked local neurotoxicity (in IM use) in the last decade, the risk of GI bleeding and -due to the sodium content - exacerbations of heart failure and hypertension, and therefore, its use has been considerably reduced.

Paracetamol has been promoted as a safe alternative to NSAIDs, but the agent has well-established causal links with liver damage or toxicity for decades. In other words, paracetamol is a treatment that can cause problems if posology is not considered. Therefore, NSAIDs can be used with caution after paracetamol if necessary (Belgium, 2020, Little, 2020).

## Tocilizumab as a NSAID

Tocilizumab (TCZ) is an anti-IL-6 receptor monoclonal antibody, widely used in the treatment of autoimmune diseases and has been approved by the FDA to reduce cytokine release due to CD19-specific chimeric antigen receptor T cell therapy in acute lymphoblastic leukemia (Santomasso *et al*, 2018). In COVID-19, it is used as an IL-6 inhibitor at high serum IL-6 levels in patients with bilateral diffuse pulmonary infiltrations or in severe and critical groups with cytokine storm. Mechanisms of effect attributed to anti-IL-6 receptor antibodies at the cellular level have been illustrated in Fig. (**3**).

There are contradicting reports on efficacy of TCZ in patients with COVID-19. In September 2020, Lan *et al*, published a meta-analysis and demonstrated that TCZ had no effect on mortality, ICU admission and risk of requirement for MV (Fig. **4**) (Lan, 2020).

TCZ treatment was administered in 21 patients who were diagnosed with severe or critical COVID-19. As a result of the study, it was reported that TCZ effectively improves clinical symptoms and suppresses the deterioration of patients with COVID-19 (Xu *et al*, 2020). In another study, TCZ was used in 15 patients with COVID-19 whose mean IL-6 level was 111.05 pg / mL (range 5-15 pg / mL). 47% of them were critical, 40% severe and 13% moderate. After the treatment, a decrease in IL-6 level was observed in 11 patients, along with clinical improvement. However, a steady increase in IL-6 level was observed in four critically ill patients in whom treatment was not successful (Luo *et al*, 2020).

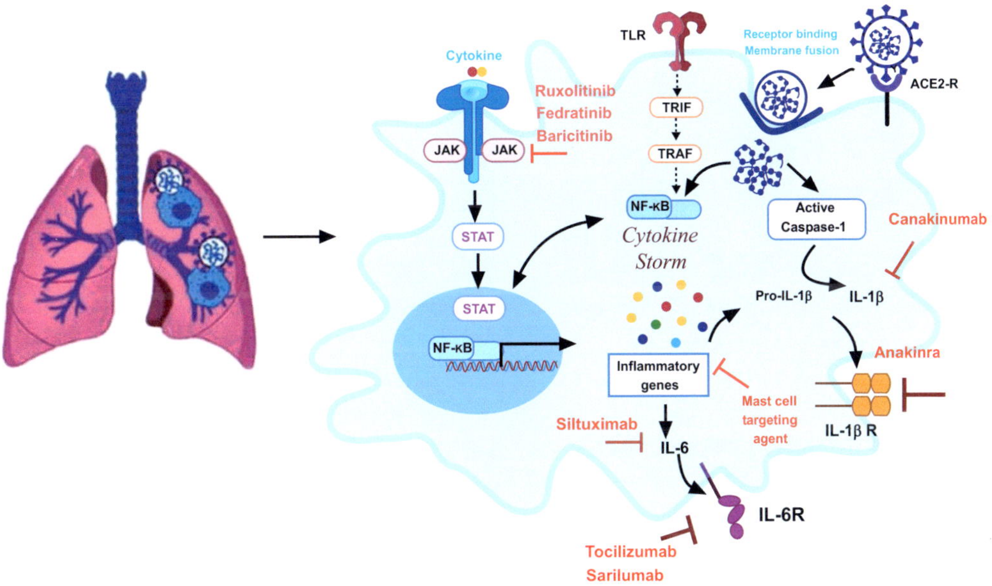


**Fig. (3).** Mechanisms of effect attributed to anti-IL-6 receptor antibodies tocilizumab and siltuximab at the cellular chemistry level.

In another study, 100 patients with COVID-19 pneumonia and ARDS requiring ventilatory support were given IV TCZ in addition to the conventional treatment, empirically considering that they had high IL-6 levels. 24-72 hours after TCZ administration, 58 patients (58%) showed a rapid clinical and respiratory improvement, 37 (37%) were stabilized clinically, 5 (5%) deteriorated and 4 of these died (Toniati *et al*, 2020). In the largest registry study conducted to date, 544 patients with severe COVID-19 pneumonia were retrospectively examined, and IV or SC treatment with TCZ was found to be associated with reduced risk of mechanical ventilation and death (adjusted hazard ratio 0 61, 95% CI 0 · 40--092; p = 0 020) (Guaraldi *et al*, 2020).

| Study or Subgroup | Tocilizumab Events | Tocilizumab Total | Control Events | Control Total | Weight | Risk Ratio M-H, Random, 95% CI |
|---|---|---|---|---|---|---|
| Capra *et al*, 2020 | 2 | 63 | 11 | 23 | 11.7% | 0.07 [0.02, 0.28] |
| Colaneri *et al* (SMACOREtrial), 2020 | 5 | 21 | 19 | 91 | 17.4% | 1.14 [0.48, 2.70] |
| Klopfenstein *et al*, 2020 | 5 | 20 | 12 | 25 | 17.4% | 0.52 [0.22, 1.23] |
| Quartucciol *et al*, 2020 | 4 | 42 | 0 | 69 | 4.5% | 14.65 [0.81, 265.46] |
| Ramaswamy *et al*, 2020 | 3 | 21 | 8 | 65 | 13.5% | 1.16 [0.34, 3.98] |
| Roumier *et al*, 2020 | 3 | 30 | 9 | 29 | 13.8% | 0.32 [0.10, 1.07] |
| Wadud *et al*, 2020 | 17 | 44 | 26 | 50 | 21.7% | 0.74 [0.47, 1.17] |
| Total (95% CI) | | 241 | | 352 | 100.0% | 0.61 [0.31, 1.22] |
| Total events | 39 | | 85 | | | |

Heterogeneity: Tau² = 0.51; Chi² =18.64, df = 6(P = 0.005); I² = 68%
Test for overall effect; Z = 140 (P = 0.16)

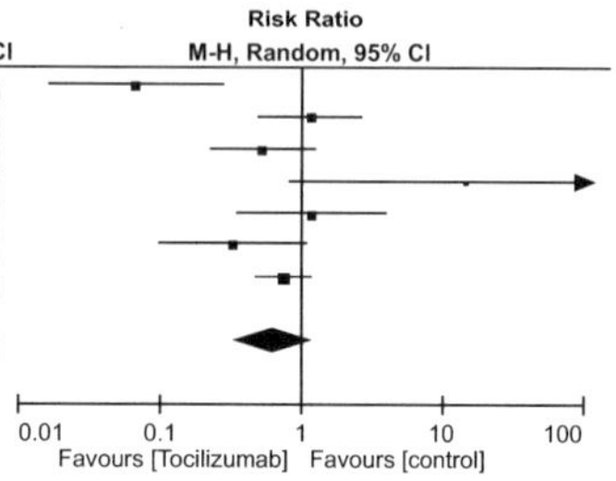


| Study or Subgroup | Tocilizumab Events | Tocilizumab Total | Control Events | Control Total | Weight | Risk Ratio M-H, Random, 95% CI |
|---|---|---|---|---|---|---|
| Colaneri *et al* (SMACOREtrial), 2020 | 3 | 21 | 12 | 91 | 22.8% | 1.08 [0.34, 3.50] |
| Klopfenstein *et al*, 2020 | 0 | 20 | 11 | 25 | 13.9% | 0.05 [0.00, 0.86] |
| Quartucciol *et al*, 2020 | 27 | 42 | 0 | 69 | 13.9% | 89.53 [5.60, 1430.27] |
| Ramaswamy *et al*, 2020 | 10 | 21 | 8 | 65 | 24.6% | 3.87 [1.76, 8.52] |
| Roumier *et al*, 2020 | 7 | 30 | 13 | 29 | 24.7% | 0.52 [0.24, 1.12] |
| Total (95% CI) | | 134 | | 279 | 100.0% | 1.51 [0.33, 6.78] |
| Total events | 47 | | 44 | | | |

Heterogeneity: Tau² = 2.23; Chi² =28.84, df = 4(P < 0.00001); I² = 86%
Test for overall effect; Z = 0.53 (P = 0.59)

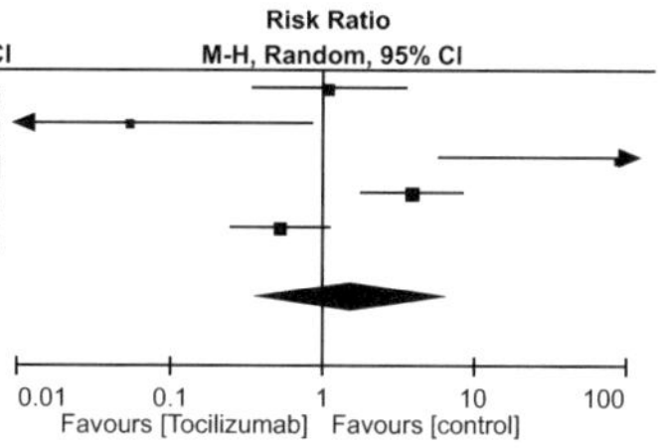


| Study or Subgroup | Tocilizumab Events | Tocilizumab Total | Control Events | Control Total | Weight | Risk Ratio M-H, Random, 95% CI |
|---|---|---|---|---|---|---|
| Colaneri *et al* (SMACOREtrial), 2020 | 3 | 21 | 12 | 91 | 22.8% | 1.08 [0.34, 3.50] |
| Klopfenstein *et al*, 2020 | 0 | 20 | 11 | 25 | 13.9% | 0.05 [0.00, 0.86] |
| Quartucciol *et al*, 2020 | 27 | 42 | 0 | 69 | 13.9% | 89.53 [5.60, 1430.27] |
| Ramaswamy *et al*, 2020 | 10 | 21 | 8 | 65 | 24.6% | 3.87 [1.76, 8.52] |
| Roumier *et al*, 2020 | 7 | 30 | 13 | 29 | 24.7% | 0.52 [0.24, 1.12] |
| Total (95% CI) | | 134 | | 279 | 100.0% | 1.51 [0.33, 6.78] |
| Total events | 47 | | 44 | | | |

Heterogeneity: Tau² = 2.23; Chi² =28.84, df = 4(P < 0.00001); I² = 86%
Test for overall effect; Z = 0.53 (P = 0.59)

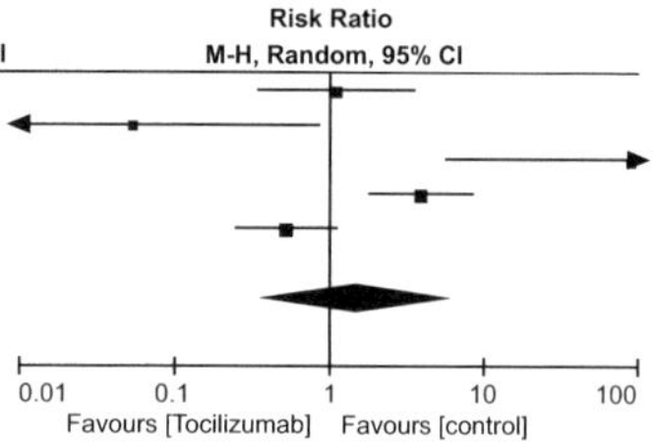


**Fig. (4).** Tocilizumab was found ineffective on mortality **(A)**, ICU admission **(B)** and risk of requirement for MV **(C)** in a meta-analytic study by Lan *et al*, 2020.

The initial dose of TCZ is 4 to 8 mg / kg. The recommended starting dose is 400 mg, diluted to 100 ml with 0.9% normal saline and given as IV infusion in 1 hour. Patients who do not show a significant improvement after the first dose, the same dose is repeated a second time after 12 hours. The maximum single dose should not exceed 800 mg. Attention should be paid to allergic reactions. TCZ is not used in patients with active infections such as tuberculosis (Diagnosis and Treatment Protocol for Novel Coronavirus Pneumonia. Trial Version 7).

In an academic medical center, Meleveedu *et al*, described outcomes in severely ill patients with cytokine release syndrome (CRS) due to COVID-19 following treatment with anti-IL-6/IL-6-Receptor (anti-IL-6/IL-6-R) therapy, including tocilizumab or siltuximab. They have reported that clinical responses to anti-I-

-6/IL-6-R therapy were accompanied by significant decreases in temperature, oxygen requirement, CRP, IL-6, and IL-10 levels.

There are numerous ongoing well-designed research projects tocilizumab and sarilumab such as COVACTA and SARCOVID, respectively (https://clinicaltrials.gov/ct2/show/NCT04320615, Garcia-Vicuña

Pearl: There are definitely COVID-19 cases where NSAIDs would not be appropriate to use, such as those who are prone to GI bleeding. However, a scientific basis for not using them in other cases has not been established.

As with many drugs, questions to be asked before prescribing in optimizing the safety profile of NSAIDs are shown in the Table **10**.

**Table 10. As with many drugs, questions to be asked before prescribing in optimizing the safety profile of NSAIDs. With this six-item approach, which can be called the "3W2H1C system", a safer profile will be created for patients.**

| Q | Explanation |
|---|---|
| **To Whom?** | Make sure it is given to the right patient |
| **Why?** | With what indication? |
| **Which drug?** | Choose the agent with the best profile of effect/adverse events |
| **How much?** | In what dosage? |
| **How?** | IV / oral route |
| **Caution!** | Drug interactions and allergies |

In conclusion, the use of NSAIDs as antipyretic, analgesic and anti-inflammatory agents appears to be indicated in viral infections such as COVID-19, also during pandemic periods. There is no evidence to support NSAIDs not to be used in COVID-19 infections due to their side effects. NSAIDs are used after paracetamol, if necessary, to manage the symptoms of COVID-19.

## IS VITAMIN C EFFECTIVE IN THE TREATMENT OF COVID-19, SEPSIS AND ARDS?

Ascorbic acid (AscA), also known as "vitamin C", is found naturally in many foods, especially in fruits. It is an acidic substance and has a pH between 2.1 and 2.6 (Padayatty, 2004). When isolated, it has a powder or yellowish crystal appearance, in a colorless, odorless and soluble structure. AscA is necessary for many biochemical reactions in the body to occur normally. Since it is not produced in the body, it is necessary to provide this absolute need from the outside, orally or parenterally. Pharmacological concentrations can only be reached after intravenous (IV) administration.

## Antioxidant AscA

Parenteral AscA is known for its antioxidant properties without showing pro-oxidant effects. AscA is a molecule that readily functions as one or two electron-reducing agents for many radicals and oxidants. It functions as an antioxidant by inhibiting hydrogen peroxide-induced cell death and DNA damage triggered by oxidizing stress (Tyml, 2017). It protects the body's cells and tissues from oxidizing damage and dysfunction by removing harmful reactive oxygen species. This vitamin also has many important properties that support immunity in the body. Since it is involved in the formation of a protective barrier against infections and viruses, its consumption in the body increases during infection. Therefore, the need for AscA increases in proportion to the severity of the infection (Lowes, 2010; Carr, Crit Care 2017).

## AscA in Sepsis

AscA affects the immune system, for example the function of phagocytes, the transformation of T lymphocytes, and the production of interferon (INF). In some studies, a significantly lower rate of pneumonia was recorded in groups receiving AscA (Carr, Nutrients 2017). As a result of the reduction of plasma free iron (Fe), removal of free radicals and the consumption of its oxidizing form, dehydroascorbic acid (DHA), plasma AscA concentrations in sepsis gradually decrease; and eventually it can run out. AscA deficiency due to sepsis allows uncontrolled oxidizing activity that increases tissue damage (Wilson, 2009).

AscA is effective as a protective factor against sepsis syndromes, and appears to be inversely correlated with multi-organ failure and mortality rate (Wilson, 2009; Borrelli, 1996). In the experimental sepsis model created by injecting pathogenic bacteria to rodents, the existing AscA in the organism was depleted and the survival rate decreased (Gaut, 2006). It has been shown in another study that AscA administration reverses the deficiency in capillary circulation which ensues due to sepsis (Tyml, 2008).

The adhesion of leukocytes and platelets to the endothelium precipitates blood clots during sepsis which stops blood flow in certain areas. IV AscA can potentially reverse the adhesion by increasing bioavailability of NO, decreasing the secretion of P-selectin protein, and preventing platelet adhesion (Tyml, 2011). IV AscA replacement contributes to the effective and safe resolution of inflammation and to prevent the release of neutrophil granule enzymes that cause cytotoxicity and hydrolysis which may cause tissue damage (Tyml, 2017). It has been reported that IV AscA therapy could potentially relieve sepsis-related vascular inflammation (Wilson, 2009) (Table **11**).

**Table 11. Effects of AscA in experimental studies: (Adapted from Armour, 2001; Wu, 2004; Tyml, 2005; Kim, 2006).**

| |
|---|
| 1. Prevents endotoxin-induced hypotension, |
| 2. Augments the ability of capillary arteries to respond to hypotension by partially correcting the basal arterial pressure, |
| 3. Escalates endothelial NO production with vasodilator efficacy, which protects from hypersensitivity against vasoconstriction in the arterioles, |
| 4. Increases capillary blood flow, |
| 5. Reduces the growth of bacteria, |
| 6. Prevents hydrogen peroxide-induced damage in cultured capillary tissue cells, |
| 7. Protects against capillary dysfunction in skeletal muscle of septic animals, |
| 8. Increases survival rate after treatment in experimental sepsis model, |
| 9. Protects liver functions |

## AscA in ARDS

In an earlier study, it was reported that the mortality rate decreased by 50% when high dose IV AscA and tocopherol, N-acetyl-cysteine and selenium antioxidants were administered to patients with ARDS (Sawyer, 1989).

Later, Tanaka *et al*, administered AscA IV at a dose and rate of 66 mg / kg / hour continuously for the first 24 hours in patients with surface area burns covering more than 50% of body area (Tanaka, 2000). After 96 hours, the patients had a reduction in the fluid volume requirement and had significantly reduced wound edema. In addition, a decrease in the severity of respiratory dysfunction was observed in these patients. Nathens *et al*, administered α-tocopherol and AscA as antioxidants for 28 days to 595 patients who were surgically treated in the ICU (Nathens, 2002). When compared with 155 patients who did not receive antioxidants, the rate of organ failure and the duration of stay in ICU was decreased in patients who were treated with antioxidants .

One study in septic patients showed that medical AscA therapy reduced the severity of multiorgan failure and levels of circulating injury biomarkers. Patients treated with AscA had rapid and sustained decreases in SOFA scores during the 4-day treatment regimen, in contrast to the placebo controls. The decrease in SOFA score was observed most prominently in patients receiving high dose IV AscA (Fowler, 2014).

Intracellular AscA inhibits TNF-α-induced Nuclear Factor-kappa B (NF-κB) activation in human cell lines in a dose-dependent manner in primary tissue cells. AscA may affect inflammatory, neoplastic, and programmed cellular death processes through inhibition of NF-κB activation. In this way, it could potentially weaken the cytokine storm that occurs in sepsis (Carcamo, 2002). The effects of AscA in some systemic and septic infections are shown in the Table **12**.

**Table 12. Effects of Vitamin C (AscA) on some systemic and septic infections.**

| Systemic Effects | Effects in Critical Care: ARDS and Septic Infections |
|---|---|
| **1. Antioxidant Effect:**<br>• Prevents cell death and DNA damage<br>• Increases the scavenging of reactive oxygen ($O_2$) radicals.<br>**2. Anti-inflammatory Effect:**<br>• Creating a protective barrier against infections<br>• Increasing nitric oxide (NO) production<br>• Reducing platelet adhesion<br>• Increasing the content of tetrahydrobiopterin in platelets<br>• reducing the secretion of P-selectin protein<br>• Preventing the release of cytotoxic and hydrophilic neutrophil granule enzymes<br>**3. Immune System Effects:**<br>• Increasing the function of phagocytes<br>• Increasing the turnover of T lymphocytes<br>• Increasing interferon (INF) production and activity<br>• Increasing the production of immunological thymic hormones | **1. ARDS:**<br>• Decrease in death rate<br>• Decrease in fluid volume requirements and wound edema<br>• Decrease in the severity of respiratory dysfunction in patients<br>**2. ICU and critical surgery patients:**<br>**Effects on Septic Infections**<br>• Prevention of endotoxin-induced hypotension by increasing capillary arteriolar responsiveness,<br>• Increased endothelial NO production with vasodilator efficacy, which protects from hypersensitivity against vasoconstriction in the arterioles.<br>• Increase in capillary blood flow,<br>• Bacteriostatic effect,<br>• Preventing hydrogen peroxide damage to capillary tissue cells,<br>• Increase in survival rate after treatment,<br>• Protection in liver functions<br>**3. Sepsis:**<br>• Increase in survival rate<br>• Protective factor against precipitation of sepsis<br>• Reversing capillary circulation disorder<br>• Increase in capillary blood flow and strengthen permeability barrier<br>• Relieving sepsis-associated vascular inflammation<br>**4. ALI:**<br>• Reducing the pulmonary proinflammatory response<br>• To reduce the accumulation of polymorphonuclear neutrophils (PMN) in certain tissues<br>• Preventing the destruction of Na + -K + -ATPase pump in lung alveolar tissue cells<br>• To restore the viscosity of blood to normal<br>• Maintain tissue cellular permeability to ions and small molecules by normalizing the expression of 'Tight junctions' (TJ) proteins<br>• Correcting prothrombin time (PT) and activated partial thromboplastin time (aPTT)<br>• To reverse signs of sepsis-induced bleeding coagulation disorders<br>**5. COVID-19:**<br>• There is no evidence supported by adequate clinical studies. |

The largest study evaluating the use of high-dose AscA in patients with sepsis and ARDS in recent years is the vitamin C infusion (CITRIS-ALI) study for patients with sepsis and severe acute respiratory failure (Fowler, 2019). This clinical study is a comparative, double-blind, controlled, multicenter study conducted in 7 ICUs in the USA, and enrolled patients with sepsis and ARDS. Patients were randomized to receive IV AscA (50 mg / kg in 5% dextrose solution, n = 84) or distilled water (n = 83) IV every 6 hours for 96 hours. Among patients with sepsis and ARDS, it has been reported that 96-hour high-dose vitamin C IV treatment did not significantly reduce organ failure scores or improve biomarker levels at 168 hours. However, it has been shown that the mortality rate can be reduced in these patients. It has been reported that more research is needed to evaluate the role of AscA in sepsis and ARDS.

## AscA in The Treatment of Acute Lung Injury (ALI)

In an experimental study, IV AscA was administered after polymicrobial peritonitis was induced in mice. The administration of IV AscA significantly reduced both the preinflammatory response of the lungs and the accumulation of polymorphonuclear neutrophils (PMN) in certain tissues without homogenous distribution in the body. Thus, IV AscA treatment preserved lung barrier function in septic mice. In addition, it has been reported that AscA prevents the degradation of the $Na^+$-$K^+$-ATPase pump in lung alveolar cells.

AscA preserved tissue cellular permeability to ions and small molecules by normalizing the release of tight junctions (TJ) proteins into the environment. AscA vascular therapy eliminated the coagulation abnormalities found in septic mice (Fisher, 2012). The regulation of pre-coagulation, anti-coagulation and clot-dissolving pathways can explain the main regulatory effects of AscA on peritonitis-mediated ALI-related coagulation abnormalities. These experimental data show that parenterally administered AscA accumulates in the cell and increases the lung barrier cell function and structure. In this study, it is shown that AscA alleviates ALI precipitated by sepsis by increasing the integrity of the epithelial barrier of the lung alveoli. AscA also up regulated the secretion of ion channels and pumps that play a critical role in improving lung alveolar fluid drainage.

## Effect on Coagulation Disorders

In addition, significant changes were observed in viscosity and clot properties of septic mouse blood. IV AscA treatment in septic mice completely normalized bleeding coagulation disorders (Fisher, 2012). It has been shown that AscA improves almost all symptoms of sepsis-induced coagulation disorders, prothrombin time (PT) and activated partial thromboplastin time (aPTT) in the endotoxin-induced sepsis model (Fisher, 2011).

## High Dose Vitamin C (AscA) Treatment in COVID-19

Currently, there is no specific treatment with proven reliability and efficacy for COVID-19 infection, which may develop pneumonia, sepsis, ARDS, multiple organ failure and death in severe cases. Treatment options are based on information obtained within the framework of comparative controlled studies and other scientific research. One of these treatment options is supportive high dose vitamin C, namely AscA treatment. The basis for this treatment is based on the aforementioned efficacy that has been reported in many studies published previously.

Ready-to-use 15 g (500 mg / ml) AscA vials are available in 50 ml water solution for injection (Fig. **5**). IV treatment is administered at a dose of 50 mg / kg, qid (4 times a day) (Carr, 2018). Although there is no clear data on the duration of treatment, it was given to patients in the ICU for 4 days in CITRIS-ALI study (Fowler, 2019). Although no negative results have been reported regarding its safety and short-term adverse effects, the issue of high-dose AscA treatment duration and undesirable long-term effects should be investigated with larger studies.

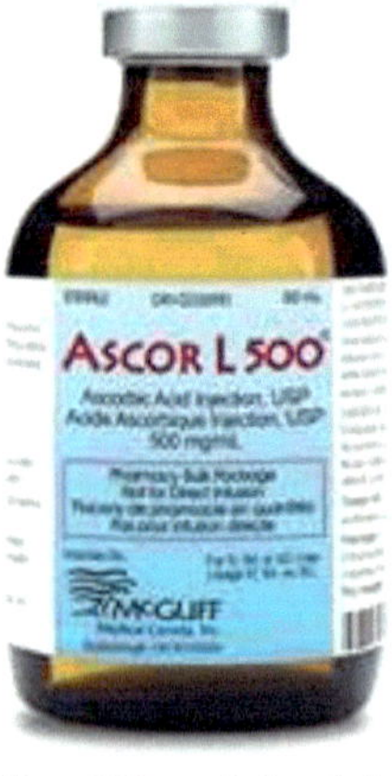


**Fig. (5).** Vitamin C vial for injection, including 500 mg l-AscA / mL.

In conclusion, AscA has positive contributions to the inflammatory process with various effects and mechanisms. The use of high-dose AscA may be considered in the supportive treatment of COVID-19, as it has been reported in the previous studies. It has been reported to significantly reduce the degree of multi-organ failure, organ damage, especially acute lung injury, and reduce the severity of respiratory dysfunction and mortality. Experiences with high-dose AscA treatment in the COVID-19 pandemic will be a guiding resource in the future in overcoming the uncertainties. However, for now, it cannot be said that AscA treatment is absolutely beneficial and indicated in the management of COVID-19.

## VITAMIN D AND COVID-19: A REAL TREATMENT?

Vitamin D (DV), known as the sunshine vitamin, is an important molecule for healthy bones, teeth and muscles. Vitamin D2 is synthesized by plants, while vitamin D3 is produced in our skin. The active form of DV (1,25-dihydroxyvitamin D / calcitriol) is thought to be effective in many inflammatory, infectious diseases. DV deficiency leads to rickets in children, bone softening in adults or diseases called 'ostoemalacia'.

DV is transformed from the passive form to the active form in the skin by ultraviolet radiation. Therefore, it is known that physical activity in the open air under the sun can effectively increase DV levels (Carter *et al*, 2020). It has been shown that DV synthesis is less active in blacks, which is due to the fact that melanin pigment absorbs less ultraviolet (UV) rays (Nair *et al*, 2012).

### Is COVID-19 related to vitamin D?

Yes and no. COVID-19 has been linked to DV as well as everything else. It is confusing that COVID-19 is more common and more deadly in the northern hemisphere, in winter, in the black race and in the elderly. DV levels in the body tend to decrease with age. Case fatality rates caused by COVID-19 also increase with age (Novel, C.P.E.R.E. 2020).

Cannell *et al*, report that the winter peak in infections is partially linked to the time period when solar UV radiation doses and thus DV concentrations are lowest in most mid- and high-latitude countries (Cannell *et al*, 2006). A study recruiting 198 healthy adults in the autumn and winter of 2009-2010 in Connecticut examined the relationship between serum DV concentration and the incidence of acute lower respiratory tract infection (LRTI). Throughout the study, 45% of those with DV levels below 38 ng / mL developed LRTI while the disease ensued in only 17% of those who had DV above 38 ng / mL. Concentrations of a DV level of 38 ng / mL or more were associated with a two-fold reduction in the risk of developing LRTI ($p < 0.0001$) and a significant reduction in the patient days (Sabetta *et al*, 2010).

There are significant differences between countries in mortality rates caused by COVID-19. During the outbreak, countries in the southern hemisphere experienced a relatively low mortality rate. "Thirty-five degrees North" is latitude where human being does not get enough sunlight to maintain adequate vitamin D levels during the winter months. This suggests a possible role of vitamin D in determining outcomes from COVID-19. There is little evidence that DV can protect against infection. It is important to note that the hypothesis is not that DV will protect against SARS-CoV-2 infection but may be very important in the prevention of cytokine storm and subsequent LRTI that causes mortality. Large-scale studies are urgently needed to assess whether there is a relationship between DV and COVID-19 disease severity (Garg *et al*, 2020).

## What are The Claims Related to Infections and DV?

In fact, there seems to be no serious evidence that DV supports the immune system. Still, some studies have shown that DV deficiency increases the susceptibility to viral diseases such as flu and colds. The effects of DV related to infections are listed in Table **13**.

**Table 13. Effects of DV related to infections.**

| |
|---|
| 1. It takes part in the regulation and suppression of the inflammatory cytokine response of respiratory epithelial cells and macrophages against various pathogens. |
| 2. Reducing the risk or severe respiratory infections; resulting from increased expression and secretion of pro-inflammatory cytokines and chemokines. |
| 3. Protective effect from lipopolysaccharide-induced lung injury by modulating ACE-I and II expression |
| 4. Reduced risk of microbial infection and death through physical barrier and cellular innate immune mechanisms. |
| 5. Increases expression of antioxidation-related genes with antimicrobial activities, which prevent the consumption of AscA (C vit) utilized for the prevention and treatment of COVID-19 |
| 6. Antiviral effect |
| 7. It alleviates acute lung injury with immunomodulatory effect, including down-regulation of pro-inflammatory cytokines. |

ACE: Angiotensin-converting enzyme, AscA: Ascorbic acid

There are outstanding experimental data showing that DV is important in regulating and suppressing the inflammatory cytokine response via respiratory epithelial cells and macrophages against various pathogens, including respiratory viruses (Greiller *et al*, 2015).

Respiratory monocytes / macrophages and epithelial cells protect against respiratory tract infections by expressing the DV receptor. DV and DV receptor agonists significantly reduce the pro-inflammatory response to antigen challenge in cystic fibrosis airway epithelial cells *in vitro*. Some studies suggest that low DV levels may increase the risk or severity of respiratory viral infections, in relation with increased expression and secretion of pro-inflammatory cytokines and chemokines. Therapeutic administration of DV reduces the inflammatory response to viral infections in the airway epithelium. This suggests that adequate DV level will contribute to mitigated inflammation severity in individuals infected with respiratory syncytial virus (RSV) (Hansdottir *et al*, 2010).

DV has been experimentally shown to exert protective effects from lipopolysaccharide-induced lung damage by modulating the expression of ACE-I and II. ACE-II is the host receptor for the entry of SARS-CoV-2 into intestinal and alveolar cells. Later, dysregulation of the renin-angiotensin system can lead to large-scale cytokine activation leading to acute respiratory distress syndrome (ARDS), which can be fatal (Xu *et al*, 2017).

In some publications, it has been reported that DV reduces the risk of microbial infection and death and provides this with physical barrier and cellular innate immune mechanisms (Rondanelli *et al*, 2018). It suppresses responses mediated by T helper type 1 (Thl) cells, primarily by inhibiting the production of inflammatory cytokines IL-2 and interferon gamma (INF- γ). It also promotes cytokine production by T helper type 2 (Th2) cells, which helps to increase the indirect suppression of Th1 cells. It increases the induction of T regulatory cells. Thus, DV has been claimed to inhibit inflammatory processes.

DV also increases the expression of genes associated with antioxidation (glutathione reductase and glutamate-cysteine ligase modifier subunit), and then increased glutathione production, has prevent consumption of AscA (C vit), which has antimicrobial activities and also proposed for treatment and prevention of COVID-19.

Teymoori-Rad has also suggested that DV, which can act as an immunomodulator and anti-inflammatory, has antiviral activity with many different mechanisms (Teymoori-Rad *et al*, 2019). DV has been reported to be associated with cytokine hyperproduction and ARDS and has recently been recommended as a drug for lung damage caused by influenza A H5N1 virus due to its protective effect. Again, some studies show the effectiveness of DV as an adjuvant treatment with antiretroviral agents in patients infected with human immunodeficiency virus (HIV). In addition, DV pretreatment is beneficial in animal models of ARDS and reduces lung permeability by modulation of the renin-angiotensin system activity and ACE2 expression (Xu *et al*, 2017).

DV has immunomodulatory properties, including down-regulation of pro-inflammatory cytokines, and has been shown to mitigate lipopolysaccharide-induced acute lung injury by the renin-angiotensin pathway in mice by inhibiting effects on angiopoietin (Ang)-2-Tie-2 signaling. In another study conducted on DV's replication of rotavirus both *in vitro* and *in vivo*, it was claimed that 4000 IU / day DV supplementation reduced Dengue virus infection (Arboleda *et al*, 2019).

In population-based studies, it has been stated that COVID-19 infection is more common and more severe in people with DV deficiency, blacks and other ethnic minorities in Western societies (Khunti *et al*, 2020). For example, only 13% of the UK society consists of ethnic minorities, but 1/3 of the patients with COVID-19 hospitalized in hospitals are from these minorities. It was written in the Washington Post that in the United States, the risk of black people getting COVID-19 is 3 times higher and the risk of death is 6 times higher than the others. However, the reason for the relationship between ethnicity and DV deficiency is not fully clarified yet. The fact that DV deficiency was more common in these groups was postulated to be a potential explanation (Thebault *et al*, 2020).

## Immune Modulatory Effect and Vitamin D

DV is a modulator of adaptive immunity, and it has been suggested that it can help manage the proinflammatory environment or "cytokine storm" observed in COVID-19 patients (Grant *et al*, 2020). It has been claimed to show immunomodulatory activity with IL-6 antagonist activity similar to tocilizumab, and it even provides cyclicity of seasonal flu (Silberstein, 2020). Urashima *et al*, It showed that DV level is directly related to susceptibility to influenza disease. The authors suggested that DV therapy, rather than tocilizumab, could be used more economically to manage COVID-19. It has been shown that giving DV at regular intervals in the elderly can protect against respiratory infections. Higher doses may be required in the treatment of those with COVID-19 (Urashima *et al*, 2010).

## Who are The Risk Groups?

Obese individuals, pregnant women, those with chronic diseases and the elderly are at high risk for DV deficiency. It has been suggested that the link between obesity and the severe course of COVID-19 stems from DV deficiency. It has been reported that DV deficiency is also effective in the development of ARDS in those with COVID-19 (Han *et al*, 2016). The fact that advanced age and the presence of comorbidity, which are factors in COVID-19 deaths, also accompany DV deficiency make it difficult to realize which is the main factor (Pilz *et al*, 2018). Taking all these into consideration, Grant *et al*, He recommended that people in risk groups take 10,000 IU / day for a few weeks and then 5,000 IU / day of vitamin D3 to reduce the risk of COVID-19 and other infections. The goal is to rise DV level above 40–60 ng / mL (100–150 nmol / L) (Grant *et al*, 2020).

## Smoking, Men, and vitamin D: a Bad Trio?

Yes. It has also been suggested that the higher mortality rate due to COVID-19 in men is the result of higher smoking in men and the decrease in DV level of smoking (Grant *et al*, 2020; Brot *et al*, 1999).

## Vitamin D in Intensive Care

In 2016, it has been shown that administration of high doses of DV to patients with DV deficiency (N = 31) among the patients in ICU on mechanical ventilation in Atlanta decreased deaths (Han *et al*, 2016).

## What Should Be Considered When Getting DV?

Patients receiving DV are also recommended to consume magnesium and calcium, which help activation and act together in bone metabolism. One of the most comprehensive clinical studies on this subject has been conducted and recently published in England. Blood (25 (OH) D) level has been associated with risk of COVID-19 among UK Biobank participants (502,624 people, 37-73 years old). It has also been investigated for its relationship to increased risk in ethnic minorities. Indeed, DV deficiency appears to be associated with inflicted by COVID-19. However, when 'confounding factors' such as low socioeconomic status, malnutrition etc. are discarded, the "statistically significant relationship" disappears (OR = 1.00; 95% CI = 0.998-1.01; p = 0.208). In other words, DV is not directly and independently associated with COVID-19 as a risk factor. Interestingly, being black and of South Asian origin directly increases the risk of COVID (OR values 5.3 and 2.6, respectively, p <0.001 and p <0.001) (Hastie *et al*, 2020).

# CONCLUSION

Vitamin D (DV) is an important molecule for healthy bones, teeth and muscles. A deficiency of DV leads to rickets in children, pathological bone softening in adults or diseases called 'osteomalacia'. Its active form (1,25-dihydroxyvitamin D / calcitriol) is considered to be effective against many inflammatory, infectious diseases. It is involved in regulation and suppression of the inflammatory cytokine response of respiratory epithelial cells and macrophages to various pathogens.

By modulating ACE-I and II expression, it prevents lipopolysaccharide-induced pulmonary damage, reducing the risk of microbial infection and death by physical barrier and cellular natural immune mechanisms.

It has been demonstrated that the level of DV is not associated with the risk of COVID-19, nor is it a source of increased risk in ethnic minorities. Other comorbid diseases and malnutrition will need to be more common in these groups and socioeconomic factors should be emphasized. Data so far suggest that it is appropriate to give DV to elderly people with DV deficiency and those with comorbid diseases, not everyone should have DV. Nevertheless, multi-center, community-based, well-designed studies seem necessary to clarify the DV-COVID-19 relationship.

## REFERENCES

Abella, BS, Jolkovsky, EL & Biney, BT (2020) Efficacy and safety of hydroxychloroquine *vs* placebo for pre-exposure SARS-CoV-2 prophylaxis among healthcare workers. *JAMA Intern Med,* e206319.

Adisasmito, W, Chan, PK, Lee, N, Oner, AF, Gasimov, V, Aghayev, F, Zaman, M, Bamgboye, E, Dogan, N, Coker, R, Starzyk, K, Dreyer, NA & Toovey, S (2010) Effectiveness of antiviral treatment in human influenza A(H5N1) infections: analysis of a Global Patient Registry. *J Infect Dis,* 202, 1154-60. [http://dx.doi.org/10.1086/656316] [PMID: 20831384]

Andreou, A, Trantza, S, Filippou, D, Sipsas, N & Tsiodras, S (2020) COVID-19: The Potential Role of Copper and N-acetylcysteine (NAC) in a Combination of Candidate Antiviral Treatments Against SARS-CoV-2. *In Vivo,* 34 (Suppl.), 1567-88. [http://dx.doi.org/10.21873/invivo.11946] [PMID: 32503814]

Arabi, YM, Alothman, A, Balkhy, HH, Al-Dawood, A, AlJohani, S, Al Harbi, S, Kojan, S, Al Jeraisy, M, Deeb, AM, Assiri, AM, Al-Hameed, F, AlSaedi, A, Mandourah, Y, Almekhlafi, GA, Sherbeeni, NM, Elzein, FE, Memon, J, Taha, Y, Almotairi, A, Maghrabi, KA, Qushmaq, I, Al Bshabshe, A, Kharaba, A, Shalhoub, S, Jose, J, Fowler, RA, Hayden, FG & Hussein, MA And the MIRACLE trial group (2018) Treatment of Middle East Respiratory Syndrome with a combination of lopinavir-ritonavir and interferon-β1b (MIRACLE trial): study protocol for a randomized controlled trial. *Trials,* 19, 81. [http://dx.doi.org/10.1186/s13063-017-2427-0] [PMID: 29382391]

Arabi, YM, Alothman, A, Balkhy, HH, Al-Dawood, A, AlJohani, S, Al Harbi, S, Kojan, S, Al Jeraisy, M, Deeb, AM, Assiri, AM, Al-Hameed, F, AlSaedi, A, Mandourah, Y, Almekhlafi, GA, Sherbeeni, NM, Elzein, FE, Memon, J, Taha, Y, Almotairi, A, Maghrabi, KA, Qushmaq, I, Al Bshabshe, A, Kharaba, A, Shalhoub, S, Jose, J, Fowler, RA, Hayden, FG & Hussein, MA And the MIRACLE trial group (2018) Treatment of Middle East Respiratory Syndrome with a combination of lopinavir-ritonavir and interferon-β1b (MIRACLE trial): study protocol for a randomized controlled trial. *Trials,* 19, 81. [http://dx.doi.org/10.1186/s13063-017-2427-0] [PMID: 29382391]

Arboleda, JF, Fernandez, GJ & Urcuqui-Inchima, S (2019) Vitamin D-mediated attenuation of miR-155 in human macrophages infected with dengue virus: Implications for the cytokine response. *Infect Genet Evol,* 69, 12-21. [http://dx.doi.org/10.1016/j.meegid.2018.12.033] [PMID: 30639520]

Armour, J, Tyml, K, Lidington, D & Wilson, JX (2001) Ascorbate prevents microvascular dysfunction in the skeletal muscle of the septic rat. *J Appl Physiol (1985),* 90, 795-803. [http://dx.doi.org/10.1152/jappl.2001.90.3.795] [PMID: 11181585]

Barnes, BJ, Adrover, JM, Baxter-Stoltzfus, A, Borczuk, A, Cools-Lartigue, J, Crawford, JM, Daßler-Plenker, J, Guerci, P, Huynh, C, Knight, JS, Loda, M, Looney, MR, McAllister, F, Rayes, R, Renaud, S, Rousseau, S, Salvatore, S, Schwartz, RE, Spicer, JD, Yost, CC, Weber, A, Zuo, Y & Egeblad, M (2020) Targeting potential drivers of COVID-19: Neutrophil extracellular traps. *J Exp Med,* 217, e20200652. [http://dx.doi.org/10.1084/jem.20200652] [PMID: 32302401]

Basille, D, Plouvier, N, Trouve, C, Duhaut, P, Andrejak, C & Jounieaux, V (2017) Nonsteroidal anti-inflammatory drugs may worsen the course of community acquired pneumonia: a cohort study. *Lung,* 195, 201-8. [http://dx.doi.org/10.1007/s00408-016-9973-1] [PMID: 28005149]

Bassetti, M, Giacobbe, DR, Aliberti, S, Barisione, E, Centanni, S, De Rosa, FG, Di Marco, F, Gori, A, Granata, G, Mikulska, M, Petrosillo, N, Richeldi, L, Santus, P, Tascini, C, Vena, A, Viale, P & Blasi, F Italian Society of Anti-infective Therapy (SITA) and the Italian Society of Pulmonology (SIP) (2020) Balancing evidence and frontline experience in the early phases of the COVID-19 pandemic: current position of the Italian Society of Anti-infective Therapy (SITA) and the Italian Society of Pulmonology (SIP). *Clin Microbiol Infect,* 26, 880-94.
[http://dx.doi.org/10.1016/j.cmi.2020.04.031] [PMID: 32360444]

Beigel, JH, Nam, HH, Adams, PL, Krafft, A, Ince, WL, El-Kamary, SS & Sims, AC (2019) Advances in respiratory virus therapeutics - A meeting report from the 6th isirv Antiviral Group conference. *Antiviral Res,* 167, 45-67.
[http://dx.doi.org/10.1016/j.antiviral.2019.04.006] [PMID: 30974127]

Beigel, JH, Tomashek, KM & Dodd, LE (2020) Remdesivir for the Treatment of Covid-19 — Preliminary Report. *N Engl J Med.* NEJMoa2007764.

Beigel, JH, Nam, HH, Adams, PL, Krafft, A, Ince, WL, El-Kamary, SS & Sims, AC (2019) Advances in respiratory virus therapeutics - A meeting report from the 6th isirv Antiviral Group conference. *Antiviral Res,* 167, 45-67.
[http://dx.doi.org/10.1016/j.antiviral.2019.04.006] [PMID: 30974127]

Bengoechea, JA & Bamford, CGG (2020) SARS-CoV-2, bacterial co-infections, and AMR: the deadly trio in COVID-19? *EMBO Mol Med,* 12, e12560.
[http://dx.doi.org/10.15252/emmm.202012560] [PMID: 32453917]

Beović, B, Doušak, M, Ferreira-Coimbra, J, Nadrah, K, Rubulotta, F, Belliato, M, Berger-Estilita, J, Ayoade, F, Rello, J & Erdem, H (2020) Antibiotic use in patients with COVID-19: a 'snapshot' Infectious Diseases International Research Initiative (ID-IRI) survey. *J Antimicrob Chemother,* 75, 3386-90.
[http://dx.doi.org/10.1093/jac/dkaa326] [PMID: 32766706]

Bhala, N, Emberson, J, Merhi, A, Abramson, S, Arber, N, Baron, JA, Bombardier, C, Cannon, C, Farkouh, ME, FitzGerald, GA, Goss, P, Halls, H, Hawk, E, Hawkey, C, Hennekens, C, Hochberg, M, Holland, LE, Kearney, PM, Laine, L, Lanas, A, Lance, P, Laupacis, A, Oates, J, Patrono, C, Schnitzer, TJ, Solomon, S, Tugwell, P, Wilson, K, Wittes, J & Baigent, C Coxib and traditional NSAID Trialists' (CNT) Collaboration (2013) Vascular and upper gastrointestinal effects of non-steroidal anti-inflammatory drugs: meta-analyses of individual participant data from randomised trials. *Lancet,* 382, 769-79.
[http://dx.doi.org/10.1016/S0140-6736(13)60900-9] [PMID: 23726390]

Bleibtreu, A, Jaureguiberry, S, Houhou, N, Boutolleau, D, Guillot, H, Vallois, D, Lucet, JC, Robert, J, Mourvillier, B, Delemazure, J, Jaspard, M, Lescure, FX, Rioux, C, Caumes, E & Yazdanapanah, Y (2018) Clinical management of respiratory syndrome in patients hospitalized for suspected Middle East respiratory syndrome coronavirus infection in the Paris area from 2013 to 2016. *BMC Infect Dis,* 18, 331.
[http://dx.doi.org/10.1186/s12879-018-3223-5] [PMID: 30012113]

Bolay, H, Gül, A & Baykan, B (2020) COVID-19 is a Real Headache! *Headache,* 60, 1415-21.
[http://dx.doi.org/10.1111/head.13856] [PMID: 32412101]

Borges do Nascimento, IJ, Cacic, N, Abdulazeem, HM, von Groote, TC, Jayarajah, U, Weerasekara, I, Esfahani, MA, Civile, VT, Marusic, A, Jeroncic, A, Carvas Junior, N, Pericic, TP, Zakarija-Grkovic, I, Meirelles Guimarães, SM, Luigi Bragazzi, N, Bjorklund, M, Sofi-Mahmudi, A, Altujjar, M, Tian, M, Arcani, DMC, O'Mathúna, DP & Marcolino, MS (2020) Coronavirus infection (COVID-19) in humans: A scoping review and meta-analysis. *J Clin Med,* 9, 941.
[http://dx.doi.org/10.3390/jcm9040941] [PMID: 32235486]

Borrelli, E, Roux-Lombard, P, Grau, GE, Girardin, E, Ricou, B, Dayer, J & Suter, PM (1996) Plasma concentrations of cytokines, their soluble receptors, and antioxidant vitamins can predict the development of multiple organ failure in patients at risk. *Crit Care Med,* 24, 392-7.
[http://dx.doi.org/10.1097/00003246-199603000-00006] [PMID: 8625625]

Bosseboeuf, E, Aubry, M & Nhan, T (2018) Azithromycin inhibits the replication Zika virus. *J Antivir*

*Antiretrovir,* 10, 6-11.
[http://dx.doi.org/10.4172/1948-5964.1000173]

Boulware, DR, Pullen, MF, Bangdiwala, AS, Pastick, KA, Lofgren, SM, Okafor, EC, Skipper, CP, Nascene, AA, Nicol, MR, Abassi, M, Engen, NW, Cheng, MP, LaBar, D, Lother, SA, MacKenzie, LJ, Drobot, G, Marten, N, Zarychanski, R, Kelly, LE, Schwartz, IS, McDonald, eg, Rajasingham, R, Lee, TC & Hullsiek, KH (2020) A randomized trial of hydroxychloroquine as postexposure prophylaxis for COVID-19. *N Engl J Med,* 383, 517-25.
[http://dx.doi.org/10.1056/NEJMoa2016638] [PMID: 32492293]

*British National Formulary,* (2014 ed.,) British Medical Association, London 686-8. March 2014-September 2014

Brot, C, Jorgensen, NR & Sorensen, OH (1999) The influence of smoking on vitamin D status and calcium metabolism. *Eur J Clin Nutr,* 53, 920-6.
[http://dx.doi.org/10.1038/sj.ejcn.1600870] [PMID: 10602348]

Brown, AJ, Won, JJ, Graham, RL, Dinnon, KH, III, Sims, AC, Feng, JY, Cihlar, T, Denison, MR, Baric, RS & Sheahan, TP (2019) Broad spectrum antiviral remdesivir inhibits human endemic and zoonotic deltacoronaviruses with a highly divergent RNA dependent RNA polymerase. *Antiviral Res,* 169, 104541.
[http://dx.doi.org/10.1016/j.antiviral.2019.104541] [PMID: 31233808]

Cai, Q, Yang, M, Liu, D, Chen, J, Shu, D, Xia, J, Liao, X, Gu, Y, Cai, Q, Yang, Y, Shen, C, Li, X, Peng, L, Huang, D, Zhang, J, Zhang, S, Wang, F, Liu, J, Chen, L, Chen, S, Wang, Z, Zhang, Z, Cao, R, Zhong, W, Liu, Y & Liu, L (2020) Experimental Treatment with Favipiravir for COVID-19: An Open-Label Control Study. *Engineering (Beijing),* 6, 1192-8.
[http://dx.doi.org/10.1016/j.eng.2020.03.007] [PMID: 32346491]

Cannell, JJ, Vieth, R, Umhau, JC, Holick, MF, Grant, WB, Madronich, S, Garland, CF & Giovannucci, E (2006) Epidemic influenza and vitamin D. *Epidemiol Infect,* 134, 1129-40.
[http://dx.doi.org/10.1017/S0950268806007175] [PMID: 16959053]

Cao, B, Wang, Y, Wen, D, Liu, W, Wang, J, Fan, G, Ruan, L, Song, B, Cai, Y, Wei, M, Li, X, Xia, J, Chen, N, Xiang, J, Yu, T, Bai, T, Xie, X, Zhang, L, Li, C, Yuan, Y, Chen, H, Li, H, Huang, H, Tu, S, Gong, F, Liu, Y, Wei, Y, Dong, C, Zhou, F, Gu, X, Xu, J, Liu, Z, Zhang, Y, Li, H, Shang, L, Wang, K, Li, K, Zhou, X, Dong, X, Qu, Z, Lu, S, Hu, X, Ruan, S, Luo, S, Wu, J, Peng, L, Cheng, F, Pan, L, Zou, J, Jia, C, Wang, J, Liu, X, Wang, S, Wu, X, Ge, Q, He, J, Zhan, H, Qiu, F, Guo, L, Huang, C, Jaki, T, Hayden, FG, Horby, PW, Zhang, D & Wang, C (2020) A trial of lopinavir–ritonavir in adults hospitalized with severe Covid-19. *N Engl J Med,* 382, 1787-99.
[http://dx.doi.org/10.1056/NEJMoa2001282] [PMID: 32187464]

Cao, Y, Li, L & Feng, Z (2020) Comparative genetic analysis of the novel coronavirus (2019-nCoV/SAR--CoV-2) receptor ACE2 in different populations. *Cell Discov,* 6, 11.
[http://dx.doi.org/10.1038/s41421-020-0147-1]

Cárcamo, JM, Pedraza, A, Bórquez-Ojeda, O & Golde, DW (2002) Vitamin C suppresses TNF alpha-induced NF kappa B activation by inhibiting I kappa B alpha phosphorylation. *Biochemistry,* 41, 12995-3002.
[http://dx.doi.org/10.1021/bi0263210] [PMID: 12390026]

Carr, A, Wohlrab, C, Young, P & Bellomo, R (2018) Stability of intravenous vitamin C solutions: a technical report. *Crit Care Resusc,* 20, 180-1.
[PMID: 30153779]

Carr, AC & Maggini, S (2017) Vitamin C and Immune Function. *Nutrients,* 9, 1211.
[http://dx.doi.org/10.3390/nu9111211] [PMID: 29099763]

Carr, AC, Rosengrave, PC, Bayer, S, Chambers, S, Mehrtens, J & Shaw, GM (2017) Hypovitaminosis C and vitamin C deficiency in critically ill patients despite recommended enteral and parenteral intakes. *Crit Care,* 21, 300.
[http://dx.doi.org/10.1186/s13054-017-1891-y] [PMID: 29228951]

Carter, SJ, Baranauskas, MN & Fly, AD (2020) Considerations for Obesity, Vitamin D, and Physical Activity

Amid the COVID-19 Pandemic. *Obesity (Silver Spring),* 28, 1176-7.
[http://dx.doi.org/10.1002/oby.22838] [PMID: 32299148]

Cavalcanti, AB, Zampieri, FG, Rosa, RG, Azevedo, LCP, Veiga, VC, Avezum, A, Damiani, LP, Marcadenti, A, Kawano-Dourado, L, Lisboa, T, Junqueira, DLM, de Barros E Silva, PGM, Tramujas, L, Abreu-Silva, EO, Laranjeira, LN, Soares, AT, Echenique, LS, Pereira, AJ, Freitas, FGR, Gebara, OCE, Dantas, VCS, Furtado, RHM, Milan, EP, Golin, NA, Cardoso, FF, Maia, IS, Hoffmann Filho, CR, Kormann, APM, Amazonas, RB, Bocchi de Oliveira, MF, Serpa-Neto, A, Falavigna, M, Lopes, RD, Machado, FR & Berwanger, O Coalition Covid-19 Brazil I Investigators (2020) Hydroxychloroquine with or without azithromycin in mild-t--moderate COVID-19. *N Engl J Med,* 383, 2041-52.
[http://dx.doi.org/10.1056/NEJMoa2019014] [PMID: 32706953]

Centers for Disease Control and Prevention. (2020) *Updated guidance on evaluating and testing persons for coronavirus disease 2019 (COVID 19).* https://www.cdc.gov/csels/dls/locs/2020/updated_guidance_on_testing_persons_for_covid-19.html

Chan, KS, Lai, ST, Chu, CM, Tsui, E, Tam, CY, Wong, MM, Tse, MW, Que, TL, Peiris, JS, Sung, J, Wong, VC & Yuen, KY (2003) Treatment of severe acute respiratory syndrome with lopinavir/ritonavir: a multicentre retrospective matched cohort study. *Hong Kong Med J,* 9, 399-406.
[PMID: 14660806]

Chen, C, Pan, K & Wu, B (2020) Safety of hydroxychloroquine in COVID-19 and other diseases: a systematic review and meta-analysis of 53 randomized trials. *Eur J Clin Pharmacol,* 1-12.
[http://dx.doi.org/10.1007/s00228-020-02962-5] [PMID: 32780229]

Chen, T, Wu, D, Chen, H, Yan, W, Yang, D, Chen, G, Ma, K, Xu, D, Yu, H, Wang, H, Wang, T, Guo, W, Chen, J, Ding, C, Zhang, X, Huang, J, Han, M, Li, S, Luo, X, Zhao, J & Ning, Q (2020) Clinical characteristics of 113 deceased patients with coronavirus disease 2019: retrospective study. *BMJ,* 368, m1091.
[http://dx.doi.org/10.1136/bmj.m1091] [PMID: 32217556]

Chloroquine Side Effects (2019) *Medically reviewed by Drugscom.* https://www.drugs.com/sfx/chloroquine-side-effects.html Last updated on Jul 30, 2019

Chu, CM, Cheng, VCC, Hung, IFN, Wong, MM, Chan, KH, Chan, KS, Kao, RY, Poon, LL, Wong, CL, Guan, Y, Peiris, JS & Yuen, KY HKU/UCH SARS Study Group (2004) Role of lopinavir/ritonavir in the treatment of SARS: initial virological and clinical findings. *Thorax,* 59, 252-6.
[http://dx.doi.org/10.1136/thorax.2003.012658] [PMID: 14985565]

Chu, CM, Cheng, VCC, Hung, IFN, Wong, MM, Chan, KH, Chan, KS, Kao, RY, Poon, LL, Wong, CL, Guan, Y, Peiris, JS & Yuen, KY HKU/UCH SARS Study Group (2004) Role of lopinavir/ritonavir in the treatment of SARS: initial virological and clinical findings. *Thorax,* 59, 252-6.
[http://dx.doi.org/10.1136/thorax.2003.012658] [PMID: 14985565]

Chu, CM, Cheng, VCC, Hung, IFN, Wong, MM, Chan, KH, Chan, KS, Kao, RY, Poon, LL, Wong, CL, Guan, Y, Peiris, JS & Yuen, KY HKU/UCH SARS Study Group (2004) Role of lopinavir/ritonavir in the treatment of SARS: initial virological and clinical findings. *Thorax,* 59, 252-6.
[http://dx.doi.org/10.1136/thorax.2003.012658] [PMID: 14985565]

Russell, CD, Millar, JE & Baillie, JK (2020) Clinical evidence does not support corticosteroid treatment for 2019-nCoV lung injury. *Lancet,* 395, 473-5.
[http://dx.doi.org/10.1016/S0140-6736(20)30317-2] [PMID: 32043983]

Conner, EM & Grisham, MB (1996) Inflammation, free radicals, and antioxidants. *Nutrition,* 12, 274-7.
[http://dx.doi.org/10.1016/S0899-9007(96)00000-8] [PMID: 8862535]

de Girolamo, L, Peretti, GM, Maffulli, N & Brini, AT (2020) Covid-19-The real role of NSAIDs in Italy. *J Orthop Surg Res,* 15, 165.
[http://dx.doi.org/10.1186/s13018-020-01682-x] [PMID: 32366317]

Delang, L, Abdelnabi, R & Neyts, J (2018) Favipiravir as a potential countermeasure against neglected and emerging RNA viruses. *Antiviral Res,* 153, 85-94.

[http://dx.doi.org/10.1016/j.antiviral.2018.03.003] [PMID: 29524445]

Deng, L, Li, C, Zeng, Q, Liu, X, Li, X, Zhang, H, Hong, Z & Xia, J (2020) Arbidol combined with LPV/r versus LPV/r alone against Corona Virus Disease 2019: A retrospective cohort study. *J Infect,* 81, e1-5. [http://dx.doi.org/10.1016/j.jinf.2020.03.002] [PMID: 32171872]

Deppe, S, Böger, RH, Weiss, J & Benndorf, RA (2010) Telmisartan: a review of its pharmacodynamic and pharmacokinetic properties. *Expert Opin Drug Metab Toxicol,* 6, 863-71. [http://dx.doi.org/10.1517/17425255.2010.494597] [PMID: 20509777]

Diagnosis and Treatment Protocol for Novel Coronavirus Pneumonia.Trial Version 7. *Released by National Health Commission & State Administration of Traditional Chinese Medicine.*

Diagnosis and Treatment Protocol for Novel Coronavirus Pneumonia.Trial Version 7. *Released by National Health Commission & State Administration of Traditional Chinese Medicine.*

Diagnosis and Treatment Protocol for Novel Coronavirus Pneumonia.Trial Version 7. *Released by National Health Commission & State Administration of Traditional Chinese Medicine.*

Edalatifard, M, Akhtari, M, Salehi, M, Naderi, Z, Jamshidi, A, Mostafaei, S, Najafizadeh, SR, Farhadi, E, Jalili, N, Esfahani, M, Rahimi, B, Kazemzadeh, H, Mahmoodi Aliabadi, M, Ghazanfari, T, Sattarian, M, Ebrahimi Louyeh, H, Raeeskarami, SR, Jamalimoghadamsiahkali, S, Khajavirad, N, Mahmoudi, M & Rostamian, A (2020) Intravenous methylprednisolone pulse as a treatment for hospitalised severe COVID-19 patients: results from a randomised controlled clinical trial. *Eur Respir J,* 56, 2002808. [http://dx.doi.org/10.1183/13993003.02808-2020] [PMID: 32943404]

Fernandez-Cruz, A, Ruiz-Antoran, B & Munoz-Gomez, A (2020) *A retrospective controlled cohort study of the impact of glucocorticoid treatment in SARS-CoV-2 Infection mortality Antimicrob Agents Chemother,* 64, e01168-20.

Fisher, BJ, Kraskauskas, D, Martin, EJ, Farkas, D, Wegelin, JA, Brophy, D, Ward, KR, Voelkel, NF, Fowler, AA, III & Natarajan, R (2012) Mechanisms of attenuation of abdominal sepsis induced acute lung injury by ascorbic acid. *Am J Physiol Lung Cell Mol Physiol,* 303, L20-32. [http://dx.doi.org/10.1152/ajplung.00300.2011] [PMID: 22523283]

Fisher, BJ, Seropian, IM, Kraskauskas, D, Thakkar, JN, Voelkel, NF, Fowler, AA, III & Natarajan, R (2011) Ascorbic acid attenuates lipopolysaccharide-induced acute lung injury. *Crit Care Med,* 39, 1454-60. [http://dx.doi.org/10.1097/CCM.0b013e3182120cb8] [PMID: 21358394]

Fowler, AA, III, Syed, AA, Knowlson, S, Sculthorpe, R, Farthing, D, DeWilde, C, Farthing, CA, Larus, TL, Martin, E, Brophy, DF, Gupta, S, Fisher, BJ & Natarajan, R Medical Respiratory Intensive Care Unit Nursing (2014) Phase I safety trial of intravenous ascorbic acid in patients with severe sepsis. *J Transl Med,* 12, 32. [http://dx.doi.org/10.1186/1479-5876-12-32] [PMID: 24484547]

Fowler, AA, III, Truwit, JD, Hite, RD, Morris, PE, DeWilde, C, Priday, A, Fisher, B, Thacker, LR, II, Natarajan, R, Brophy, DF, Sculthorpe, R, Nanchal, R, Syed, A, Sturgill, J, Martin, GS, Sevransky, J, Kashiouris, M, Hamman, S, Egan, KF, Hastings, A, Spencer, W, Tench, S, Mehkri, O, Bindas, J, Duggal, A, Graf, J, Zellner, S, Yanny, L, McPolin, C, Hollrith, T, Kramer, D, Ojielo, C, Damm, T, Cassity, E, Wieliczko, A & Halquist, M (2019) Effect of Vitamin C Infusion on Organ Failure and Biomarkers of Inflammation and Vascular Injury in Patients With Sepsis and Severe Acute Respiratory Failure: The CITRIS-ALI Randomized Clinical Trial. *JAMA,* 322, 1261-70. [http://dx.doi.org/10.1001/jama.2019.11825] [PMID: 31573637]

Furuhashi, M, Moniwa, N, Mita, T, Fuseya, T, Ishimura, S, Ohno, K, Shibata, S, Tanaka, M, Watanabe, Y, Akasaka, H, Ohnishi, H, Yoshida, H, Takizawa, H, Saitoh, S, Ura, N, Shimamoto, K & Miura, T (2015) Urinary angiotensin-converting enzyme 2 in hypertensive patients may be increased by olmesartan, an angiotensin II receptor blocker. *Am J Hypertens,* 28, 15-21. [http://dx.doi.org/10.1093/ajh/hpu086] [PMID: 24842388]

Furuta, Y, Komeno, T & Nakamura, T (2017) Favipiravir (T-705), a broad spectrum inhibitor of viral RNA polymerase. *Proc Jpn Acad, Ser B, Phys Biol Sci,* 93, 449-63.

[http://dx.doi.org/10.2183/pjab.93.027] [PMID: 28769016]

Furuta, Y, Takahashi, K, Kuno-Maekawa, M, Sangawa, H, Uehara, S, Kozaki, K, Nomura, N, Egawa, H & Shiraki, K (2005) Mechanism of action of T-705 against influenza virus. *Antimicrob Agents Chemother,* 49, 981-6.
[http://dx.doi.org/10.1128/AAC.49.3.981-986.2005] [PMID: 15728892]

Garg, M, Al-Ani, A, Mitchell, H, Hendy, P & Christensen, B (2020) Editorial: low population mortality from COVID-19 in countries south of latitude 35 degrees North-supports vitamin D as a factor determining severity. Authors' reply. *Aliment Pharmacol Ther,* 51, 1438-9.
[http://dx.doi.org/10.1111/apt.15796] [PMID: 32352178]

Gaut, JP, Belaaouaj, A, Byun, J, Roberts, LJ, II, Maeda, N, Frei, B & Heinecke, JW (2006) Vitamin C fails to protect amino acids and lipids from oxidation during acute inflammation. *Free Radic Biol Med,* 40, 1494-501.
[http://dx.doi.org/10.1016/j.freeradbiomed.2005.12.013] [PMID: 16632110]

Gautret, P, Lagier, JC, Parola, P, Hoang, VT, Meddeb, L, Sevestre, J, Mailhe, M, Doudier, B, Aubry, C, Amrane, S, Seng, P, Hocquart, M, Eldin, C, Finance, J, Vieira, VE, Tissot-Dupont, HT, Honoré, S, Stein, A, Million, M, Colson, P, La Scola, B, Veit, V, Jacquier, A, Deharo, JC, Drancourt, M, Fournier, PE, Rolain, JM, Brouqui, P & Raoult, D (2020) Clinical and microbiological effect of a combination of hydroxychloroquine and azithromycin in 80 COVID-19 patients with at least a six-day follow up: A pilot observational study. *Travel Med Infect Dis,* 34, 101663.
[http://dx.doi.org/10.1016/j.tmaid.2020.101663] [PMID: 32289548]

Gautret, P, Lagier, JC, Parola, P, Hoang, VT, Meddeb, L, Mailhe, M, Doudier, B, Courjon, J, Giordanengo, V, Vieira, VE, Tissot Dupont, H, Honoré, S, Colson, P, Chabrière, E, La Scola, B, Rolain, JM, Brouqui, P & Raoult, D (2020) Hydroxychloroquine and azithromycin as a treatment of COVID-19: results of an open-label non-randomized clinical trial. *Int J Antimicrob Agents,* 56, 105949.
[http://dx.doi.org/10.1016/j.ijantimicag.2020.105949] [PMID: 32205204]

Gov.UK (2020) *Commission on human medicines advice on ibuprofen and coronavirus (COVID-19).*https://www.gov.uk/government/news/commission-on-human-medicines-advi-e-on-ibuprofen-and-coronavirus- covid-19

Grant, WB, Lahore, H, McDonnell, SL, Baggerly, CA, French, CB, Aliano, JL & Bhattoa, HP (2020) Evidence that Vitamin D Supplementation Could Reduce Risk of Influenza and COVID-19 Infections and Deaths. *Nutrients,* 12, E988.
[http://dx.doi.org/10.3390/nu12040988] [PMID: 32252338]

Greiller, CL & Martineau, AR (2015) Modulation of the immune response to respiratory viruses by vitamin D. *Nutrients,* 7, 4240-70.
[http://dx.doi.org/10.3390/nu7064240] [PMID: 26035247]

Guan, WJ, Ni, ZY, Hu, Y, Liang, WH, Ou, CQ, He, JX, Liu, L, Shan, H, Lei, CL, Hui, DSC, Du, B, Li, LJ, Zeng, G, Yuen, KY, Chen, RC, Tang, CL, Wang, T, Chen, PY, Xiang, J, Li, SY, Wang, JL, Liang, ZJ, Peng, YX, Wei, L, Liu, Y, Hu, YH, Peng, P, Wang, JM, Liu, JY, Chen, Z, Li, G, Zheng, ZJ, Qiu, SQ, Luo, J, Ye, CJ, Zhu, SY & Zhong, NS China Medical Treatment Expert Group for Covid-19 (2020) Clinical Characteristics of Coronavirus Disease 2019 in China. *N Engl J Med,* 382, 1708-20.
[http://dx.doi.org/10.1056/NEJMoa2002032] [PMID: 32109013]

Guaraldi, G, Meschiari, M, Cozzi-Lepri, A, Milic, J, Tonelli, R, Menozzi, M, Franceschini, E, Cuomo, G, Orlando, G, Borghi, V, Santoro, A, Di Gaetano, M, Puzzolante, C, Carli, F, Bedini, A, Corradi, L, Fantini, R, Castaniere, I, Tabbì, L, Girardis, M, Tedeschi, S, Giannella, M, Bartoletti, M, Pascale, R, Dolci, G, Brugioni, L, Pietrangelo, A, Cossarizza, A, Pea, F, Clini, E, Salvarani, C, Massari, M, Viale, PL & Mussini, C (2020) Tocilizumab in patients with severe COVID-19: a retrospective cohort study. *Lancet Rheumatol,* 2, e474-84.
[http://dx.doi.org/10.1016/S2665-9913(20)30173-9] [PMID: 32835257]

Habib, AMG, Ali, MAE, Zouaoui, BR, Taha, MAH, Mohammed, BS & Saquib, N (2019) Clinical outcomes among hospital patients with Middle East respiratory syndrome coronavirus (MERS-CoV) infection. *BMC Infect Dis,* 19, 870.

[http://dx.doi.org/10.1186/s12879-019-4555-5] [PMID: 31640578]

Han, JE, Jones, JL, Tangpricha, V, Brown, MA, Brown, LAS, Hao, L, Hebbar, G, Lee, MJ, Liu, S, Ziegler, TR & Martin, GS (2016) High Dose Vitamin D Administration in Ventilated Intensive Care Unit Patients: A Pilot Double Blind Randomized Controlled Trial. *J Clin Transl Endocrinol,* 4, 59-65. [http://dx.doi.org/10.1016/j.jcte.2016.04.004] [PMID: 27419080]

Hansdottir, S, Monick, MM, Lovan, N, Powers, L, Gerke, A & Hunninghake, GW (2010) Vitamin D decreases respiratory syncytial virus induction of NF-kappaB-linked chemokines and cytokines in airway epithelium while maintaining the antiviral state. *J Immunol,* 184, 965-74. [http://dx.doi.org/10.4049/jimmunol.0902840] [PMID: 20008294]

Hartmann, W, Brunn, ML, Stetter, N, Gagliani, N, Muscate, F, Stanelle-Bertram, S, Gabriel, G & Breloer, M (2019) Helminth Infections Suppress the Efficacy of Vaccination against Seasonal Influenza. *Cell Rep,* 29, 2243-2256.e4. [http://dx.doi.org/10.1016/j.celrep.2019.10.051] [PMID: 31747598]

Hastie, CE, Mackay, DF, Ho, F, Celis-Morales, CA, Katikireddi, SV, Niedzwiedz, CL, Jani, BD, Welsh, P, Mair, FS, Gray, SR, O'Donnell, CA, Gill, JM, Sattar, N & Pell, JP (2020) Vitamin D concentrations and COVID-19 infection in UK Biobank. *Diabetes Metab Syndr,* 14, 561-5. [http://dx.doi.org/10.1016/j.dsx.2020.04.050] [PMID: 32413819]

Horby, P, Lim, WS & Emberson, JR (2020) Dexamethasone in Hospitalized Patients with Covid-19 - Preliminary Report. *N Engl J Med.* NEJMoa2021436

Hsieh, HP & Hsu, JT (2007) Strategies of development of antiviral agents directed against influenza virus replication. *Curr Pharm Des,* 13, 3531-42. [http://dx.doi.org/10.2174/138161207782794248] [PMID: 18220789]

Huang, M, Tang, T, Pang, P, Li, M, Ma, R, Lu, J, Shu, J, You, Y, Chen, B, Liang, J, Hong, Z, Chen, H, Kong, L, Qin, D, Pei, D, Xia, J, Jiang, S & Shan, H (2020) Treating COVID-19 with Chloroquine. *J Mol Cell Biol,* 12, 322-5. [http://dx.doi.org/10.1093/jmcb/mjaa014] [PMID: 32236562]

Hulseberg, CE, Fénéant, L, Szymańska-de Wijs, KM, Kessler, NP, Nelson, EA, Shoemaker, CJ, Schmaljohn, CS, Polyak, SJ & White, JM (2019) Arbidol and other low-molecular-weight drugs that inhibit Lassa and Ebola viruses. *J Virol,* 93, e02185-18. [http://dx.doi.org/10.1128/JVI.02185-18] [PMID: 30700611]

Imai, Y, Kuba, K, Rao, S, Huan, Y, Guo, F, Guan, B, Yang, P, Sarao, R, Wada, T, Leong-Poi, H, Crackower, MA, Fukamizu, A, Hui, CC, Hein, L, Uhlig, S, Slutsky, AS, Jiang, C & Penninger, JM (2005) Angiotensin-converting enzyme 2 protects from severe acute lung failure. *Nature,* 436, 112-6. [http://dx.doi.org/10.1038/nature03712] [PMID: 16001071]

*Interim Clinical Guidance for Adults with Suspected or Confirmed COVID-19 in Belgium.* 16 mars Version 3.

*Interim Clinical Guidance For Patients Suspected of/Confirmed With COVID-19 in Belgium.* 16 Mars Version 3

*Interim Clinical Guidance For Patients Suspected of/Confirmed With COVID-19 in Belgium.* 16 Mars Version 3

Ishiyama, Y, Gallagher, PE, Averill, DB, Tallant, EA, Brosnihan, KB & Ferrario, CM (2004) Upregulation of angiotensin-converting enzyme 2 after myocardial infarction by blockade of angiotensin II receptors. *Hypertension,* 43, 970-6. [http://dx.doi.org/10.1161/01.HYP.0000124667.34652.1a] [PMID: 15007027]

Izmirly, PM, Costedoat-Chalumeau, N, Pisoni, CN, Khamashta, MA, Kim, MY, Saxena, A, Friedman, D, Llanos, C, Piette, JC & Buyon, JP (2012) Maternal use of hydroxychloroquine is associated with a reduced risk of recurrent anti-SSA/Ro-antibody-associated cardiac manifestations of neonatal lupus. *Circulation,* 126, 76-82. [http://dx.doi.org/10.1161/CIRCULATIONAHA.111.089268] [PMID: 22626746]

Jin, YH, Cai, L, Cheng, ZS, Cheng, H, Deng, T, Fan, YP, Fang, C, Huang, D, Huang, LQ, Huang, Q, Han, Y, Hu, B, Hu, F, Li, BH, Li, YR, Liang, K, Lin, LK, Luo, LS, Ma, J, Ma, LL, Peng, ZY, Pan, YB, Pan, ZY, Ren, XQ, Sun, HM, Wang, Y, Wang, YY, Weng, H, Wei, CJ, Wu, DF, Xia, J, Xiong, Y, Xu, HB, Yao, XM, Yuan, YF, Ye, TS, Zhang, XC, Zhang, YW, Zhang, YG, Zhang, HM, Zhao, Y, Zhao, MJ, Zi, H, Zeng, XT, Wang, YY & Wang, XH for the Zhongnan Hospital of Wuhan University Novel Coronavirus Management and Research Team, Evidence-Based Medicine Chapter of China International Exchange and Promotive Association for Medical and Health Care (CPAM) (2020) A rapid advice guideline for the diagnosis and treatment of 2019 novel coronavirus (2019-nCoV) infected pneumonia (standard version). *Mil Med Res,* 7, 4.
[http://dx.doi.org/10.1186/s40779-020-0233-6] [PMID: 32029004]

Joseph, C, Togawa, Y & Shindo, N (2013) Bacterial and viral infections associated with influenza. *Influenza Other Respir Viruses,* 7 (Suppl. 2), 105-13.
[http://dx.doi.org/10.1111/irv.12089] [PMID: 24034494]

Joshi, S, Parkar, J, Ansari, A, Tiwaskar, M & Patil, S (2020) Role of favipiravir in the treatment of COVID-19. *Int J Infect Dis*
[http://dx.doi.org/10.1016/j.ijid.2020.10.069] [PMID: 33130203]

Kakodkar, P, Kaka, N & Baig, MN (2020) A Comprehensive Literature Review on the Clinical Presentation, and Management of the Pandemic Coronavirus Disease 2019 (COVID-19). *Cureus,* 12, e7560.
[http://dx.doi.org/10.7759/cureus.7560] [PMID: 32269893]

Khunti, K, Singh, AK, Pareek, M & Hanif, W (2020) Is ethnicity linked to incidence or outcomes of covid-19? *BMJ,* 369, m1548.
[http://dx.doi.org/10.1136/bmj.m1548] [PMID: 32312785]

Kim, JY & Lee, SM (2006) Vitamins C and E protect hepatic cytochrome P450 dysfunction induced by polymicrobial sepsis. *Eur J Pharmacol,* 534, 202-9.
[http://dx.doi.org/10.1016/j.ejphar.2006.01.015] [PMID: 16483564]

Klein, EY, Monteforte, B, Gupta, A, Jiang, W, May, L, Hsieh, YH & Dugas, A (2016) The frequency of influenza and bacterial coinfection: a systematic review and meta-analysis. *Influenza Other Respir Viruses,* 10, 394-403.
[http://dx.doi.org/10.1111/irv.12398] [PMID: 27232677]

Klimas, J, Olvedy, M & Ochodnicka-Mackovicova, K (2015) Perinatally admin- istered losartan augments renal ACE2 expression but not cardiac or renal Mas receptor in spontaneously hypertensive rats. *Journal of Cel- lular and Molecular Medicine,* 19, 1965-74.https://doi.org/10

Kuba, K, Imai, Y, Rao, S, Gao, H, Guo, F, Guan, B, Huan, Y, Yang, P, Zhang, Y, Deng, W, Bao, L, Zhang, B, Liu, G, Wang, Z, Chappell, M, Liu, Y, Zheng, D, Leibbrandt, A, Wada, T, Slutsky, AS, Liu, D, Qin, C, Jiang, C & Penninger, JM (2005) A crucial role of angiotensin converting enzyme 2 (ACE2) in SARS coronavirus-induced lung injury. *Nat Med,* 11, 875-9.
[http://dx.doi.org/10.1038/nm1267] [PMID: 16007097]

Kwiatkowski, S, Borowski, D, Kajdy, A, Poon, LC, Rokita, W & Wielgos, M (2020) Why we should not stop giving aspirin to pregnant women during the COVID-19 pandemic. *Ultrasound Obstet Gynecol,* 55, 841-3.
[http://dx.doi.org/10.1002/uog.22049] [PMID: 32304612]

Siemieniuk, R, Rochwerg, B, Agoritsas, T, Lamontagne, F, Leo, YS, Macdonald, H, Agarwal, A, Zeng, L, Lytvyn, L, Appiah, JA, Amin, W, Arabi, Y, Blumberg, L, Burhan, E, Bausch, FJ, Calfee, CS, Cao, B, Cecconi, M, Chanda, D, Cooke, G, Du, B, Dunning, J, Geduld, H, Gee, P, Hashimi, M, Hui, DS, Kabra, S, Kanda, S, Kawano-Dourado, L, Kim, YJ, Kissoon, N, Kwizera, A, Laake, JH, Machado, FR, Mahaka, I, Manai, H, Mino, G, Nsutedu, E, Pshenichnaya, N, Qadir, N, Sabzwari, S, Sarin, R, Sharland, M, Shen, Y, Sri Ranganathan, S, Souza, J, Ugarte, S, Venkatapuram, S, Quoc Dat, V, Vuyiseka, D, Stegemann, M, Wijewickrama, A, Maguire, B, Zeraatkar, D, Bartoszko, J, Ge, L, Brignardello-Petersen, R, Owen, A, Guyatt, G, Diaz, J, Jacobs, M & Vandvik, PO (2020) A living WHO guideline on drugs for covid-19. *BMJ,* 370, m3379.
[http://dx.doi.org/10.1136/bmj.m3379] [PMID: 32887691]

Lan, SH, Lai, CC, Huang, HT, Chang, SP, Lu, LC & Hsueh, PR (2020) Tocilizumab for severe COVID-19: a systematic review and meta-analysis. *Int J Antimicrob Agents,* 56, 106103. [http://dx.doi.org/10.1016/j.ijantimicag.2020.106103] [PMID: 32712333]

Lansbury, L, Lim, B, Baskaran, V & Lim, WS (2020) Co-infections in people with COVID-19: a systematic review and meta-analysis. *J Infect,* 81, 266-75. [http://dx.doi.org/10.1016/j.jinf.2020.05.046] [PMID: 32473235]

Lee, N, Allen Chan, KC, Hui, DS, Ng, EK, Wu, A, Chiu, RW, Wong, VW, Chan, PK, Wong, KT, Wong, E, Cockram, CS, Tam, JS, Sung, JJ & Lo, YM (2004) Effects of early corticosteroid treatment on plasma SARS-associated Coronavirus RNA concentrations in adult patients. *J Clin Virol,* 31, 304-9. [http://dx.doi.org/10.1016/j.jcv.2004.07.006] [PMID: 15494274]

Lee, N, Hui, D, Wu, A, Chan, P, Cameron, P, Joynt, GM, Ahuja, A, Yung, MY, Leung, CB, To, KF, Lui, SF, Szeto, CC, Chung, S & Sung, JJ (2003) A major outbreak of severe acute respiratory syndrome in Hong Kong. *N Engl J Med,* 348, 1986-94. [http://dx.doi.org/10.1056/NEJMoa030685] [PMID: 12682352]

Lee, N, Wong, CK, Chan, MCW, Yeung, ESL, Tam, WWS, Tsang, OTY, Choi, KW, Chan, PKS, Kwok, A, Lui, GCY, Leung, WS, Yung, IMH, Wong, RYK, Cheung, CSK & Hui, DSC (2017) Anti-inflammatory effects of adjunctive macrolide treatment in adults hospitalized with influenza: A randomized controlled trial. *Antiviral Res,* 144, 48-56. [http://dx.doi.org/10.1016/j.antiviral.2017.05.008] [PMID: 28535933]

Lendermon, EA, Coon, TA, Bednash, JS, Weathington, NM, McDyer, JF & Mallampalli, RK (2017) Azithromycin decreases NALP3 mRNA stability in monocytes to limit inflammasome-dependent inflammation. *Respir Res,* 18, 131. [http://dx.doi.org/10.1186/s12931-017-0608-8] [PMID: 28659178]

Leneva, IA, Burtseva, EI, Yatsyshina, SB, Fedyakina, IT, Kirillova, ES, Selkova, EP, Osipova, E & Maleev, VV (2016) Virus susceptibility and clinical effectiveness of anti-influenza drugs during the 2010-2011 influenza season in Russia. *Int J Infect Dis,* 43, 77-84. [http://dx.doi.org/10.1016/j.ijid.2016.01.001] [PMID: 26775570]

Leneva, IA, Fediakina, IT & Gus'kova, TA (2005) Sensitivity of various influenza virus strains to arbidol. Influence of arbidol combination with different antiviral drugs on reproduction of influenza virus A. Terapevticheskii Arkhiv (Russian translation). ИЗДАТЕЛЬСТВО. *МЕДИЦИНА,* 77, 84-8.

Lim, J, Jeon, S & Shin, HY (2020) Case of the Index Patient Who Caused Tertiary Transmission of Coronavirus Disease 2019 in Korea: the Application of Lopinavir/Ritonavir for the Treatment of COVID-19 Pneumonia Monitored by Quantitative RT-PCR. *J Korean Med Sci,* 35, e79. [http://dx.doi.org/10.3346/jkms.2020.35.e79] [PMID: 32056407]

Baden, LR & Rubin, EJ (2020) Covid-19 - The Search for Effective Therapy. *N Engl J Med,* 382, 1851-2. [http://dx.doi.org/10.1056/NEJMe2005477] [PMID: 32187463]

Lisney, AR, Szelinski, F, Reiter, K, Burmester, GR, Rose, T & Dörner, T (2017) High maternal expression of SIGLEC1 on monocytes as a surrogate marker of a type I interferon signature is a risk factor for the development of autoimmune congenital heart block. *Ann Rheum Dis,* 76, 1476-80. [http://dx.doi.org/10.1136/annrheumdis-2016-210927] [PMID: 28501799]

Little, P (2020) Non-steroidal anti-inflammatory drugs and covid-19. *BMJ,* 368, m1185. [http://dx.doi.org/10.1136/bmj.m1185] [PMID: 32220865]

Morse, JS, Lalonde, T, Xu, S & Liu, WR (2020) Learning from the Past: Possible Urgent Prevention and Treatment Options for Severe Acute Respiratory Infections Caused by 2019-nCoV. *ChemBioChem,* 21, 730-8. [http://dx.doi.org/10.1002/cbic.202000047] [PMID: 32022370]

Lotteau, V, Teyton, L, Peleraux, A, Nilsson, T, Karlsson, L, Schmid, SL, Quaranta, V & Peterson, PA (1990) Intracellular transport of class II MHC molecules directed by invariant chain. *Nature,* 348, 600-5.

[http://dx.doi.org/10.1038/348600a0] [PMID: 2250716]

Lowes, DA, Webster, NR & Galley, HF (2010) Dehydroascorbic acid as pre-conditioner: protection from lipopolysaccharide induced mitochondrial damage. *Free Radic Res,* 44, 283-92.
[http://dx.doi.org/10.3109/10715760903468766] [PMID: 20166893]

Lu, H (2020) Drug treatment options for the 2019-new coronavirus (2019-nCoV). *Biosci Trends,* 14, 69-71.
[http://dx.doi.org/10.5582/bst.2020.01020] [PMID: 31996494]

Lu, R, Zhao, X, Li, J, Niu, P, Yang, B, Wu, H, Wang, W, Song, H, Huang, B, Zhu, N, Bi, Y, Ma, X, Zhan, F, Wang, L, Hu, T, Zhou, H, Hu, Z, Zhou, W, Zhao, L, Chen, J, Meng, Y, Wang, J, Lin, Y, Yuan, J, Xie, Z, Ma, J, Liu, WJ, Wang, D, Xu, W, Holmes, EC, Gao, GF, Wu, G, Chen, W, Shi, W & Tan, W (2020) Genomic characterisation and epidemiology of 2019 novel coronavirus: implications for virus origins and receptor binding. *Lancet,* 395, 565-74.
[http://dx.doi.org/10.1016/S0140-6736(20)30251-8] [PMID: 32007145]

Lund, LC, Kristensen, KB, Reilev, M, Christensen, S, Thomsen, RW, Christiansen, CF, Støvring, H, Johansen, NB, Brun, NC, Hallas, J & Pottegård, A (2020) Adverse outcomes and mortality in users of non-steroidal anti-inflammatory drugs who tested positive for SARS-CoV-2: A Danish nationwide cohort study. *PLoS Med,* 17, e1003308.
[http://dx.doi.org/10.1371/journal.pmed.1003308] [PMID: 32898149]

Luo, P, Liu, Y, Qiu, L, Liu, X, Liu, D & Li, J (2020) Tocilizumab treatment in COVID-19: A single center experience. *J Med Virol,* 92, 814-8.
[http://dx.doi.org/10.1002/jmv.25801] [PMID: 32253759]

MaassenVanDenBrink, A, de Vries, T & Danser, AHJ (2020) Headache medication and the COVID-19 pandemic. *J Headache Pain,* 21, 38.
[http://dx.doi.org/10.1186/s10194-020-01106-5] [PMID: 32334535]

Madrid, PB, Panchal, RG, Warren, TK, Shurtleff, AC, Endsley, AN, Green, CE, Kolokoltsov, A, Davey, R, Manger, ID, Gilfillan, L, Bavari, S & Tanga, MJ (2015) Evaluation of Ebola virus inhibitors for drug repurposing. *ACS Infect Dis,* 1, 317-26.
[http://dx.doi.org/10.1021/acsinfecdis.5b00030] [PMID: 27622822]

Marmor, MF, Kellner, U, Lai, TYY, Melles, RB & Mieler, WF American Academy of Ophthalmology (2016) Recommendations on Screening for Chloroquine and Hydroxychloroquine Retinopathy (2016 Revision). *Ophthalmology,* 123, 1386-94.
[http://dx.doi.org/10.1016/j.ophtha.2016.01.058] [PMID: 26992838]

Martinez, MA (2020) Compounds with therapeutic potential against novel respiratory 2019 coronavirus. *Antimicrob Agents Chemother,* 64, e00399-20.
[http://dx.doi.org/10.1128/AAC.00399-20] [PMID: 32152082]

Marty, FM, Vidal-Puigserver, J, Clark, C, Gupta, SK, Merino, E, Garot, D, Chapman, MJ, Jacobs, F, Rodriguez-Noriega, E, Husa, P, Shortino, D, Watson, HA, Yates, PJ & Peppercorn, AF (2017) Intravenous zanamivir or oral oseltamivir for hospitalised patients with influenza: an international, randomised, double-blind, double-dummy, phase 3 trial. *Lancet Respir Med,* 5, 135-46.
[http://dx.doi.org/10.1016/S2213-2600(16)30435-0] [PMID: 28094141]

Mata, M, Morcillo, E, Gimeno, C & Cortijo, J (2011) N-acetyl-L-cysteine (NAC) inhibit mucin synthesis and pro-inflammatory mediators in alveolar type II epithelial cells infected with influenza virus A and B and with respiratory syncytial virus (RSV). *Biochem Pharmacol,* 82, 548-55.
[http://dx.doi.org/10.1016/j.bcp.2011.05.014] [PMID: 21635874]

McKee, DL, Sternberg, A, Stange, U, Laufer, S & Naujokat, C (2020) Candidate drugs against SARS-CoV-2 and COVID-19. *Pharmacol Res,* 157, 104859.
[http://dx.doi.org/10.1016/j.phrs.2020.104859] [PMID: 32360480]

Mehta, P, McAuley, DF, Brown, M, Sanchez, E, Tattersall, RS & Manson, JJ HLH Across Speciality Collaboration, UK (2020) COVID-19: consider cytokine storm syndromes and immunosuppression. *Lancet,* 395, 1033-4.

[http://dx.doi.org/10.1016/S0140-6736(20)30628-0] [PMID: 32192578]

Meleveedu, KS, Miskovsky, J, Meharg, J, Abdelrahman, A, Tandon, R, Moody, AE, Dasilva, P, Masse, G, LaPorte, J, Saied Calvino, A, Allen, G, El-Bizri, R, Roberts, T, Armenio, V & Katz, SC (2020) Tocilizumab for severe COVID-19 related illness - A community academic medical center experience. *Cytokine X,* 2, 100035.
[http://dx.doi.org/10.1016/j.cytox.2020.100035] [PMID: 32895645]

Micallef, J, Soeiro, T & Jonville-Béra, AP French Society of Pharmacology, Therapeutics (SFPT) (2020) Non-steroidal anti-inflammatory drugs, pharmacology, and COVID-19 infection. *Therapie,* 75, 355-62.
[http://dx.doi.org/10.1016/j.therap.2020.05.003] [PMID: 32418728]

Mifsud, EJ, Hayden, FG & Hurt, AC (2019) Antivirals targeting the polymerase complex of influenza viruses. *Antiviral Res,* 169, 104545.
[http://dx.doi.org/10.1016/j.antiviral.2019.104545] [PMID: 31247246]

multicenter collaboration group of Department of Science and Technology of Guangdong Province and Health Commission of Guangdong Province for chloroquine in the treatment of novel coronavirus pneumonia (2020) Expert consensus on chloroquine phosphate for the treatment of novel coronavirus pneumonia. *Zhonghua Jie He He Hu Xi Za Zhi,* 43, 185-8.
[PMID: 32164085]

Muthuri, SG, Venkatesan, S, Myles, PR, Leonardi-Bee, J, Al Khuwaitir, TS, Al Mamun, A, Anovadiya, AP, Azziz-Baumgartner, E, Báez, C, Bassetti, M, Beovic, B, Bertisch, B, Bonmarin, I, Booy, R, Borja-Aburto, VH, Burgmann, H, Cao, B, Carratala, J, Denholm, JT, Dominguez, SR, Duarte, PA, Dubnov-Raz, G, Echavarria, M, Fanella, S, Gao, Z, Gérardin, P, Giannella, M, Gubbels, S, Herberg, J, Iglesias, AL, Hoger, PH, Hu, X, Islam, QT, Jiménez, MF, Kandeel, A, Keijzers, G, Khalili, H, Knight, M, Kudo, K, Kusznierz, G, Kuzman, I, Kwan, AM, Amine, IL, Langenegger, E, Lankarani, KB, Leo, YS, Linko, R, Liu, P, Madanat, F, Mayo-Montero, E, McGeer, A, Memish, Z, Metan, G, Mickiene, A, Mikić, D, Mohn, KG, Moradi, A, Nymadawa, P, Oliva, ME, Ozkan, M, Parekh, D, Paul, M, Polack, FP, Rath, BA, Rodríguez, AH, Sarrouf, EB, Seale, AC, Sertogullarindan, B, Siqueira, MM, Skręt-Magierło, J, Stephan, F, Talarek, E, Tang, JW, To, KK, Torres, A, Törün, SH, Tran, D, Uyeki, TM, Van Zwol, A, Vaudry, W, Vidmar, T, Yokota, RT, Zarogoulidis, P & Nguyen-Van-Tam, JS PRIDE Consortium Investigators (2014) Effectiveness of neuraminidase inhibitors in reducing mortality in patients admitted to hospital with influenza A H1N1pdm09 virus infection: a meta-analysis of individual participant data. *Lancet Respir Med,* 2, 395-404.
[http://dx.doi.org/10.1016/S2213-2600(14)70041-4] [PMID: 24815805]

Nagata, T, Lefor, AK, Hasegawa, M & Ishii, M (2015) Favipiravir: a new medication for the Ebola virus disease pandemic. *Disaster Med Public Health Prep,* 9, 79-81.
[http://dx.doi.org/10.1017/dmp.2014.151] [PMID: 25544306]

Nair, R, Maseeh, A & Vitamin, D (2012) Vitamin D: The "sunshine" vitamin. *J Pharmacol Pharmacother,* 3, 118-26.
[PMID: 22629085]

Nathens, AB, Neff, MJ, Jurkovich, GJ, Klotz, P, Farver, K, Ruzinski, JT, Radella, F, Garcia, I & Maier, RV (2002) Randomized, prospective trial of antioxidant supplementation in critically ill surgical patients. *Ann Surg,* 236, 814-22.
[http://dx.doi.org/10.1097/00000658-200212000-00014] [PMID: 12454520]

NHS England (2020) *Ibuprofen for adults* . https://www. nhs. uk/ medicines/

Nishimura, H & Yamaya, M (2015) A synthetic serine protease inhibitor, Nafamostat Mesilate, is a drug potentially applicable to the treatment of ebola virus disease. *Tohoku J Exp Med,* 237, 45-50.
[http://dx.doi.org/10.1620/tjem.237.45] [PMID: 26346967]

Novel, CPERE Epidemiology Working Group for NCIP Epidemic Response, Chinese Center for Disease Control and Prevention (2020) The epidemiological characteristics of an outbreak of 2019 novel coronavirus diseases (COVID-19) in China. *Zhonghua Liu Xing Bing Xue Za Zhi,* 41, 145-51.
[PMID: 32064853]

Online March 17 (2020) COVID-19: Guidance for triage of non-emergent surgical procedures. *American College of Surgeons.* www.facs.org/covid-19/clinicalguidance/triage

Osborne, LC, Monticelli, LA, Nice, TJ, Sutherland, TE, Siracusa, MC, Hepworth, MR, Tomov, VT, Kobuley, D, Tran, SV, Bittinger, K, Bailey, AG, Laughlin, AL, Boucher, JL, Wherry, EJ, Bushman, FD, Allen, JE, Virgin, HW & Artis, D (2014) Coinfection. Virus-helminth coinfection reveals a microbiota-independent mechanism of immunomodulation. *Science,* 345, 578-82.
[http://dx.doi.org/10.1126/science.1256942] [PMID: 25082704]

Padayatty, SJ, Sun, H, Wang, Y, Riordan, HD, Hewitt, SM, Katz, A, Wesley, RA & Levine, M (2004) Vitamin C pharmacokinetics: implications for oral and intravenous use. *Ann Intern Med,* 140, 533-7.
[http://dx.doi.org/10.7326/0003-4819-140-7-200404060-00010] [PMID: 15068981]

Pécheur, EI, Borisevich, V, Halfmann, P, Morrey, JD, Smee, DF, Prichard, M, Mire, CE, Kawaoka, Y, Geisbert, TW & Polyak, SJ (2016) The synthetic antiviral drug arbidol inhibits globally prevalent pathogenic viruses. *J Virol,* 90, 3086-92.
[http://dx.doi.org/10.1128/JVI.02077-15] [PMID: 26739045]

Peiris, JSM, Chu, CM, Cheng, VCC, Chan, KS, Hung, IF, Poon, LL, Law, KI, Tang, BS, Hon, TY, Chan, CS, Chan, KH, Ng, JS, Zheng, BJ, Ng, WL, Lai, RW, Guan, Y & Yuen, KY HKU/UCH SARS Study Group (2003) Clinical progression and viral load in a community outbreak of coronavirus-associated SARS pneumonia: a prospective study. *Lancet,* 361, 1767-72.
[http://dx.doi.org/10.1016/S0140-6736(03)13412-5] [PMID: 12781535]

Pergolizzi, JV, Jr, Varrassi, G, Magnusson, P, LeQuang, JA, Paladini, A, Taylor, R, Wollmuth, C, Breve, F & Christo, P (2020) COVID-19 and NSAIDS: A Narrative Review of Knowns and Unknowns. *Pain Ther,* 9, 353-8. [published online ahead of print, 2020 May 24].
[http://dx.doi.org/10.1007/s40122-020-00173-5] [PMID: 32447629]

Pilkington, V, Pepperrell, T & Hill, A (2020) A review of the safety of favipiravir - a potential treatment in the COVID-19 pandemic? *J Virus Erad,* 6, 45-51.
[http://dx.doi.org/10.1016/S2055-6640(20)30016-9] [PMID: 32405421]

Pilz, S, März, W, Cashman, KD, Kiely, ME, Whiting, SJ, Holick, MF, Grant, WB, Pludowski, P, Hiligsmann, M, Trummer, C, Schwetz, V, Lerchbaum, E, Pandis, M, Tomaschitz, A, Grübler, MR, Gaksch, M, Verheyen, N, Hollis, BW, Rejnmark, L, Karras, SN, Hahn, A, Bischoff-Ferrari, HA, Reichrath, J, Jorde, R, Elmadfa, I, Vieth, R, Scragg, R, Calvo, MS, van Schoor, NM, Bouillon, R, Lips, P, Itkonen, ST, Martineau, AR, Lamberg-Allardt, C & Zittermann, A (2018) Rationale and Plan for Vitamin D Food Fortification: A Review and Guidance Paper. *Front Endocrinol (Lausanne),* 9, 373.
[http://dx.doi.org/10.3389/fendo.2018.00373] [PMID: 30065699]

Poutanen, SM, Low, DE, Henry, B, Finkelstein, S, Rose, D, Green, K, Tellier, R, Draker, R, Adachi, D, Ayers, M, Chan, AK, Skowronski, DM, Salit, I, Simor, AE, Slutsky, AS, Doyle, PW, Krajden, M, Petric, M, Brunham, RC & McGeer, AJ National Microbiology Laboratory, Canada; (2003) Canadian Severe Acute Respiratory Syndrome Study Team (2003) Identification of severe acute respiratory syndrome in Canada. *N Engl J Med,* 348, 1995-2005.
[http://dx.doi.org/10.1056/NEJMoa030634] [PMID: 12671061]

Qiao, W, Wang, C, Chen, B, Zhang, F, Liu, Y, Lu, Q, Guo, H, Yan, C, Sun, H, Hu, G & Yin, X (2015) Ibuprofen attenuates cardiac fibrosis in streptozotocin-induced diabetic rats. *Cardiology,* 131, 97-106.
[http://dx.doi.org/10.1159/000375362] [PMID: 25896805]

Rajoli, RK, Pertinez, H & Arshad, U (2020) Dose prediction for repurposing nitazoxanide in SARS-CoV-2 treatment or chemoprophylaxis. *Preprint medRxiv.*

Rawson, TM, Moore, LSP & Zhu, N (2020) Bacterial and fungal co-infection in individuals with coronavirus: A rapid review to support COVID-19 antimicrobial prescribing. *Clin Infect Dis,* ciaa530.

Rodrigo, C, Leonardi-Bee, J, Nguyen-Van-Tam, J & Lim, WS (2016) Corticosteroids as adjunctive therapy in the treatment of influenza. *Cochrane Database Syst Rev,* 3, CD010406.

[http://dx.doi.org/10.1002/14651858.CD010406.pub2] [PMID: 26950335]

Rondanelli, M, Miccono, A, Lamburghini, S, Avanzato, I, Riva, A, Allegrini, P, Faliva, MA, Peroni, G, Nichetti, M & Perna, S (2018) Self-Care for Common Colds: The Pivotal Role of Vitamin D, Vitamin C, Zinc, and *Echinacea* in Three Main Immune Interactive Clusters (Physical Barriers, Innate and Adaptive Immunity) Involved during an Episode of Common Colds-Practical Advice on Dosages and on the Time to Take These Nutrients/Botanicals in order to Prevent or Treat Common Colds. *Evid Based Complement Alternat Med,* 2018, 5813095.
[http://dx.doi.org/10.1155/2018/5813095] [PMID: 29853961]

Rossignol, JF (2016) Nitazoxanide, a new drug candidate for the treatment of Middle East respiratory syndrome coronavirus. *J Infect Public Health,* 9, 227-30.
[http://dx.doi.org/10.1016/j.jiph.2016.04.001] [PMID: 27095301]

Rossignol, JF (2014) Nitazoxanide: a first-in-class broad-spectrum antiviral agent. *Antiviral Res,* 110, 94-103.
[http://dx.doi.org/10.1016/j.antiviral.2014.07.014] [PMID: 25108173]

Ruan, SY, Lin, HH, Huang, CT, Kuo, PH, Wu, HD & Yu, CJ (2014) Exploring the heterogeneity of effects of corticosteroids on acute respiratory distress syndrome: a systematic review and meta-analysis. *Crit Care,* 18, R63.
[http://dx.doi.org/10.1186/cc13819] [PMID: 24708846]

Ruiz-Irastorza, G, Ramos-Casals, M, Brito-Zeron, P & Khamashta, MA (2010) Clinical efficacy and side effects of antimalarials in systemic lupus erythematosus: a systematic review. *Ann Rheum Dis,* 69, 20-8.
[http://dx.doi.org/10.1136/ard.2008.101766] [PMID: 19103632]

Russell, CD, Millar, JE & Baillie, JK (2020) Clinical evidence does not support corticosteroid treatment for 2019-nCoV lung injury. *Lancet,* 395, 473-5.
[http://dx.doi.org/10.1016/S0140-6736(20)30317-2] [PMID: 32043983]

Sabetta, JR, DePetrillo, P, Cipriani, RJ, Smardin, J, Burns, LA & Landry, ML (2010) Serum 25-hydroxyvitamin d and the incidence of acute viral respiratory tract infections in healthy adults. *PLoS One,* 5, e11088.
[http://dx.doi.org/10.1371/journal.pone.0011088] [PMID: 20559424]

Sadowska, AM, Manuel-Y-Keenoy, B & De Backer, WA (2007) Antioxidant and anti-inflammatory efficacy of NAC in the treatment of COPD: discordant *in vitro* and in vivo dose-effects: a review. *Pulm Pharmacol Ther,* 20, 9-22.
[http://dx.doi.org/10.1016/j.pupt.2005.12.007] [PMID: 16458553]

Sanguinetti, CM (2016) N-acetylcysteine in COPD: why, how, and when? *Multidiscip Respir Med,* 11, 8.
[http://dx.doi.org/10.1186/s40248-016-0039-2] [PMID: 26855777]

Santomasso, BD, Park, JH, Salloum, D, Riviere, I, Flynn, J, Mead, E, Halton, E, Wang, X, Senechal, B, Purdon, T, Cross, JR, Liu, H, Vachha, B, Chen, X, DeAngelis, LM, Li, D, Bernal, Y, Gonen, M, Wendel, HG, Sadelain, M & Brentjens, RJ (2018) Clinical and biological correlates of neurotoxicity associated with CAR T-cell therapy in patients with B-cell acute lymphoblastic leukemia. *Cancer Discov,* 8, 958-71.
[http://dx.doi.org/10.1158/2159-8290.CD-17-1319] [PMID: 29880584]

Savarino, A, Boelaert, JR, Cassone, A, Majori, G & Cauda, R (2003) Effects of chloroquine on viral infections: an old drug against today's diseases? *Lancet Infect Dis,* 3, 722-7.
[http://dx.doi.org/10.1016/S1473-3099(03)00806-5] [PMID: 14592603]

Sawyer, MAJ, Mike, JJ & Chavin, K (1989) Antioxidant therapy and survival in ARDS. *Crit Care Med,* 17, S153. [abstract].

Schrezenmeier, E & Dörner, T (2020) Mechanisms of action of hydroxychloroquine and chloroquine: implications for rheumatology. *Nat Rev Rheumatol,* 16, 155-66.
[http://dx.doi.org/10.1038/s41584-020-0372-x] [PMID: 32034323]

Schwartz, C, Hams, E & Fallon, PG (2018) Helminth modulation of lung inflammation. *Trends Parasitol,* 34, 388-403.

[http://dx.doi.org/10.1016/j.pt.2017.12.007] [PMID: 29339033]

Self, WH, Semler, MW, Leither, LM, Casey, JD, Angus, DC, Brower, RG, Chang, SY, Collins, SP, Eppensteiner, JC, Filbin, MR, Files, DC, Gibbs, KW, Ginde, AA, Gong, MN, Harrell, FE, Jr, Hayden, DL, Hough, CL, Johnson, NJ, Khan, A, Lindsell, CJ, Matthay, MA, Moss, M, Park, PK, Rice, TW, Robinson, BRH, Schoenfeld, DA, Shapiro, NI, Steingrub, JS, Ulysse, CA, Weissman, A, Yealy, DM, Thompson, BT, Brown, SM, Steingrub, J, Smithline, H, Tiru, B, Tidswell, M, Kozikowski, L, Thornton-Thompson, S, De Souza, L, Hou, P, Baron, R, Massaro, A, Aisiku, I, Fredenburgh, L, Seethala, R, Johnsky, L, Riker, R, Seder, D, May, T, Baumann, M, Eldridge, A, Lord, C, Shapiro, N, Talmor, D, O'Mara, T, Kirk, C, Harrison, K, Kurt, L, Schermerhorn, M, Banner-Goodspeed, V, Boyle, K, Dubosh, N, Filbin, M, Hibbert, K, Parry, B, Lavin-Parsons, K, Pulido, N, Lilley, B, Lodenstein, C, Margolin, J, Brait, K, Jones, A, Galbraith, J, Peacock, R, Nandi, U, Wachs, T, Matthay, M, Liu, K, Kangelaris, K, Wang, R, Calfee, C, Yee, K, Hendey, G, Chang, S, Lim, G, Qadir, N, Tam, A, Beutler, R, Levitt, J, Wilson, J, Rogers, A, Vojnik, R, Roque, J, Albertson, T, Chenoweth, J, Adams, J, Pearson, S, Juarez, M, Almasri, E, Fayed, M, Hughes, A, Hillard, S, Huebinger, R, Wang, H, Vidales, E, Patel, B, Ginde, A, Moss, M, Baduashvili, A, McKeehan, J, Finck, L, Higgins, C, Howell, M, Douglas, I, Haukoos, J, Hiller, T, Lyle, C, Cupelo, A, Caruso, E, Camacho, C, Gravitz, S, Finigan, J, Griesmer, C, Park, P, Hyzy, R, Nelson, K, McDonough, K, Olbrich, N, Williams, M, Kapoor, R, Nash, J, Willig, M, Ford, H, Gardner-Gray, J, Ramesh, M, Moses, M, Ng Gong, M, Aboodi, M, Asghar, A, Amosu, O, Torres, M, Kaur, S, Chen, JT, Hope, A, Lopez, B, Rosales, K, Young You, J, Mosier, J, Hypes, C, Natt, B, Borg, B, Salvagio Campbell, E, Hite, RD, Hudock, K, Cresie, A, Alhasan, F, Gomez-Arroyo, J, Duggal, A, Mehkri, O, Hastings, A, Sahoo, D, Abi Fadel, F, Gole, S, Shaner, V, Wimer, A, Meli, Y, King, A, Terndrup, T, Exline, M, Pannu, S, Robart, E, Karow, S, Hough, C, Robinson, B, Johnson, N, Henning, D, Campo, M, Gundel, S, Seghal, S, Katsandres, S, Dean, S, Khan, A, Krol, O, Jouzestani, M, Huynh, P, Weissman, A, Yealy, D, Scholl, D, Adams, P, McVerry, B, Huang, D, Angus, D, Schooler, J, Moore, S, Files, C, Miller, C, Gibbs, K, LaRose, M, Flores, L, Koehler, L, Morse, C, Sanders, J, Langford, C, Nanney, K, MdalaGausi, M, Yeboah, P, Morris, P, Sturgill, J, Seif, S, Cassity, E, Dhar, S, de Wit, M, Mason, J, Goodwin, A, Hall, G, Grady, A, Chamberlain, A, Brown, S, Bledsoe, J, Leither, L, Peltan, I, Starr, N, Fergus, M, Aston, V, Montgomery, Q, Smith, R, Merrill, M, Brown, K, Armbruster, B, Harris, E, Middleton, E, Paine, R, Johnson, S, Barrios, M, Eppensteiner, J, Limkakeng, A, McGowan, L, Porter, T, Bouffler, A, Leahy, JC, deBoisblanc, B, Lammi, M, Happel, K, Lauto, P, Self, W, Casey, J, Semler, M, Collins, S, Harrell, F, Lindsell, C, Rice, T, Stubblefield, W, Gray, C, Johnson, J, Roth, M, Hays, M, Torr, D, Zakaria, A, Schoenfeld, D, Thompson, T, Hayden, D, Ringwood, N, Oldmixon, C, Ulysse, C, Morse, R, Muzikansky, A, Fitzgerald, L, Whitaker, S, Lagakos, A, Brower, R, Reineck, L, Aggarwal, N, Bienstock, K, Freemer, M, Maclawiw, M, Weinmann, G, Morrison, L, Gillespie, M, Kryscio, R, Brodie, D, Zareba, W, Rompalo, A, Boeckh, M, Parsons, P, Christie, J, Hall, J, Horton, N, Zoloth, L, Dickert, N & Diercks, D National Heart, Lung, and Blood Institute PETAL Clinical Trials Network (2020) Effect of hydroxychloroquine on clinical status at 14 days in hospitalized patients with COVID-19. *JAMA,* 324, 2165-76.
[http://dx.doi.org/10.1001/jama.2020.22240] [PMID: 33165621]

Sheahan, TP, Sims, AC, Graham, RL, Menachery, VD, Gralinski, LE, Case, JB, Leist, SR, Pyrc, K, Feng, JY, Trantcheva, I, Bannister, R, Park, Y, Babusis, D, Clarke, MO, Mackman, RL, Spahn, JE, Palmiotti, CA, Siegel, D, Ray, AS, Cihlar, T, Jordan, R, Denison, MR & Baric, RS (2017) Broad-spectrum antiviral GS-5734 inhibits both epidemic and zoonotic coronaviruses. *Sci Transl Med,* 9, eaal3653.
[http://dx.doi.org/10.1126/scitranslmed.aal3653] [PMID: 28659436]

Sheahan, TP, Sims, AC, Leist, SR, Schäfer, A, Won, J, Brown, AJ, Montgomery, SA, Hogg, A, Babusis, D, Clarke, MO, Spahn, JE, Bauer, L, Sellers, S, Porter, D, Feng, JY, Cihlar, T, Jordan, R, Denison, MR & Baric, RS (2020) Comparative therapeutic efficacy of remdesivir and combination lopinavir, ritonavir, and interferon beta against MERS-CoV. *Nat Commun,* 11, 222.
[http://dx.doi.org/10.1038/s41467-019-13940-6] [PMID: 31924756]

Shibasaki, Y, Mori, Y, Tsutumi, Y, Masaki, H, Sakamoto, K, Murasawa, S, Maruyama, K, Moriguchi, Y, Tanaka, Y, Iwasaka, T, Inada, M & Matsubara, H (1999) Differential kinetics of circulating angiotensin IV and II after treatment with angiotensin II type 1 receptor antagonist and their plasma levels in patients with chronic renal failure. *Clin Nephrol,* 51, 83-91.
[PMID: 10069643]

Shrestha, DB, Budhathoki, P, Khadka, S, Shah, PB, Pokharel, N & Rashmi, P (2020) Favipiravir versus other

antiviral or standard of care for COVID-19 treatment: a rapid systematic review and meta-analysis. *Virol J,* 17, 141.
[http://dx.doi.org/10.1186/s12985-020-01412-z] [PMID: 32972430]

Silberstein, M & Vitamin, D (2020) Vitamin D: A simpler alternative to tocilizumab for trial in COVID-19? *Med Hypotheses,* 140, 109767.
[http://dx.doi.org/10.1016/j.mehy.2020.109767] [PMID: 32353742]

Sun, ML, Yang, JM, Sun, YP & Su, GH (2020) Inhibitors of RAS might be a good choice for the therapy of COVID-19 pneumonia. *Zhonghua Jie He He Hu Xi Za Zhi,* 43, E014.
[PMID: 32061198]

Sun, S, Liu, D, Zhang, H, Zhang, X & Wan, B (2019) Effect of different doses and time-courses of corticosteroid treatment in patients with acute respiratory distress syndrome: A meta-analysis. *Exp Ther Med,* 18, 4637-44.
[http://dx.doi.org/10.3892/etm.2019.8167] [PMID: 31807150]

Sağlık Bakanlığı, TC (2020) COVID-19 (SARS-CoV-2 Enfeksiyonu) Ağır pnömoni. *ARDS, sepsis ve septik şok yönetimi 7 Kasım.* https://covid19.saglik.gov.tr/Eklenti/39297/0/covid-19rehberiagirpnomoniardsseps isveseptiksokyontemipdf.pdf

Tanaka, H, Matsuda, T, Miyagantani, Y, Yukioka, T, Matsuda, H & Shimazaki, S (2000) Reduction of resuscitation fluid volumes in severely burned patients using ascorbic acid administration: a randomized, prospective study. *Arch Surg,* 135, 326-31.
[http://dx.doi.org/10.1001/archsurg.135.3.326] [PMID: 10722036]

Tang, W, Cao, Z, Han, M, Wang, Z, Chen, J, Sun, W, Wu, Y, Xiao, W, Liu, S, Chen, E, Chen, W, Wang, X, Yang, J, Lin, J, Zhao, Q, Yan, Y, Xie, Z, Li, D, Yang, Y, Liu, L, Qu, J, Ning, G, Shi, G & Xie, Q (2020) Hydroxychloroquine in patients with mainly mild to moderate coronavirus disease 2019: open label, randomised controlled trial. *BMJ,* 369, m1849.
[http://dx.doi.org/10.1136/bmj.m1849] [PMID: 32409561]

Teymoori-Rad, M, Shokri, F, Salimi, V & Marashi, SM (2019) The interplay between vitamin D and viral infections. *Rev Med Virol,* 29, e2032.
[http://dx.doi.org/10.1002/rmv.2032] [PMID: 30614127]

Thebault, R, Tran, AB & Williams, V (2020) *The coronavirus is infecting and killing black Americans at an alarmingly high rate*Washington Post.

Thebault, R, Tran, AB & Williams, V (2020) *The coronavirus is infecting and killing black Americans at an alarmingly high rate*https://www.washingtonpost.com/nation/2020/04/07/coronavirus-is-infecting-kill-ng-black-americans-an-alarm inglyhigh-rate-post-analysis-shows

Thindwa, D, Garcia Quesada, M, Liu, Y, Bennett, J, Cohen, C, Knoll, MD, von Gottberg, A, Hayford, K & Flasche, S (2020) Use of seasonal influenza and pneumococcal polysaccharide vaccines in older adults to reduce COVID-19 mortality. *Vaccine,* 38, 5398-401.
[http://dx.doi.org/10.1016/j.vaccine.2020.06.047] [PMID: 32600911]

Tian, X, Li, C & Huang, A (2020) A potent binding of 2019-nCoV spike protein by a SARS-CoV specific human monoclonal antibody. *Emerg Microbes Infect,* 9, 382-5.
[http://dx.doi.org/10.1080/22221751.2020.1729069] [PMID: 32065055]

Toniati, P, Piva, S, Cattalini, M, Garrafa, E, Regola, F, Castelli, F, Franceschini, F, Airò, P, Bazzani, C, Beindorf, EA, Berlendis, M, Bezzi, M, Bossini, N, Castellano, M, Cattaneo, S, Cavazzana, I, Contessi, GB, Crippa, M, Delbarba, A, De Peri, E, Faletti, A, Filippini, M, Filippini, M, Frassi, M, Gaggiotti, M, Gorla, R, Lanspa, M, Lorenzotti, S, Marino, R, Maroldi, R, Metra, M, Matteelli, A, Modina, D, Moioli, G, Montani, G, Muiesan, ML, Odolini, S, Peli, E, Pesenti, S, Pezzoli, MC, Pirola, I, Pozzi, A, Proto, A, Rasulo, FA, Renisi, G, Ricci, C, Rizzoni, D, Romanelli, G, Rossi, M, Salvetti, M, Scolari, F, Signorini, L, Taglietti, M, Tomasoni, G, Tomasoni, LR, Turla, F, Valsecchi, A, Zani, D, Zuccalà, F, Zunica, F, Focà, E, Andreoli, L & Latronico, N (2020) Tocilizumab for the treatment of severe COVID-19 pneumonia with hyperinflammatory syndrome and acute respiratory failure: A single center study of 100 patients in Brescia, Italy. *Autoimmun Rev,* 19,

102568.
[http://dx.doi.org/10.1016/j.autrev.2020.102568] [PMID: 32376398]

*Türk Toraks Derneği' nin COVID-19' da hidroksiklorokin kullanımına ilişkin görüşü.* https://www.toraks.org.tr/site/community/news/5955

Tyml, K, Li, F & Wilson, JX (2005) Delayed ascorbate bolus protects against maldistribution of microvascular blood flow in septic rat skeletal muscle. *Crit Care Med,* 33, 1823-8.
[http://dx.doi.org/10.1097/01.CCM.0000172548.34622.DE] [PMID: 16096461]

Tyml, K, Li, F & Wilson, JX (2008) Septic impairment of capillary blood flow requires nicotinamide adenine dinucleotide phosphate oxidase but not nitric oxide synthase and is rapidly reversed by ascorbate through an endothelial nitric oxide synthase-dependent mechanism. *Crit Care Med,* 36, 2355-62.
[http://dx.doi.org/10.1097/CCM.0b013e31818024f6] [PMID: 18596627]

Tyml, K (2011) Critical role for oxidative stress, platelets, and coagulation in capillary blood flow impairment in sepsis. *Microcirculation,* 18, 152-62.
[http://dx.doi.org/10.1111/j.1549-8719.2010.00080.x] [PMID: 21199094]

Tyml, K (2017) Vitamin C and Microvascular Dysfunction in Systemic Inflammation. *Antioxidants,* 6, 49.
[http://dx.doi.org/10.3390/antiox6030049] [PMID: 28661424]

Unger, T (2000) Neurohormonal modulation in cardiovascular disease. *Am Heart J,* 139, S2-8.
[http://dx.doi.org/10.1067/mhj.2000.102901] [PMID: 10618581]

Urashima, M, Segawa, T, Okazaki, M, Kurihara, M, Wada, Y & Ida, H (2010) Randomized trial of vitamin D supplementation to prevent seasonal influenza A in schoolchildren. *Am J Clin Nutr,* 91, 1255-60.
[http://dx.doi.org/10.3945/ajcn.2009.29094] [PMID: 20219962]

Uyeki, TM, Bernstein, HH, Bradley, JS, Englund, JA, File, TM, Fry, AM, Gravenstein, S, Hayden, FG, Harper, SA, Hirshon, JM, Ison, MG, Johnston, BL, Knight, SL, McGeer, A, Riley, LE, Wolfe, CR, Alexander, PE & Pavia, AT (2019) Clinical practice guidelines by the infectious diseases society of America: 2018 update on diagnosis, treatment, chemoprophylaxis, and institutional outbreak management of seasonal influenzaa. *Clin Infect Dis,* 68, 895-902.
[http://dx.doi.org/10.1093/cid/ciy874] [PMID: 30834445]

van den Borne, BE, Dijkmans, BA, de Rooij, HH, le Cessie, S & Verweij, CL (1997) Chloroquine and hydroxychloroquine equally affect tumor necrosis factor-alpha, interleukin 6, and interferon-gamma production by peripheral blood mononuclear cells. *J Rheumatol,* 24, 55-60.
[PMID: 9002011]

Vincent, MJ, Bergeron, E, Benjannet, S, Erickson, BR, Rollin, PE, Ksiazek, TG, Seidah, NG & Nichol, ST (2005) Chloroquine is a potent inhibitor of SARS coronavirus infection and spread. *Virol J,* 2, 69.
[http://dx.doi.org/10.1186/1743-422X-2-69] [PMID: 16115318]

Voiriot, G, Chalumeau, M, Messika, J, Basille, D, Philippe, B, Ricard, JD, Andrejak, C, Jounieaux, V, Sanchez, O & Fartoukh, M (2018) [Risks associated with the use of non-steroidal anti-inflammatory drugs during pneumonia]. *Rev Mal Respir,* 35, 430-40.
[http://dx.doi.org/10.1016/j.rmr.2017.12.003] [PMID: 29754841]

Wan, Y, Shang, J, Graham, R, Baric, RS & Li, F (2020) Receptor recognition by novelcoronavirus from Wuhan: An analysis based on decade-long structural studies of SARS. *J Virol,* 94, e00127-20.
[http://dx.doi.org/10.1128/JVI.00127-20] [PMID: 31996437]

Wang, M, Cao, R, Zhang, L, Yang, X, Liu, J, Xu, M, Shi, Z, Hu, Z, Zhong, W & Xiao, G (2020) Remdesivir and chloroquine effectively inhibit the recently emerged novel coronavirus (2019-nCoV) *in vitro*. *Cell Res,* 30, 269-71.
[http://dx.doi.org/10.1038/s41422-020-0282-0] [PMID: 32020029]

Wang, PH & Cheng, Y (2020) Increasing Host Cellular Receptor—Angiotensin-Converting Enzyme 2 (ACE2) Expression by Coronavirus may Facilitate 2019-nCoV Infection. *J Med Virol*
[http://dx.doi.org/10.1002/jmv.26139]

Wang, Q, Wu, J, Wang, H, Gao, Y, Liu, Q, Mu, A, Ji, W, Yan, L, Zhu, Y, Zhu, C, Fang, X, Yang, X, Huang, Y, Gao, H, Liu, F, Ge, J, Sun, Q, Yang, X, Xu, W, Liu, Z, Yang, H, Lou, Z, Jiang, B, Guddat, LW, Gong, P & Rao, Z (2020) Structural Basis for RNA Replication by the SARS-CoV-2 Polymerase. *Cell,* 182, 417-428.e13.
[http://dx.doi.org/10.1016/j.cell.2020.05.034] [PMID: 32526208]

Wang, Y, Guo, Q, Yan, Z, Zhou, D, Zhang, W, Zhou, S, Li, YP, Yuan, J, Uyeki, TM, Shen, X, Wu, W, Zhao, H, Wu, YF, Shang, J, He, Z, Yang, Y, Zhao, H, Hong, Y, Zhang, Z, Wu, M, Wei, T, Deng, X, Deng, Y, Cai, LH, Lu, W, Shu, H, Zhang, L, Luo, H, Ing Zhou, Y, Weng, H, Song, K, Yao, L, Jiang, M, Zhao, B, Chi, R, Guo, B, Fu, L, Yu, L, Min, H, Chen, P, Chen, S, Hong, L, Mao, W, Huang, X, Gu, L, Li, H, Wang, C & Cao, B CAP-China Network (2018) Factors associated with prolonged viral shedding in patients with avian influenza A(H7N9) virus infection. *J Infect Dis,* 217, 1708-17.
[http://dx.doi.org/10.1093/infdis/jiy115] [PMID: 29648602]

Wang, Y, Zhang, D, Du, G, Du, R, Zhao, J, Jin, Y, Fu, S, Gao, L, Cheng, Z, Lu, Q, Hu, Y, Luo, G, Wang, K, Lu, Y, Li, H, Wang, S, Ruan, S, Yang, C, Mei, C, Wang, Y, Ding, D, Wu, F, Tang, X, Ye, X, Ye, Y, Liu, B, Yang, J, Yin, W, Wang, A, Fan, G, Zhou, F, Liu, Z, Gu, X, Xu, J, Shang, L, Zhang, Y, Cao, L, Guo, T, Wan, Y, Qin, H, Jiang, Y, Jaki, T, Hayden, FG, Horby, PW, Cao, B & Wang, C (2020) Remdesivir in adults with severe COVID-19: a randomised, double-blind, placebo-controlled, multicentre trial. *Lancet,* 395, 1569-78.
[http://dx.doi.org/10.1016/S0140-6736(20)31022-9] [PMID: 32423584]

Wang, Z, Yang, B, Li, Q, Wen, L & Zhang, R (2020) Clinical Features of 69 Cases With Coronavirus Disease 2019 in Wuhan, China. *Clin Infect Dis,* 71, 769-77.
[http://dx.doi.org/10.1093/cid/ciaa272] [PMID: 32176772]

Wen, YC, Hsiao, FY, Chan, KA, Lin, ZF, Shen, LJ & Fang, CC (2017) Acute respiratory infection and use of nonsteroidal anti-inflammatory drugs on risk of acute myocardial infarction: a nationwide case-crossover study. *J Infect Dis,* 215, 503-9.
[http://dx.doi.org/10.1093/infdis/jiw603] [PMID: 28158479]

Wen, YC, Hsiao, FY, Lin, ZF, Fang, CC & Shen, LJ (2018) Risk of stroke associated with use of nonsteroidal anti-inflammatory drugs during acute respiratory infection episode. *Pharmacoepidemiol Drug Saf,* 27, 645-51.
[http://dx.doi.org/10.1002/pds.4428] [PMID: 29659118]

Meta-analysis, A (2020) *JAMA,* 324, 1330-41. WHO Rapid Evidence Appraisal for COVID-19 Therapies REACT Working Group, Sterne JAC, Murthy S, Diaz JV, *et al*, Association Between Administration of Systemic Corticosteroids and Mortality Among Critically Ill Patients With COVID-19:
[http://dx.doi.org/10.1001/jama.2020.17023] [PMID: 32876694]

WHO (2020) *Clinical management of severe acute respiratory infection when novel coronavirus (nCoV) infection is suspected.* https://www.who.int/docs/default-source/coronaviruse/clinical-management-of-n-vel-cov. pdf

Wiersinga, WJ, Rhodes, A, Cheng, AC, Peacock, SJ & Prescott, HC (2020) Pathophysiology, Transmission, Diagnosis, and Treatment of Coronavirus Disease 2019 (COVID-19): A Review. *JAMA,* 324, 782-93.
[http://dx.doi.org/10.1001/jama.2020.12839] [PMID: 32648899]

Wilson, JX (2009) Mechanism of action of vitamin C in sepsis: ascorbate modulates redox signaling in endothelium. *Biofactors,* 35, 5-13.
[http://dx.doi.org/10.1002/biof.7] [PMID: 19319840]

Wu, C, Chen, X, Cai, Y, Xia, J, Zhou, X, Xu, S, Huang, H, Zhang, L, Zhou, X, Du, C, Zhang, Y, Song, J, Wang, S, Chao, Y, Yang, Z, Xu, J, Zhou, X, Chen, D, Xiong, W, Xu, L, Zhou, F, Jiang, J, Bai, C, Zheng, J & Song, Y (2020) Risk factors associated with acute respiratory distress syndrome and death in patients with coronavirus disease 2019 pneumonia inWuhan, China. *JAMA Intern Med,* 180, 934-43.
[http://dx.doi.org/10.1001/jamainternmed.2020.0994] [PMID: 32167524]

Wu, F, Wilson, JX & Tyml, K (2004) Ascorbate protects against impaired arteriolar constriction in sepsis by inhibiting inducible nitric oxide synthase expression. *Free Radic Biol Med,* 37, 1282-9.

[http://dx.doi.org/10.1016/j.freeradbiomed.2004.06.025] [PMID: 15451067]

Wu, J, Liu, L & Zhao, X (2020) Hydroxychloroquine inhibits CD154 expression in CD4(!) T lymphocytes of systemic lupus erythema- tosus through NFAT, but not STAT5, signaling. *Arthritis Res Ther,* 19, 183.

Wu, SF, Chang, CB, Hsu, JM, Lu, MC, Lai, NS, Li, C & Tung, CH (2017) Hydroxychloroquine inhibits CD154 expression in $CD4^+$ T lymphocytes of systemic lupus erythematosus through NFAT, but not STAT5, signaling. *Arthritis Res Ther,* 19, 183.
[http://dx.doi.org/10.1186/s13075-017-1393-y] [PMID: 28793932]

Wu, Z & McGoogan, JM (2020) Characteristics of and Important Lessons From the Coronavirus Disease 2019 (COVID-19) Outbreak in China: Summary of a Report of 72 314 Cases From the Chinese Center for Disease Control and Prevention. *JAMA,* 323, 1239-42.
[http://dx.doi.org/10.1001/jama.2020.2648] [PMID: 32091533]

Xu, J, Yang, J, Chen, J, Luo, Q, Zhang, Q & Zhang, H (2017) Vitamin D alleviates lipopolysaccharide□induced acute lung injury via regulation of the renin□angiotensin system. *Mol Med Rep,* 16, 7432-8.
[http://dx.doi.org/10.3892/mmr.2017.7546] [PMID: 28944831]

Xu, X, Chen, P, Wang, J, Feng, J, Zhou, H, Li, X, Zhong, W & Hao, P (2020) Evolution of the novel coronavirus from the ongoing Wuhan outbreak and modeling of its spike protein for risk of human transmission. *Sci China Life Sci,* 63, 457-60.
[http://dx.doi.org/10.1007/s11427-020-1637-5] [PMID: 32009228]

Xu, X, Han, M, Li, T, Sun, W, Wang, D, Fu, B, Zhou, Y, Zheng, X, Yang, Y, Li, X, Zhang, X, Pan, A & Wei, H (2020) Effective treatment of severe COVID-19 patients with tocilizumab. *Proc Natl Acad Sci USA,* 117, 10970-5.
[http://dx.doi.org/10.1073/pnas.2005615117] [PMID: 32350134]

Xu, XW, Wu, XX, Jiang, XG, Xu, KJ, Ying, LJ, Ma, CL, Li, SB, Wang, HY, Zhang, S, Gao, HN, Sheng, JF, Cai, HL, Qiu, YQ & Li, LJ (2020) Clinical findings in a group of patients infected with the 2019 novel coronavirus (SARS-Cov-2) outside of Wuhan, China: retrospective case series. *BMJ,* 368, m606.
[http://dx.doi.org/10.1136/bmj.m606] [PMID: 32075786]

Yao, X, Ye, F, Zhang, M, Cui, C, Huang, B, Niu, P, Liu, X, Zhao, L, Dong, E, Song, C, Zhan, S, Lu, R, Li, H, Tan, W & Liu, D (2020) *In vitro* Antiviral Activity and Projection of Optimized Dosing Design of Hydroxychloroquine for the Treatment of Severe Acute Respiratory Syndrome Coronavirus 2 (SARS-Co--2). *Clin Infect Dis,* 71, 732-9.
[http://dx.doi.org/10.1093/cid/ciaa237] [PMID: 32150618]

Young, BE, Ong, SWX, Kalimuddin, S, Low, JG, Tan, SY, Loh, J, Ng, OT, Marimuthu, K, Ang, LW, Mak, TM, Lau, SK, Anderson, DE, Chan, KS, Tan, TY, Ng, TY, Cui, L, Said, Z, Kurupatham, L, Chen, MI, Chan, M, Vasoo, S, Wang, LF, Tan, BH, Lin, RTP, Lee, VJM, Leo, YS & Lye, DC Singapore 2019 Novel Coronavirus Outbreak Research Team (2020) Epidemiologic Features and Clinical Course of Patients Infected With SARS-CoV-2 in Singapore. *JAMA,* 323, 1488-94.
[http://dx.doi.org/10.1001/jama.2020.3204] [PMID: 32125362]

Yu, CM, Wong, RS, Wu, EB, Kong, SL, Wong, J, Yip, GW, Soo, YO, Chiu, ML, Chan, YS, Hui, D, Lee, N, Wu, A, Leung, CB & Sung, JJ (2006) Cardiovascular complications of severe acute respiratory syndrome. *Postgrad Med J,* 82, 140-4.
[http://dx.doi.org/10.1136/pgmj.2005.037515] [PMID: 16461478]

Zhang, Q, Ju, Y, Ma, Y & Wang, T (2018) N-acetylcysteine improves oxidative stress and inflammatory response in patients with community acquired pneumonia: A randomized controlled trial. *Medicine (Baltimore),* 97, e13087.
[http://dx.doi.org/10.1097/MD.0000000000013087] [PMID: 30407312]

Zhang, X, Cai, H, Hu, J, Lian, J, Gu, J, Zhang, S, Ye, C, Lu, Y, Jin, C, Yu, G, Jia, H, Zhang, Y, Sheng, J, Li, L & Yang, Y (2020) Epidemiological, clinical characteristics of cases of SARS-CoV-2 infection with abnormal imaging findings. *Int J Infect Dis,* 94, 81-7.

[http://dx.doi.org/10.1016/j.ijid.2020.03.040] [PMID: 32205284]

Zheng, W & Lau, M (2020) Clinical course and risk factors for mortality of adult inpatients with COVID-19 in Wuhan, China: a retrospective cohort study. *Lancet,* 395, 1054-62.

Zhou, F, Yu, T, Du, R, Fan, G, Liu, Y, Liu, Z, Xiang, J, Wang, Y, Song, B, Gu, X, Guan, L, Wei, Y, Li, H, Wu, X, Xu, J, Tu, S, Zhang, Y, Chen, H & Cao, B (2020) Clinical course and risk factors for mortality of adult inpatients with COVID-19 in Wuhan, China: a retrospective cohort study. *Lancet,* 395, 1054-62. [http://dx.doi.org/10.1016/S0140-6736(20)30566-3] [PMID: 32171076]

Zhou, F, Yu, T, Du, R, Fan, G, Liu, Y, Liu, Z, Xiang, J, Wang, Y, Song, B, Gu, X, Guan, L, Wei, Y, Li, H, Wu, X, Xu, J, Tu, S, Zhang, Y, Chen, H & Cao, B (2020) Clinical course and risk factors for mortality of adult inpatients with COVID-19 in Wuhan, China: a retrospective cohort study. *Lancet,* 395, 1054-62. [http://dx.doi.org/10.1016/S0140-6736(20)30566-3] [PMID: 32171076]

Zhou, S, Yang, Y, Zhang, X, Li, Z, Liu, X, Hu, C, Chen, C, Wang, D & Peng, Z (2020) Clinical Course of 195 Critically Ill COVID-19 Patients: A Retrospective Multicenter Study. *Shock,* 54, 644-51. [http://dx.doi.org/10.1097/SHK.0000000000001629] [PMID: 32826818]

Zhu, X, Ge, Y, Wu, T, Zhao, K, Chen, Y, Wu, B, Zhu, F, Zhu, B & Cui, L (2020) Co-infection with respiratory pathogens among COVID-2019 cases. *Virus Res,* 285, 198005. [http://dx.doi.org/10.1016/j.virusres.2020.198005] [PMID: 32408156]

Zolk, O, Hafner, S & Schmidt, CQ German Society for Experimental and Clinical Pharmacology and Toxicology (DGPT) (2020) COVID-19 pandemic and therapy with ibuprofen or renin-angiotensin system blockers: no need for interruptions or changes in ongoing chronic treatments. *Naunyn Schmiedebergs Arch Pharmacol,* 393, 1131-5. [http://dx.doi.org/10.1007/s00210-020-01890-6] [PMID: 32415494]

# CHAPTER 15

# Critical Care in COVID-19

**Abstract:** There are currently no recommended specific treatments for the group with severe COVID-19. Therefore , supportive treatment is essential. Expedient recognition and decisions for aggressive measures such as permanent control of the airway and positive-pressure ventilation, along with CST and t-PA administration, should be evaluated using certain selection criteria. Prone position is mostly associated with more favorable outcomes than supine position in the resuscitation of selected cases. Shock is also a catastrophic event that should be recognized and managed as early as possible for favorable outcomes. If the mean arterial pressure (MAP) cannot be kept above 65 mmHg with intravenous (IV) hydration and lactate cannot be maintained below 2 mmol/L, vasopressor support should definitely be initiated.

Extracorporeal membrane oxygenation (ECMO) therapy is used in ARDS to temporarily maintain adequate $O_2$ supply and $CO_2$ elimination and / or provide perfusion in patients with respiratory and / or heart failure who do not respond to conventional interventions and whose physiological variables are abnormal despite maximal support.

The development of coagulopathy is associated with high mortality in patients with COVID-19. Therefore, low molecular weight heparin (LMWH) should be used for prophylactic purposes. In order to reduce the incidence of VTE, it should be administered to patients with severe conditions and who are dependent on mechanical ventilation. Prophylactic LMWH will also benefit patients at high risk of VTE. The use of LMWH and anticoagulant therapy has been shown to reduce mortality in COVID-19.

The FDA has also recently approved the use of convalescent (immune) plasma therapy (CPT) in the COVID-19 era. Sera of the persons recovering from COVID-19 infection can be used in the prophylaxis or treatment of COVID-19 infection. CPT is one of the most important treatment options that can be used in pandemic COVID-19 infection. Antibody replacement by plasma infusion may be beneficial in the first 7-10 days of the disease. CPT is an important option for the prevention and treatment of COVID-19 disease in the presence of a sufficient number of people who can donate Ig-containing plasma. Patients treated with CP have a shorter hospital stay and lower mortality rates than other patients.

**Keywords:** Convalescent plasma, CPR, COVID-19, Critical care, Emergency cardiac care, Extracorporeal membrane oxygenation, Low molecular weight heparin, Positive-pressure ventilation, Prone position, Shock, Treatment.

**Ozgur KARCIOGLU, Selman YENIOCAK and Mandana HOSSEINZADEH**

## CPR, EMERGENCY CARDIAC CARE AND COVID-19: WHAT'S NEW?

It is well established that 3 to 6% of patients with COVID-19 are critically ill and some of them die. Patient factors, main strategies of the management, geographical differences, and perhaps subtypes of the virus affect these rates. Every healthcare worker (HCW) may encounter arrest status of a COVID-19 case at any time, which mandates a thorough knowledge and skills developed for each deadly scenario. For example, cardiotoxic effects of treatment agents such as hydroxychloroquine and azithromycin, which are frequently used in the treatment of COVID-19, induce QT prolongation which can trigger life-threatening arrhythmias in the vulnerable groups of patients. Main principles for protection of HCW are shown in the Table **1**.

**Table 1. Main principles for protection of HCW.**

| |
|---|
| 1. Be sure to report the COVID-19 status without transferring the patient to another team or person. |
| 2. Everyone in the team should know by heart that protection is a priority. HCW who are exposed to infection will not only be subtracted from the manpower temporarily, but they will also pose a danger as a new 'walking source of transmission'. |
| 3. Use of PPE is vital. All personnel to respond should use PPE completely. |
| 4. There should be no HCW in the intervention room without a vital task. |
| 5. Although not a sine qua non, the use of a mechanical CPR device (MCD) should be considered. It can help reduce the number of involved HCW. |

Resuscitative procedures pose the greatest risk for disease transmission. Unlike many other personnel, one of the most important problems emergency HCW face in CPR / ACLS is being unaware of the given patient's infection status or contagiousness related to COVID-19. This factor renders HCWs in primary care, EMS and EDs especially prone to be inflicted by the disease.

The use of PPE is vital in all procedures and interactions with patients in pandemic period. Applications precipitating aerosolization are primarily CPR, laryngoscopy- **endotracheal intubation (ETE)**, ventilation management, *i.e.*, NIV, PPV and other advanced airway interventions.

Take every measure to minimize the risk of aerosolization.

### Will there be any changes in the CPR?

Yes. The most important principle is to consider every arrest or pre-arrest phenomenon as COVID-19 and take precautions accordingly. One of the most important changes than before is wearing a mask for the patient and the use of MCD in the procedure. Mouth-to-mouth breathing is being abandoned eventually. Recommended steps for adult CPR amid the pandemics are summarized in the Fig. (**1**).

**Does 'ABCD' mnemonic for BLS change after COVID-19?**

Yes. Let us be ready for “PCBDI”.

- P: PPE (personal protective measures) N95, gloves, apron.
- C: Compressions (+/- MCD)
- B: Breathing, ventilation, bagging with HEPA filter
- D: Defibrillation with paddles or pads
- I: Isolated CPR room

Suggested algorithm for adult ACLS in the pandemic era is shown in the Fig. (**2**).

If endotracheal intubation (ETE) and ventilation is performed with a closed circuit, the risk of transmission is very low if a ventilator with high-efficiency particulate air (HEPA) filter is used.

- It is also helpful to use a tube with cuff for ETE.

- Before the ETE, HEPA filter bag-valve-mask (BVM) device (or T-piece in newborns) should be used, and air leakage should be prevented completely.

- The most experienced person should intubate the patient to mitigate the risk of ETE failure and thus prolonged aerosolization. Compressions should be interrupted during the attempt for ETE.

- Videolaryngoscopy (VL) can be preferred as it will increase the success of ETE.

- Before ETE, BMV device with HEPA filter should be used.

- Prevent disconnection of the circuit after closed circuit is provided in the intervention.

**How Should Cpr / Acls Be Done In Covid-19 Period?**

Some other issues may be ignored as attention focuses on saving the patient during CPR. Disease transition is one of them. It should be kept in mind that critical COVID-19 cases have a high mortality, which increases with age and comorbid CV and respiratory diseases. For this reason, the success expected from resuscitation on the basis of a single case should be balanced with the risks.

- The patient or his / her relatives should be discussed about the CPR / ACLS procedures, the patient's vital status, life expectancy, requirements, and targeted level of care.
- The EMS should prepare guidelines for the front line HCW about when CPR / ACLS interventions will be appropriate. At this point, the life expectancy should be estimated by taking into account the risk factors of the patient.
- There is insufficient data to support the effectiveness of routine ECMO administration in COVID-19 cases.

In August 2020, Australasian College for Emergency Medicine published a consensus statement on adult resuscitation. The recommendations are summarized below: (Adapted from Craig *et al*, 2020).

- In a setting of low community transmission, most cardiac arrests are not due to COVID-19.
- Early defibrillation saves lives and is not considered an aerosol
- generating procedure.
- Compression-only cardiopulmonary resuscitation is thought to be a low-risk procedure and can be safely initiated with the patient's mouth and nose covered.
- If COVID-19 significantly affects hospital resource availability, the ethics of resource allocation must be considered.
- All other resuscitative procedures are considered aerosol generating and require the use of airborne personal protective equipment (PPE).
- It is important to balance the appropriateness of resuscitation against the risk of infection.
- Methods to reduce nosocomial transmission of COVID-19 include a physical barrier such as a towel or mask over the patient's mouth and nose, appropriate use of PPE, minimising the staff involved in resuscitation, and use of mechanical chest compression devices when available.

## Out-of-Hospital Cardiac Arrest: (OHCA)

Although CPR is the golden rule in OHCA cases, it is known that the overall survival rate of these cases is as low as 7.6% (Wang, 2018). For this reason, it was suggested that the risk of disease transmission should be considered with multiple factors in on-scene CPR decisions. Cho *et al* from Korea. also stated that the resuscitation strategies should be revised rapidly, and the capacity should be managed cautiously in the use of resources in OHCA patients (Cho, 2020).

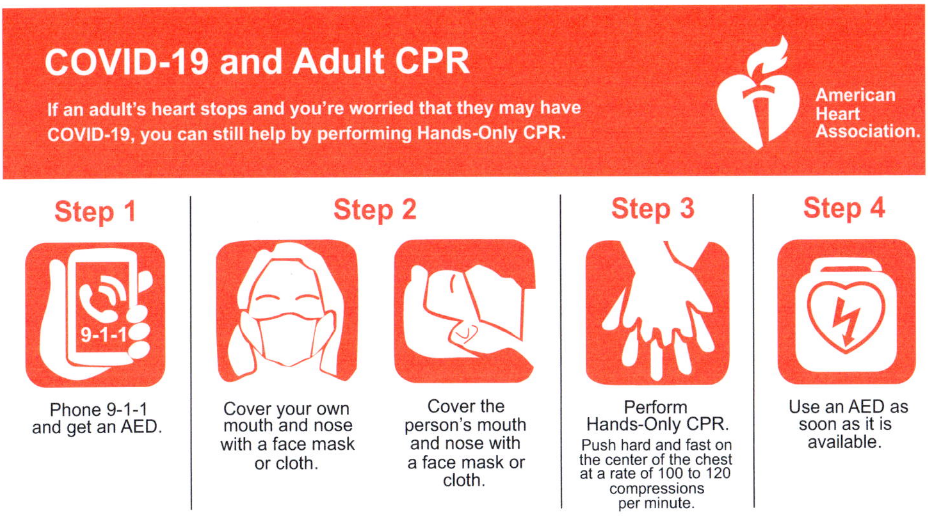


**Fig. (1).** Steps of Adult CPR in the COVID-19 era (Adapted from AHA).

Resuscitative events in patients with OHCA in New York in the period of boosted epidemic between March 1 and April 25, 2020, was analyzed (Lai, 2020). A total of 3989 OHCA patients in this period were compared to 1336 cases resuscitated in the previous year in the same region. 56% of the total 5325 OHCA cases were male and the mean age was 71. The incidence of OHCA increased 3 times when compared to the figures in the previous year. Interestingly, for example, on April 6, OHCA cases boosted 10-fold compared to the previous year.

**Mechanical Compression Device (MCD) and CPR:** These devices, which have been discussed extensively in recent years preceding COVID-19 era, come to the fore with the pandemic. In a study which enrolled 171 patients with OHCA in Korea, it was reported that MCD was performed almost as the standard procedure in OHCA cases during COVID-19 period (Cho, 2020). Compared to the historical control group in 2018, the OR value for survival and discharge decreased to 0.51 in the COVID-19 period. Characteristics of patients with OHCA in 2020 compared to the previous year are shown in the Table **2**. Randomized- controlled, population-based studies are still needed before drawing firm conclusions on the benefits with the use of MCD in OHCA.

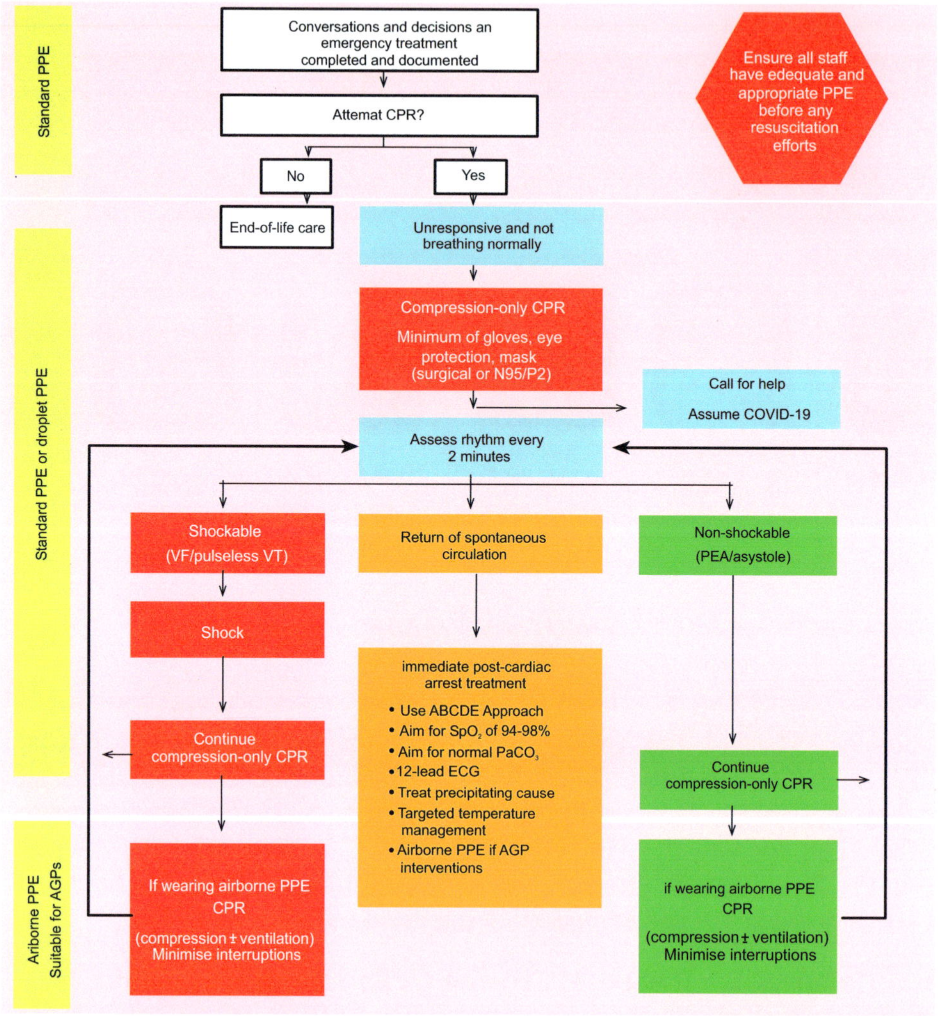


**Fig. (2).** Suggested algorithm for adult ACLS in the COVID-19 era (Adapted from Craig *et al*, 2020).

**Table 2. Features of OHCA cases in the pandemic period compared to the previous year (Lai, 2020).**

| |
|---|
| • Older (mean age 72 *vs*. 68) |
| • More from non-white groups (80% *vs* 67%) |
| • More hypertensive (53% *versus* 45%) |
| • More diabetic (36% *vs*. 26%) |

(Table 2) cont.....

| |
|---|
| • Has more physical limitations (57% *vs* 47%) |
| • More commonly presented with asystole (first rhythm detected) (OR: 3.5, p <0.001) |
| • More PEA (first rhythm detected) (OR: 1.99, p = 0.001) |
| • Less commonly gained ROSC (18% *vs*. 35%) |
| • Less commonly maintained ROSC (10.6% *vs*. 25%) |

In the EMS study in Korea, that the duration of intervention to patients reportedly increased from 6 minutes to 8 minutes (p = 0.009) after COVID-19, and the duration of stay at the scene increased from 13 minutes to 19 minutes (p <0.001) (Cho, 2020). Pre-hospital epinephrine administration and intubation rates increased significantly when compared to the figures in the year 2018. The rate of CPR with MCD also increased sharply to 78%.

## The procedures are as follows in patients with OHCA with suspected or diagnosed COVID-19

### Lay rescuers on scene:

1. As a general rule, COVID19 should be presumed in every OHCA case.
2. It is known that lay rescuers starting the CPR increases the survival. Thus, 'bystanderCPR' should be encouraged in every possible situation.
3. Lay rescuers have less protective equipment than HCW, so they carry a higher risk of transmission. This risk increases even more with the age of the rescuer and comorbidities. This risk is negligible when a household member has OHCA because the rescuer must have already taken the disease from the patient (if any).
4. Chest compressions: Lay rescuers should at least especially if someone in the household is having OHCA perform "handsonly CPR", *i.e.*, solely performing chest compressions. If the nose and mouth are closed with a face mask or a cloth, the risk of contamination is reduced significantly.
5. In pediatric OHCA, rescuers should also try to give mouthtomouth breathing.
6. AEDs should be used for defibrillation. It does not convey high risk with regard to infection.

### In Ambulance:

- Medical command (MC): EMS personnel should question every patient / relative in terms of COVID-19 diagnosis or symptoms.
- MC should warn rescuers against COVID-19 transmission and ask them to take the necessary precautions before performing CPR. MC should guide them to do

hands-only CPR.

- MC should also warn EMS personnel against COVID-19 transmission and ask them to use PPE.
- Relatives of the suspected or diagnosed patient with COVID-19 during transport should not be taken to the ambulance.

If ROSC cannot be restored despite adequate resuscitation on the scene, personnel can also evaluate withholding announcement of death of the patient on the scene and not taking him/her to the hospital following communication with MC.

**What Does ERC Say For Resuscitation?**

According to the resuscitation guide published in April 2020 (Soar, 2020):

Security is a priority. You should keep safety precautions at the highest level for

- yourself,
- your colleagues and people around,
- your patient.

Safe resuscitation is worth the time you spend.

Sequence of action in IHCA status:

1. Give a Blue Code or ask your colleagues for help for any patient who is unresponsive (unconscious) or has an unusual breathing.
2. Look for signs of life and palpate the pulse. Do not strive for LISTEN / FEEL.
3. Assign someone to bring a defibrillator.
4. If the defibrillator arrives immediately, turn it ON and insert the pads, if you notice VF / PVT, shock immediately after taking safety precautions. Start compressions if the patient remains in VF / PVT and you are already wearing PPE. If there is no PPE, wear the PPE and shock until somebody comes to help (if indicated).
5. If you are using AED, follow orders, shock if indicated, do not start compressions if there is no PPE, wait for someone wearing PPE.
6. If there is PPE, you can go on both with compressions and advanced airway interventions.
7. Drive away people who do not have a critical role. Those who exist must maintain their distance from the patient, unless they have mandatory work, *i.e.*, intubation.
8. In cases of arrest without any signs of life, continue with compressions until BVM is brought.

9. If you have time before compressions, give $O_2$ with a mask. Continue giving $O_2$ until BVM arrives.
10. When BVM arrives, maintain compression-ventilation at a 30: 2 ratios. There should be HEPA filter between bag and airway.
11. Ventilation with BVM should be accomplished by two people and should be completed in a minimal time because it conveys high risk for transmission.
12. Compressions may be interrupted while performing two ventilations.
13. The most experienced physician should attempt early intubation or insert SGA to minimize BVM duration. VL can be considered to reduce the risk of disease transmission.
14. If "reversible causes" that may cause arrest are ruled out, CPR can be terminated earlier than 'usual'.
15. MCD can be used as an alternative if CPR is to be extended - especially if the team possesses the main knowledge and is experienced in performing the technique.
16. Be cautious about contamination in removing the PPE.

## What Should We Do If The Intubated Patient Has A Cardiac Arrest?

1. Wear PPE.
2. Do not disconnect the ventilator circuit when starting CPR (this will increase the risk of aerosolization).
3. Increase $FiO_2$ to 100% and set the breathing frequency to 10 bpm.
4. Check that the ventilator and its circuit are intact and well connected, whose deficits may have caused arrest.
5. If the obligation to disconnect from the ventilator occurs, you may consider clamping the tube.
6. Use a viral filter.

**In-Hospital Cardiac Arrest (IHCA):** When **IHCA** is considered in case of suspected or diagnosed COVID-19, the procedures are as follows. These procedures are not performed in patients known to be COVID-19 (-). Nevertheless, it would be reasonable to dismiss additional (unnecessary) people around the patient resuscitated during the pandemic period.

## Prearrest Period

- Patients with COVID-19 or suspected or their relatives should be discussed on the patient's condition, requirements, and targeted level of care with CPR / ACLS from the time of admission. This should be repeated in case of sudden changes in the patient's condition.

- In order to reduce the need for urgent ETE, the patient's deterioration should be monitored in advance, and his findings such as $O_2$ saturation, respiratory and pulse rates (bpm), and blood pressure should be closely monitored.
- It may be a good idea to take the patient at risk of IHCA to a negative pressure room in advance. Thus, the risks in the intervention can be reduced.

## When IHCA Develops

- After ETE, MV with HEPA filter should be used.
- Prevent / minimize opening / disconnection of the circuit after closed circuit is provided
- Set the MV settings to allow asynchronous ventilation. $FiO_2$ is set to 1.0.
- Pressure control ventilation, 6 mL / kg is sufficient for tidal volume.

Modifications were suggested for COVID-19 era in Adult Advanced Cardiac Life Support Protocols (Fig. **3**).

Adult and pediatric BLS/ACLS guidelines were also modified in accord with the "Interim Guidance for Basic and Advanced Life Support in Adults, Children, and Neonates with Suspected or Confirmed COVID-19 from the Emergency Cardiovascular Care Committee and Get With The Guidelines-Resuscitation Adult and Pediatric Task Forces of the American Heart Association" (Fig. **3**).

Aerosol-creating sources during airway maneuvers are listed in Table **3**.

## Emergency Airway Interventions During the COVID-19 Period

In order to prevent the transmission of viruses, it is recommended that early intubation and a closed-circuit system with viral filter are started early to provide safe airway (AHA guidelines)

**Table 3. Sources That Create Aerosols During Airway Management.**

| | |
|---|---|
| Aerosol-inducing interventions and events | - Coughing / sneezing / expectoration<br>- Inadequate seal in NIV or PPV procedures (best seal is provided by tracheal intubation with a cuff)<br>- High flow nasal oxygenation, HFNO)<br>- Jet ventilation<br>- Administration of nebulized medication with simple face mask<br>- CPR (in non-intubated patient)<br>- Tracheal extubation |

*(Table 3) cont.....*

| | |
|---|---|
| Procedures with a high risk of aerosol generation | - Tracheal suction (without using closed circuit)<br>- Laryngoscopy<br>- Tracheal intubation<br>- Bronchoscopy / gastroscopy<br>- Interventions in the anterior cervical area such as tracheostomy and cricothyroidotomy |

In cases where this cannot be achieved, any airway intervention will be risky. For example, in the NIV or PPV interventions that are commonly performed in COPD and CHF cases, failure to provide a good seal causes transmission by aerosolization. The best seal is provided by tracheal intubation, which is followed by supraglottic devices, while the situation with the highest risk is the performance of NIV or PPV *via* mask (open system) (Brewster, 2020).

## Is There any Difference in RSI / Rapid Sequential Intubation Application?

- Yes. When sedative and muscle relaxant agents are given more than the usual doses, more robust and expedient management is accomplished. For example, rocuronium 1.5 mg / kg can be administered for a net muscle relaxant effect.

## What will we Do Before the Procedure for a Patient Who is Coughing and Who May Succumb to Respiratory Failure?

- Full use of PPE before close contact with the patient.
- Minimize the time it takes to remove the patient's mask and apply a mask with a viral filter and closed-circuit system.
- Check if the viral filter mask provides a good seal (also check the mask tight-fitting the face before the attempt, even if only an estimate)
- Providing complete muscle relaxation in rapid sequence intubation (RSI) application, which will prevent waste of time. Similarly, agitation should be prevented as quickly as possible.
- Management of extubation (if necessary).

## What can we Do to Ensure Mask Seal in Pre-oxygenation?

- Learn and apply "C-E" or "V-E" grip (Figs. **4A** and **B**)
- Perform manual bagging with a high-quality bag that easily collapses
- - Close monitoring of oxygenation and $CO_2$ clearance (*e.g.*, *via* pulse oximetry and $ETCO_2$ probes), which will enable real-time warning for achievement of desired level of pre-oxygenation, so that overprocessing is prevented.

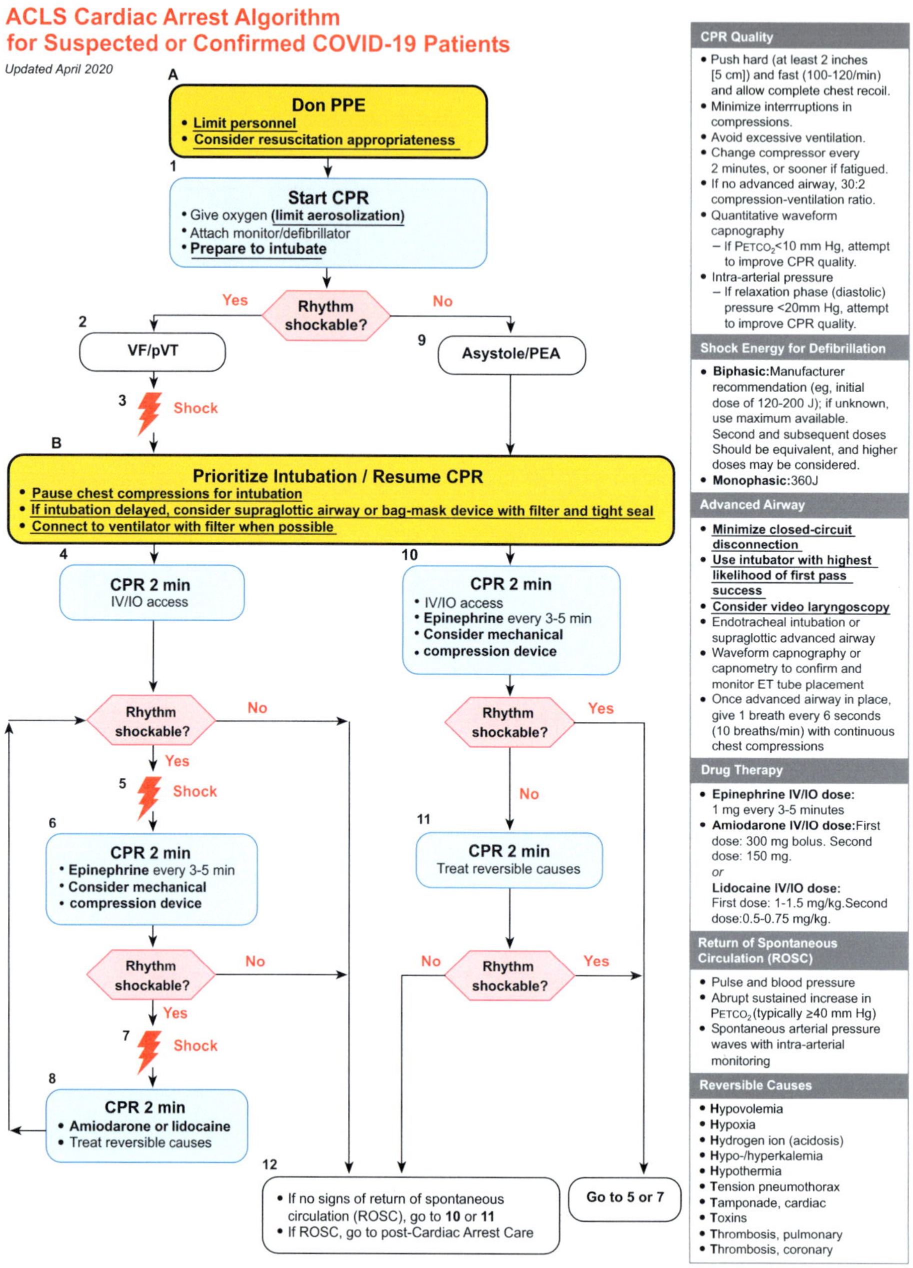


**Fig. (3).** Some modifications have been recommended for Adult Advanced Cardiac Life Support Protocols amid COVID-19. Intubation and closed-circuit ventilation have gained priority and high-risk operations have been postponed.

## Avoid Attempting PPV without A Good Seal!

What if mandatory?

1. - Use at least a second generation supraglottic device (seal pressures are higher). Make sure that this is a device fitting the patient, the cuff is well-inflated, and the depth is sufficient.
2. - ETI is a better option. In this, it is important that the cuff is below the cords and well inflated and fixed.
3. - Ventilation pressures should be kept to a minimum to ensure adequate oxygenation.
4. - Optimal paralysis and deep sedation should be achieved to preclude time losses and combat phenomenon.
5. - Airway pressures should be monitored with a manometer.

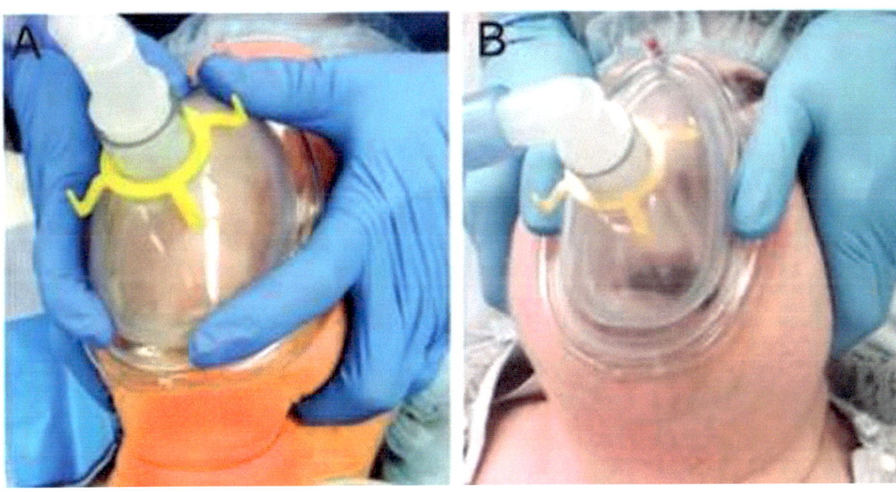


**Fig. (4).** (A/B). Drawing shows bagging *via* bimanual "vice grip".

## Videolaryngoscopy (VL)

ETI can be employed if the tube is immediately ready at the planned point. If more than one VL device is available, one should be reserved for COVID-19 patients.

Disposable VL blades should be used and disposed of when the procedure is completed.

## Aspiration

1. Unplanned, emergency and pre-hospital emergency airway management
2. These are situations that pose a great risk to HCW in many emergencies, including cardiac arrest. HCW should commence CPR immediately while protecting themselves at the highest possible level.
3. Cardiac compressions should not start without donning full PPE.
4. The number of people / employees in the resuscitation bay should be kept to a minimum. No one should be taken into the room without the PPE - including the hospital manager and the prime minister.
5. The physician should avoid close contact with the patient (especially respirations) as much as possible - (*e.g.*, lung auscultation)
6. All measures should be taken to protect the first responders during the compressions.
7. Hands-only CPR can be performed until the airway stabilization is achieved with the use of viral filter.
8. Early and expedient ETI should be performed.
9. SGD placement is a better option than a face mask, especially during cardiac compressions.
10. Performance of PPV *via* face mask should be avoided as much as possible.

### What Can We Do Else?

In a new publication from the US Navy, a safer route was proposed in regard to transmission in pre-hospital emergency intubations (Kinney, 2020).

## Case Report

A 75-year-old male patient underwent CPR in the ambulance after a call made because he had cardiac arrest. In the system presented as "Rapid outdoor non-compression intubation (RONCI)", viral filter, endotracheal tube (ETT), bag-valve-mask, inline suction (aspiration) is made ready beforehand (Fig. **5**). It is also used with VL.

**Procedure:** After the patient is brought to the emergency room with CPR, compressions are interrupted instantly and ETT was placed and the cuff was inflated. It was connected to the viral filter. CPR was continued and the lungs were ventilated with BVM. In this way, the risk of transmission was minimized. In this case, airway was secured with a 15-second interruption of CPR. In the detailed history, it was learned that the patient had flu-like complaints for 3 days.

In theory, it is known that viral infection is minimized by inflating the cuff and connecting to the viral filter.

- PPE should also be complete.
- Ambulance stretcher should be adjusted to the height to be switched to intubation immediately.
- It is necessary to ventilate the intubated environment very well.
- It is also important that there are no 'unnecessary' people in the environment who do not have any critical task.
- The RONCI technique adds to these rules as a plus, the compressions are inflated with minimal breaks in intubation and the filter connection is prepared before the patient is admitted into the emergency room.
- The fact that PPE makes it difficult for interpersonal communication when it has to be worn due to pandemics renders it necessary to prepare everything as much as possible.
- The first pass success should be the highest, thus it is important that the senior emergency HCW intubates the patient.

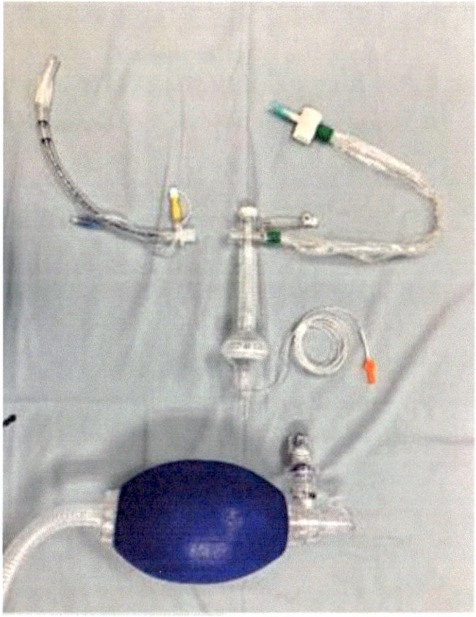

**Fig. (5).** Viral filter, endotracheal tube (ETT), bag-valve-mask, inline suction (aspiration).

## What If We Cannot Succeed With It?

If successful intubation does not occur in 10-15 seconds with RONCI, it should not be tried again, CPR should be performed, and oxygen saturation should be risen by ventilating the patient and then retried. At this stage, SGD can also be considered as an alternative.

## HYDROXYCHLOROQUINE AND CARDIAC ADVERSE EFFECTS

Hydroxychloroquine (HCQ) is one of the disease-modifying antirheumatic drugs, a powerful agent that prevents inflammation exacerbations and tissue damage. HCQ and Chloroquine (CQ) are considered as immunomodulators (Ruiz-Irastorza *et al*, 2010). The chemical structure of HCQ is very similar to CQ; it is exactly the same except for an additional hydroxyl molecule at the terminal site.

Both agents inhibit receptor binding and membrane fusion, which are the essential steps required for cell entry by SARS-CoVs. Impaired terminal glycosylation of ACE2 can reduce the binding efficiency between ACE2 and the SARS-CoV spike-protein (S) in host cells. Thus, the virus is prevented from binding to receptors on cells and the development of infection is prevented. Following entrance of HCQ and CQ into a cell, both are concentrated in low-pH organelles such as endosomes, Golgi vesicles, and lysosomes. As the virus uses endosomes as its cellular entry mechanism, increasing the pH of the endosomes with CQ therapy has a negative effect on the fusion process of the virus and the endosome. Inhibition of SARS-CoV spread has been observed in cells treated with CQ before or after infection, suggesting both the prophylactic and therapeutic advantages of CQ in combating SARS (Vincent *et al*, , 2005).

Nausea/vomiting and diarrhea are the most common side effects of CQ and HCQ. Long-term exposure to CQ can also cause serious side effects such as retinopathy, cardiovascular disorders, and cardiomyopathy (Schrezenmeier *et al*, 2020). Nonetheless, considering its safety profile during pregnancy, HCQ rather than CQ is a potential therapeutic solution for these patients (Izmirly *et al*, , 2012; Lisney *et al*, 2017).

In Summary, HCQ is Thought to be a Better Therapeutic Option Than CQ in the Treatment of COVID-19 Infection. There are Three Main Reasons for this:

- HCQ attenuates the severe progression of COVID-19 *via* inhibition of cytokine storm and reduction of CD154 expression in T cells.

- HCQ can provide a similar antiviral effect in pre- and post-infection stages found with CQ.

- HCQ has fewer side effects, safe during pregnancy.

In a study coordinated by the University of Méditerranée in Marseille, COVID-19 patients older than 12 years were divided into two groups: 24 as the HCQ treatment group and 24 as the control group (Gautret *et al*, 2020). In the treatment group, 200 mg HCQ 3 times a day for 10 days and additional azithromycin (AZT) were used if necessary. It was found to be highly and significantly effective in the clearance of the nasopharyngeal viral load measured by RT-PCR within just 3 to 6 days in the treatment group when compared to the untreated control group. A higher SARS-CoV-2 clearance rate was noted after six days of treatment with either HCQ alone or HCQ + AZT (70% *versus* 12%; $p<0.001$). AZT added to HCQ has also been reported to be significantly more effective for virus elimination. Of note, the combination of HCQ and AZT showed a synergistic effect on viral clearance. Addition of AZT to HCQ may increase the risk of QTc prolongation.

HCQ is administered orally for 5 to 10 days at the time of diagnosis or high index of suspicion, 400 mg after 12 hours, 2x200 mg up to the following 5 days. In case of It is contraindicated in those with myasthenia gravis, porphyria, retinal diseases, epilepsy and if QTc> 500 ms, (Interim Clinical Guidance for Patients Suspected of / Confirmed With COVID-19 in Belgium.16 Mars 2020; Version 3.).

## HCQ and Cardiac Adverse Effects, Ventricular Arrhythmias

In the treatment of COVID-19 infection, when HCQ is used alone or in combination with azithromycin, there is a risk of prolongation of the QT interval and ventricular arrhythmia in the ECG. QT prolongation is a predictor of torsades de pointes (TdP) and therefore VT. Female sex, structural heart diseases, congenital long QT syndromes, electrolyte disorders, hepatic / renal failure, use of QT prolonging drugs are the main factors that increase the risk of drug induced TdP. In accord with the classification published by Tisdale in 2013 and used to predict patients with drug-induced QT prolongation, a total score of $\leq 6$ represents low risk, 7 to 10 medium risk, and the score $\geq 11$ is high risk (Table **4**) (Tisdale *et al*, 2013). In the study, the specificity and NPV value of being in the moderate risk group in predicting QT prolongation was found to be 88%. Sensitivity is 67% in the medium risk group and 74% in the high-risk group.

The QT intervals of patients who were treated with HCQ / AZT due to COVID-19 was examined in the study conducted in France (Bessière *et al*, 2020). Forty patients with normal QTc found before treatment were included in the study. Eighteen (45%) of them were treated with 1x 250 mg AZT + 2x200 mg HCQ daily and 22 patients received only 2x 200 mg HCQ. Prolonged QTc was detected in 14 patients (36%) while the treatment was ongoing, between the 2nd and 6th days; however, no ventricular arrhythmia including TdP was observed. A prolongation of QTc was observed in 6 (33%) of 18 patients in the first group treated with HCQ + AZT and in 1 (5%) of 22 patients in the second group treated with HCQ alone ($p = 0.03$, $p = 0.03$).

**Table 4. Risk scoring system published by Tisdale in 2013 with respect to drug related QTc prolongation.**

| Risk Factors | Score |
|---|---|
| Age ≥ 68 | 1 |
| Female sex | 1 |
| Use of loop diuretics | 1 |
| Serum K+ ≤ 3,5 mEq/L | 2 |
| QTc ≥ 450ms on presentation | 2 |
| Acute myocardial infarction | 2 |
| Use of ≥ 2 drugs that prolongs QTc | 3 |
| Sepsis | 3 |
| Heart failure | 3 |
| Use of one drug that prolongs QTc | 3 |
| **Total score** | 21 |

Patients should be routinely screened with ECGs before starting CQ, HCQ and AZT since these drugs have the potential to prolong QTc. Concomitant use of other drugs known to prolong the QTc interval (anti-arrhythmic, anti-depressants, anti-psychotics, antihistamine, teneligliptin, ondansetron, and moxifloxacin *etc.*) should be avoided.

The most comprehensive study ever conducted on the treatment efficacy of HCQ in COVID-19 is the one by Rosenberg *et al*, (Rosenberg *et al*, 2020). In the multi-center study conducted on cases hospitalized due to COVID-19 between 15th and 28th March 2020 in 25 hospitals looking at 88.3% of COVID-19 cases in New York, 1438 patients were included and divided into four groups (Table **5**).

Hospital mortality rate was 20.3% in the whole group (95% CI, 18.2% to 22.4%). The most frequently reported adverse reactions in all groups were abnormal ECG findings and arrhythmias. Arrhythmias and ECG findings were more common in patients who received HCQ than other drugs. However, this finding was not confirmed in logistic regression models. Cardiac arrest (15.5%) and abnormal ECG findings (27%) in patients who received HCQ + AZT were similar to those who received only HCQ (13.7% and 27.3%), but higher than those who received only AZT (6.2% and 16%) (Rosenberg *et al*, 2020).

**Table 5. Study groups, number of patients, treatments, and patient mortality rates at the end of treatment (Adapted from Rosenberg *et al*, 2020.**

| Groups | # of Patients and Percentages (n/%) | Treatment | Cardiac Arrest and ECG Abnormality (%) | Mortality at the end of Treatment (n/%) |
|---|---|---|---|---|
| 1. group | 271 / 18.8 | HCQ | 13,7 / 27,3 | 54 / 19,9 |
| 2. group | 211 / 14.7 | AZT | 6,2 / 16,1 | 21 / 10,0 |
| 3. group | 735 / 51.1 | HCQ + AZT | 15,5 / 27,1 | 189 / 25,7 |
| 4. group | 221 / 15.4 | None of the study drugs were used | 6,8 / 14,0 | 28 / 12,7 |
| **Total** | **1438 / 100** | | | **292 / 20,3** |

The findings of this study sparked distrust about what is known about HCQ. This situation, which contradicts the results of previous studies, suggests that the use of HCQ in the treatment of COVID-19 patients may be unnecessary, as well as adversely affecting the patient's survival rates.

**Value of ECG monitoring in patients with COVID-19:** These patients are exposed to risk of cardiac damage caused by both direct effects of the disease on the heart and also by the toxicities of the drugs used in the treatment. Comorbid situations mostly pose a third factor, especially with the advancing age (Fig. **6**).

**QT prolongation and COVID-19:** CQ, HCQ (Zhou 2020, Gao 2020), AZT (Gautret, 2020) which takes place among the agents in the treatment of COVID-19, and antivirals (Wang 2020, Beck 2020) are often blamed for this phenomenon. Cardiotoxic agents used in the treatment of comorbid problems such as amiodarone, electrolyte abnormalities that develop secondary to diuretic use, can lead to rhythm disturbances which are further exacerbated by malnutrition.

Jain *et al*, from Yale examined 2006 ECGs obtained in 524 patients and recorded QT prolongation (QTc> 470 ms or QTc> 500 ms when QRS> 120 ms) in 103 patients (19.7%) (Jain, 2020). Patients with QT prolongation are on average 68 years old, 62% male, whose mean QTc is 507 ms and the average BMI is 28. More than half (59%) have hypertension and nearly half have diabetes.

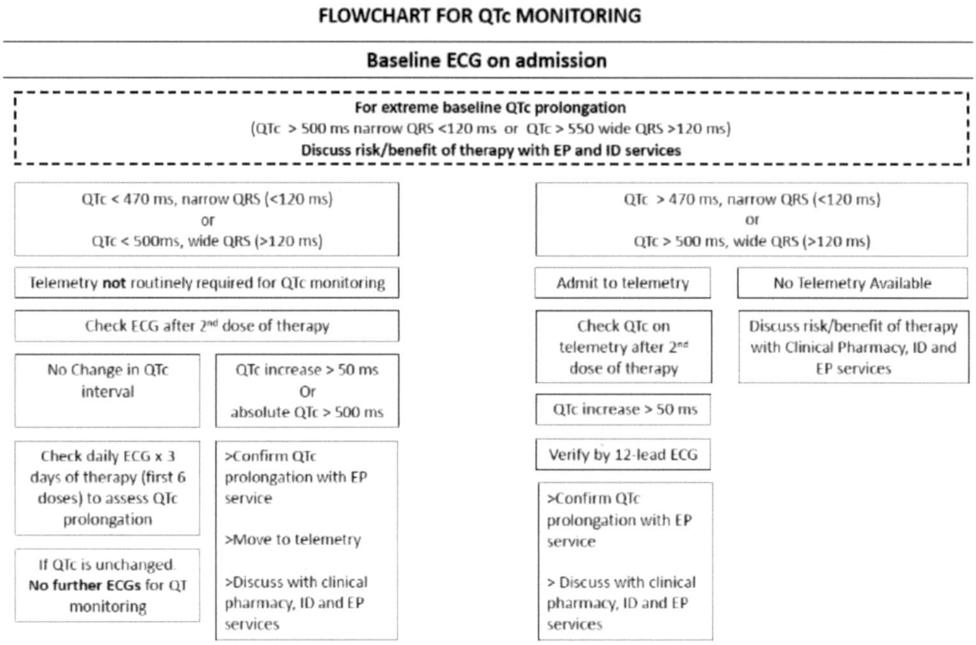


**Fig. (6).** Flowchart for QTc monitoring.

Patients with QT prolongation necessitated a higher rate of intubation than others and were hospitalized in intensive care units more commonly. Among the drugs, only tocilizumab use is more frequent in the group with QT prolongation than those without (62% *versus* 80%). Torsade de pointes or other life-threatening ventricular dysrhythmias were not observed, while only one patient with previous STEMI developed monomorphic VT.

## COVID-19 AND RESPIRATORY FAILURE (RF)

### Case presentation

52 y. male patient had been taken into isolation at home for 8 days due to fever and cough that had risen from time to time. He was brought to the ED by ambulance due to the increase in respiratory distress in the last two days.

He can speak, but his respiratory rate is 24 bpm. Peripheral $O_2$ saturation was 72%, which increased to 90% with the supplementation of $O_2$ (4 L/min). He has no fever; his cardiovascular examination is normal except for mild tachycardia.

Almost all patients who worsen with the diagnosis of COVID-19 develop acute type 1 RF. NIV is necessary in around 14% of all patients (Wu, 2020).

Preliminary indicators of RF development:

- increased respiratory rate,
- not being able to speak with long sentences,
- use of adjunctive inspiratory muscles,
- hypoxemia,
- need for additional oxygen supplementation.

**Mechanism:** Some researchers state that RF is actually triggered primarily by the pulmonary vascular injury and dysregulation and the resultant disordered gas exchange. Some patients recover within days / weeks after this stage. Those who get worse develop ARDS after this critical point. Diffuse alveolar damage and inflammatory edema develops which in turn, progresses to intubation and mechanical ventilation. Multifocal ground glass opacities and consolidations are shown in Fig. (**7**).

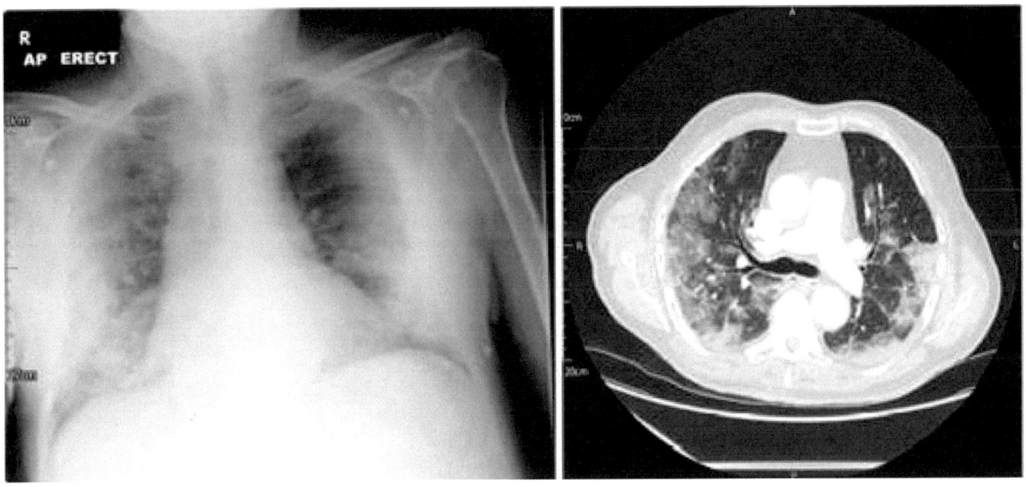


**Fig. (7).** Chest X-ray and simultaneous thoracic tomography of a patient with severe COVID-19 who eventually developed RF. Multifocal ground glass opacities and consolidations are visualized.

Algorithm for the patients with acute RF in the COVID-19 era is depicted in Algorithm **1** .

## ARDS in COVID-19

COVID-19 mainly affects the respiratory system with significantly less injury to other organs. Alveolar epithelial cell injury was the primary cause of COVID-19-related ARDS, and endothelial cells were less damaged with therefore less exudation (Li, 2020).

Many researchers pointed out that the development of ARDS in those with COVID-19 infection is a crucial factor for outcome. Histopathological hallmarks are diffuse alveolar damage caused by direct, viral cytotoxic effects on pneumocytes, and a concurrent inflammatory reaction. cytokine storm is also a pathophysiological factor in development of ARDS (Ruan, 2020).

First of all, ARDS develops in a more severe group of patients with worse physiological reserves than others. Those with ARDS had preexisting respiratory diseases more commonly than patients without ARDS (58% *versus* 42%) and were more commonly overweight or obese (83% *versus* 42%) (Dreher, 2020). They are also characterized by persistently elevated inflammatory markers such as IL-6 and CRP.

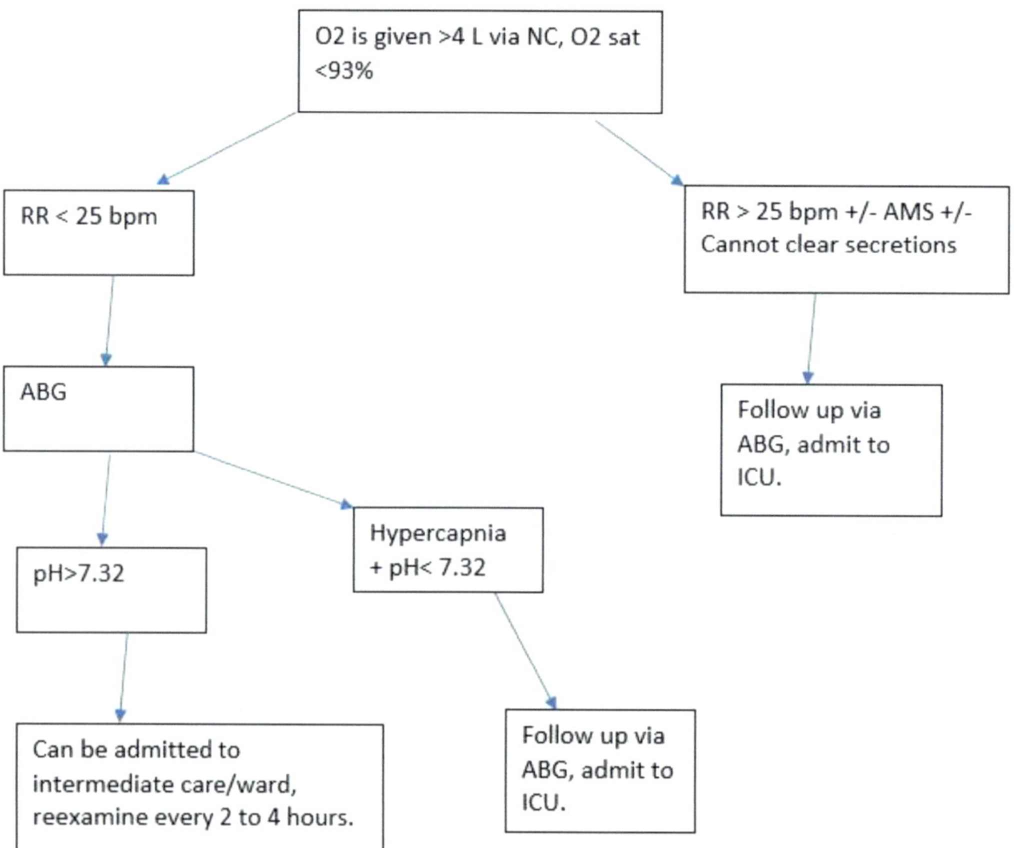


**Algorithm 1.** Scheme for the patients with acute RF in the COVID-19 era NC: nasal cannula, AMS: altered mental status, ABG: Arterial blood gas.

Studies indicated that the reported incidence of ARDS in patients with COVID-19 was 16% to 30%, higher than that of other organ injuries (Huang, 2020; Chen, 2020; Wang, 2020; Guan, 2020; Zhou, 2020). The same research cited that the most frequent respiratory symptom of COVID-19 is dry cough (60% to 80%). Sputum production is noted less commonly.

**The typical CT** findings of COVID-19 showed bilateral ground-glass opacities with a peripheral distribution (Chung, 2020). These images should not be misdiagnosed as ARDS, despite the presence of consolidation and exudation in both entities. ARDS is a condition associated with many disease processes, resulting in reduced lung compliance and severe hypoxemia (Dreher, 2020).

**Lung ultrasound score** (LUSS) was put forward by Dargent *et al*, to describe and monitor extension and severity of lung infiltrates numerically with a reproducible and validated tool (Dargent *et al*, 2020). They reported that there was a good agreement between CT-scans and LUSS as for the presence of lung consolidations. LUSS monitoring accurately reflect disease progression and indicates potential usefulness for the management of COVID-19 patients with ARDS. It might help with early recognition of ventilator-associated pneumonia (VAP), weaning from MV, and potentially reduce the need for X-ray and CT.

Based on current reports in the management of COVID-19-related ARDS, it is remarkable that there are substantial differences between COVID-19-related ARDS and ARDS caused by other factors as defined by Berlin criteria, and therefore differences in treatment.

## Management Protocols for RF in COVID-19

In terms of management in the ICU, a majority of these patients warrant a complex ventilation strategy including prone positioning (PP) and, in some cases, ECMO.

Hypoxemic RF in ARDS generally results from intrapulmonary V-P mismatch or shunt and usually prompts management with MV. HFNO reduces the need for endotracheal intubation in ARDS patients (Ou *et al*, 2020). WHO recommended that HFNO should only be used in selected patients with hypoxemic respiratory failure (WHO, 28 January 2020). Studies indicated that HFNO is more suitable for patients with mild ARDS.

**Corticosteroids (CST)** are considered a promising treatment for ARDS, especially those with severe disease, because of their efficacy in alleviating inflammation and fibrosis. However, the use of CST in ARDS patients is still controversial, thus management with CST is the only pharmacological intervention that may mitigate death rates in the course of COVID-19. Previous reports indicated that treatment with methylprednisolone were associated with shorter periods of need for invasive MV and reduced mortality in patients with ARDS (Meduri, 2018). In a recently published systematic review and meta-analysis, Ye *et al*, demonstrated that CST infusion may reduce mortality in patients with severe COVID-19 and ARDS (Ye, 2020).

The use and efficacy of CST is further discussed in the Chapter "Principles of Treatment".

## Salvage Use Of Tissue Plasminogen Activator (TPA) in The Setting Of Ards Due To COVID-19

In a well-designed analytic study for decision making in the patients in extremis, Choudhury *et al*, assigned patients with COVID-19 to either of two groups, 50.000 patients each, to simulate the life critically ill COVID-19 patients as they transitioned to either recovery or death (Choudhury, 2020). Critically ill COVID-19 patients were defined as having a refractory $PaO_2/FiO_2$ of < 60 mmHg (salvage use criteria). They reported that the 'salvage' use of tPA was associated with reduced mortality (47.6% [tPA] *vs.* 71.0% [no tPA]) for base case patients. They concluded that salvage use of tPA may improve recovery of ARDS patients, thereby reducing COVID-19-related mortality and ensuring sufficient resources to manage this pandemic.

## Resuscitation in the Prone Position (PP)

Severe COVID-19 patients are known to have improved oxygenation with PP. Although most of these patients are intubated, PP may also be beneficial in those who are not intubated. If the non-intubated patient is arrested while in PP, they should be turned supine immediately, and then CPR should be comenced. If the intubated patient has cardiac arrest, CPR can be started immediately by pressing the back. Some perfusion is achieved in this way until the patient is turned supine (Fig. **8**).

Procedure steps for PP CPR:

1. All rescuers must don PPE.
2. Apply the usual amount of pressure and depth to the middle of the scapulae. (5-6 cm and approximately twice a second)
3. Turn the patient supine if:
4. Ineffective compression: If there is arterial invasive monitoring, and a value of more than 25 mmHg could not be achieved in diastolic BP,

5. In need of intervention requiring the patient to be supine (*e.g.*, airway control),
6. if circulation was not immediately restored within minutes
7. Additional assistance will be required to turn the patient supine; you should plan ahead.
8. How to place the defibrillator paddles in the PP:
9. Anterior-posterior, or
10. Bi-axillary
11. It has been demonstrated in various studies in the recent decade that PP has a beneficial effect on survival in severe ARDS (Gattinoni, 2010; Guerin, 2013).

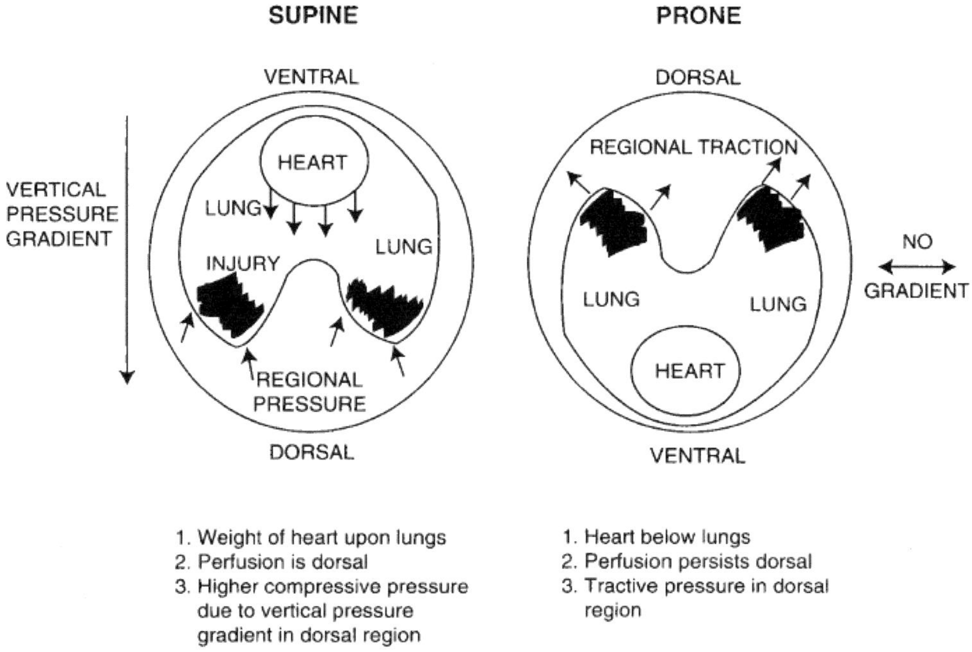


**Fig. (8).** Proposed mechanisms for efficacy of prone ventilation.

The efficacy of PP is probably most likely related to the homogeneous distribution of alveolar aeration. In addition, ventilator-associated lung injury is mitigated with PP, and stress and strain during these procedures are reduced. Meta-analyzes showed that mortality was reduced by 10% with PP, especially in patients with severe hypoxaemic ARDS (baseline $PaO_2/FiO_2$ <100 mmHg) (Sud, 2010). Of note, PP also increased $PaO_2/FiO_2$ ratio by 27-39%. It is also clear that the ICU mortality in ARDS is also decreased with PP (Abroug, 2011). In 2017, Scholten *et al*, reported that PP, which was initiated early and applied 16 hours a day by experienced HCW, would increase survival in patients with severe ARDS (Scholten, 2017).

Despite everything, the reasons why PP is not applied much in cases with ARDS or other treatments are the need for additional staff and resource use, procedure difficulties, accidental extubation, vascular access, and the need to arrange adjuncts such as drains.

**What happens when the patient is converted to PP?** It has been noted that peak and plateau airway pressures may decrease rapidly after converting to PP. Decrease in chest wall compliance and mobilization of secretions may be the reasons for this. An average increase of 10 mmHg is recorded in $PaO_2$. Beginning from the first hour of PP, signs of lung recruitment are seen, that is, a decrease in plateau pressure is recorded with the same tidal volume (Fig. **9**).

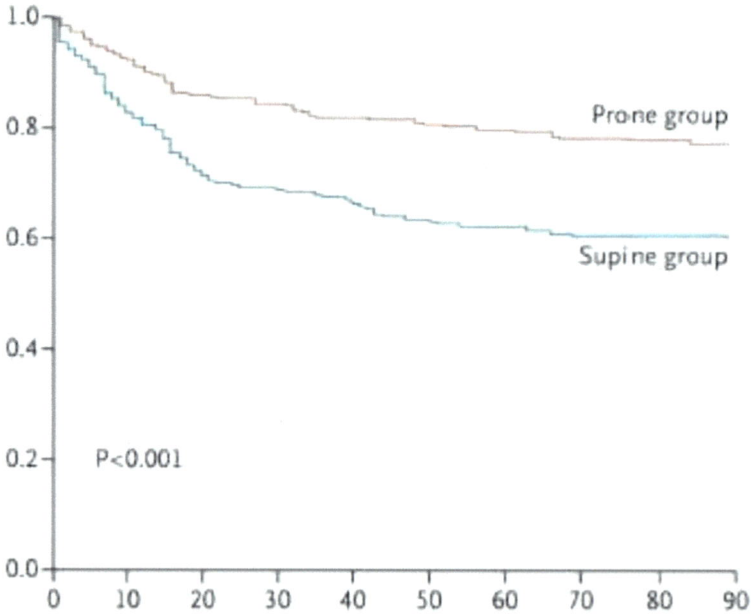


**Fig. (9).** Diagram showing that the PP affects the survival favorably in ARDS patients undergoing PEEP. The horizontal axis shows the days, the vertical axis the probability of survival.

As a result, it was revealed in the study that patients with ARDS and severe hypoxia were initiated early and benefited from the PP maintained for a long time (Guerin, 2013).

**Who are not Suitable for PP? (contraindications)**

1. Those with acute bleeding, requiring immediate intervention
2. Those in shock, prearrest condition
3. Increased intracranial pressure or decreased cerebral perfusion

4. Pregnancy
5. Spinal instability
6. Trauma, multiple fractures, femur, vertebra, or facial fractures

## Common Complications of PP

1. Nerve compression such as the brachial plexus
2. Extubation
3. Venous stasis
4. Pressure sores
5. Crush injury
6. Vomiting, arrhythmias

However, the data for use in CPR is scarce. The data flow that started with the case series in which 10 out of 22 patients survived with PP in the 2000s (Brown, 2001) continued with larger studies. It has been reported that systolic and mean arterial pressure is higher in PP- CPR (Mazer, 2003; Wei, 2006).

The role of PP- CPR should be evaluated differently in intubated and non-intubated patients. In the patient who is monitored intubated and prone, CPR should first be started prone, and the decision to turn the supine should be made only due to the decrease in pressure in clinical, arterial invasive monitoring and decreases in $ETCO_2$.

Pearl: In non-intubated patients with COVID-19, defibrilation should take priority, as the personnel wearing PPE when witnessing cardiac arrest may delay crucial steps in CPR. Ideally, in the departments where patients with a high probability of arrest are monitored, a full PPE donned beforehand will minimize these risks, and interventions including intubation will be performed more quickly.

**Turning to PP is a critical decision,** when the intubation tube should be clamped, and the optimal procedure should be managed by experienced people so that both the patient and the surrounding healthcare professionals are not injured.

In an article published in May 2020, Barker *et al*, stated the need for a guideline on CPR while intubated and non-intubated patients in PP under COVID-19 pandemic conditions (Barker, 2020).

Pearl: In AHA guidelines, PP is stated as Class IIb, (C level of evidence) which can be performed as a recommendation after securing permanent airway for the patient. It can be used in intraoperative arrests, but it is not recommended for the lay person in any arrests in or out of hospital. Providing sternal support was reminded during the application.

Team play to practice and the effects of the prone position on lung ventilation and gas exchange are shown in Figs. (**10A** and **10B**).

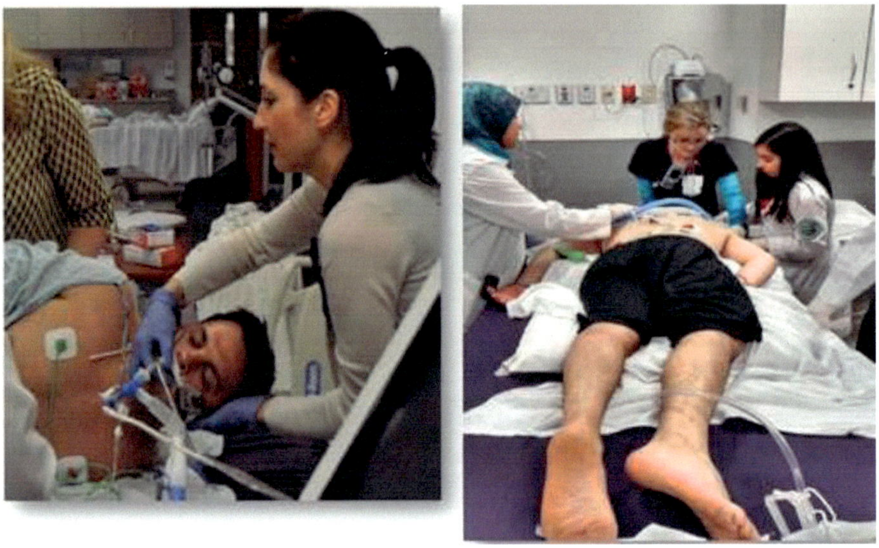

**Fig. (10A).** "Proning" on the resuscitation bay requires a team management.

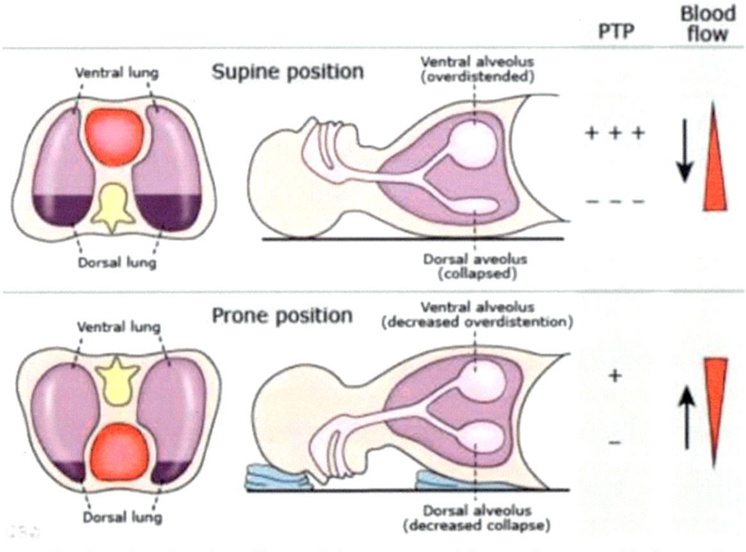


**Fig. (10B).** Schematization showing the effects of the prone position on lung ventilation and gas exchange.

COVID-19 can lead to lethal consequences, especially RF and ARDS. There are currently no recommended specific treatments for the group with severe COVID-19, therefore, supportive treatment is essential. Expedient recognition and decisions for aggressive measures such as permanent control of airway and positive-pressure ventilation, along with CST and t-PA administration, should be evaluated using certain selection criteria. PP is mostly associated with a more favorable outcomes than supine position in selected cases. Physicians and other team members should be trained on the procedure and be prepared for emergency need for such maneuvers in the resuscitation bay.

## MANAGEMENT OF SHOCK, SEPSIS, RESPIRATORY FAILURE AND ARDS

### IV Hydration

Fluid and electrolyte balance of the patient hospitalized due to COVID-19 should be evaluated. If there is a fluid or electrolyte deficiency, replacement therapy is administered along with maintenance therapy. Physiological variables such as heart rate, blood pressure, respiratory rate, body temperature and urine output should be closely monitored throughout the hospitalization period (The 3/4/2020 Chinese Health and Public Health Ministry Guideline on Novel Coronavirus Disease (COVID-19) Diagnosis and Treatment (Revision # 6)). Conservative fluid therapy should be preferred in patients with ARDS caused by sepsis, unless there are signs of hypoperfusion (Rhodes *et al*, 2017).

In adult patients with fluid deficit caused by sepsis, at least 30 ml / kg isotonic crystalloid (normal saline or Ringer's lactate) is administered for resuscitation in the first 3 hours. Most patients need 4-6 L of fluid infusion in the first 6 hours. In children, on the other hand, 20 ml / kg bolus and 40-60 ml / kg in the first hour are given rapidly. Hypotonic crystalloids, starches or gelatins are not used for resuscitation (Lamontagne *et al*, 2016). It has been found that excessive fluid treatment in sepsis impairs respiratory functions, causes organ hypoperfusion by increasing intra-abdominal pressure, triggers coagulopathy, increases the risk of cerebral edema, and consequently increases mortality. Therefore, unnecessary, and excessive fluid replacement should be avoided in these patients (Rhodes *et al*, 2017).

In adult patients for fluid deficit resuscitation caused by septic shock, at least 30 ml / kg isotonic crystalloid (normal saline or Ringer's lactate) is administered in the first 3 hours. Most patients need 4-6 L of fluid support in the first 6 hours. In children, on the other hand, 20 ml / kg bolus and 40-60 ml / kg in the first hour are given rapidly. Hypotonic crystalloids, starches or gelatins are not used for resuscitation (Lamontagne *et al*, 2016). It has been found that excessive fluid treatment in sepsis worsens respiratory functions, causes organ hypoperfusion by increasing intra-abdominal pressure, leads to coagulopathy, increases the tendency of cerebral edema, and consequently increases mortality. Therefore, unnecessary fluid replacement should be avoided in patients with this condition.

Management of patients with renal insufficiency should focus on nutritional support such as body fluids, acid-base and electrolyte balance, including nitrogen balance. "Continuous renal replacement therapy" (CRRT) can be used in this context. Indications for CRRT are hyperkalemia, acidosis, pulmonary edema or fluid overload, and fluid management in case of multiple organ dysfunction (Diagnosis and Treatment Protocol for Novel Coronavirus Pneumonia.Trial Version 7).

## Vasopressors

If there is no response to fluid loading and signs of fluid overload ensue (*e.g.*, jugular venous distension, rales in lung auscultation, pulmonary edema in imaging, or hepatomegaly in children), fluid administration should be reduced or stopped (Lamontagne *et al*, 2016).

Pearl: If COVID-19 infection is suspected or present, and the mean arterial pressure (MAP) cannot be kept above 65 mmHg with intravenous (IV) hydration and lactate cannot be maintained below 2 mmol / L, vasopressor support should definitely be initiated.

**The first option should be norepinephrine**. The infusion dose is 0.1-0.15 mcg/kg/min. The maximum dose used in refractory shock is 0.5-0.75 mcg/kg/min, and it may rarely need to be titrated up to 3.3 mcg/kg/min. In cases where an adequate response is not elicited, epinephrine 0.014 mcg/kg/min or vasopressin may be added. Low dose vasopressin is not recommended.

Pearl: If the patient has signs of myocardial dysfunction or hypoperfusion despite MAP> 65 mmHg and normovolemia is demonstrated, a positive inotropic agent should be added to vasopressor therapy.

Dobutamine is the first choice and is administered at a dose of 2-20 mcg/kg/min. Milrinone can also be used as an alternative to increase short-term cardiac output to maintain organ perfusion in cardiogenic shock resistant to other agents (Rhodes *et al*, 2017; Levy *et al*, 2018).

**Recognition of septic shock in children:** Hypotension (systolic blood pressure (SBP) <5th percentile or> 2 SD below normal for age) or 2 or 3 of the following: altered mental status; bradycardia or tachycardia (heart rate <90 / min or> 160 / min in infants and <70 / min or> 150 / min in children); hot-red skin with prolonged capillary refill (> 2 sec) or strong pulsation (vasodilation); tachypnea; mottled skin or petechial or purpuric rash; elevated lactate; oliguria; hyper- or hypothermia (Martinez, 2020).

It is preferred that vasopressors be administered *via* central venous catheters. If a central venous catheter is not available, it can be administered through a large-bore catheter in a peripheral vein. Extravasation and signs of local tissue necrosis should be closely monitored. Vasopressors can also be administered *via* intraosseous route (Loubani *et al*, 2015).

## Respiratory Support

**a) Monitor $SaO_2$ closely:** If the oxygen ($O_2$) saturation is ≤ 93%, adequate $O_2$ support needs to be provided with a face mask or high flow nasal oxygen treatment (HFNOT). You can also consider a 2/1 mixture of hydrogen (H) / $O_2$ (H / $O_2$: 66.6% / 33.3%). The patient should be intubated and mechanically ventilated if low $O_2$ saturation or relevant symptoms do not improve within 1-2 hours with noninvasive positive pressure ventilation with high flow $O_2$ procedure, or if the patient deteriorates (The 3/4/2020 Chinese Health and Public Health Ministry Guideline on Novel Coronavirus Disease (COVID-19) Diagnosis and Treatment (Revision # 6)).

**b) Invasive Ventilation:** Patients with ARDS, especially young children, obese or pregnant, can desaturate rapidly during intubation. Give oxygen with 100% $FiO_2$ 5 minutes in advance with a face mask with a reservoir bag, bag-valve mask, HFNOT or non-invasive ventilation (NIV). It is appropriate to perform rapid sequence intubation (RSI) after airway evaluation (Diagnosis and Treatment Protocol for Novel Coronavirus Pneumonia.Trial Version 7). Sedation and muscle relaxants should be used in a timely manner to avoid patient-machine asynchronization. If necessary, closed suction (vacuum) can be used depending on the condition of the airway secretions.

## Indications of Intubating The Patient With COVID-19 Infection

1. If the patient has cardiac arrest,
2. If the airway is in danger,
3. If a patient with a respiratory rate of> 30 / min or $SaO_2$ <93% and $PaO_2$ / $FiO_2$ <300 mmHg, gradually gets worse despite HFNOT or continuous positive airway pressure (CPAP) is administered for at least 2 hours,

## During Mechanical Ventilation

- Low tidal volume ventilation approach should be employed (6-8 ml/kg ideal body weight)
- Use low airway plateau pressure, ≤30 $cmH_2O$ to reduce ventilator-induced pulmonary barotrauma.
- While maintaining the airway plateau pressure ≤ 30cm $H_2O$, high “positive end

expiratory pressure" (PEEP) should be used.

- The temperature and humidity of the airway must be maintained.
- It is necessary to avoid prolonged sedation, to awaken the patient as soon as possible and to wean from MV and to start pulmonary rehabilitation.

**c) Extracorporeal membrane oxygenation (ECMO):** ECMO, also known as Extracorporeal life support (ECLS), is a form of time-saving intervention for a patient with reversible cardiac and respiratory failure to overcome this situation. During the H1N1 pandemic in 2009, ECMO treatment was used in ARDS cases and the treated patients had a low mortality (De Lange *et al*, 2013).

ECMO allows to reduce the stress on the ventilated lung at high airway pressures that can damage the lungs. Therefore, it should be recommended to patients with refractory hypoxemia or hypercapnia despite optimal ventilation.

Pearl: ECMO therapy is used in ARDS to temporarily maintain adequate $O_2$ supply and $CO_2$ elimination and / or provide perfusion in patients with respiratory and / or heart failure who do not respond to conventional ventilatory and pharmacological interventions, and whose physiological variables are abnormal despite maximal medical support.

It is performed with the principle of drawing the systemic venous blood from the patient out of the body, removing $CO_2$ from the blood through the oxygenator and delivering $O_2$, and sending blood to the body *via* a pump that acts as an artificial heart, to provide relief from the underlying disease (Combes *et al*, 2012; Brodie *et al*, , 2011). Veno-venous (VV) -ECMO for patients with respiratory failure only, and veno-arterial (VA) -ECMO mode should be used if circulatory support is needed. Weaning from ECMO may be attempted when the underlying diseases are under control and cardiopulmonary function shows signs of improvement.

Although there is little experience in using ECMO to support patients infected with COVID-19, ECMO should be considered as a rescue therapy for the disease with refractory hypoxemia despite lung-protective ventilation, according to interim guidelines published by the WHO. (WHO. Clinical management of severe acute respiratory infection when novel coronavirus (nCoV) infection is suspected. 2020).

**ECMO indications according to NHS:** ECMO is indicated in acute severe respiratory failure, if potentially reversible causes are noted. Etiologies include pneumonia, ARDS, pulmonary aspiration, major airway disease or rupture. ECMO will be the first choice in patients who cannot have lung protective ventilation. (Management of surge and escalation in critical care services: standard operating procedure for adult respiratory extra corporeal membrane oxygenation ECMO).

According to the CESAR study, the criteria for inclusion in ECMO:

1. Above 16 years old,
2. Acute severe respiratory failure with potentially reversible causes
3. Lung injury score (LIS)> 3 (If the patient worsens rapidly, Lung injury score (LIS)> 2.5) or
4. Arterial pH <7.20 accompanying hypercapnia despite conventional therapy

**The LIS or Murray Score Evaluates Lung Injury Over 4 Variables**

- Oxygenation
- Lung imaging findings (X-ray)
- PEEP level required in mechanical ventilation
- Respiratory system compliance

**Contraindications of ECMO**

1. High pressure ventilation (peak inspiratory pressure> 30 $cmH_2O$) and / or high $FiO_2$ (> 0.8) for 7 days (relative contraindication)
2. Intracranial bleeding (relative contraindication)
3. Inability to be heparinized for any reason (relative contraindication)
4. Inability to continue active treatment for any reason

ECMO indications in COVID-19

ECMO should be considered in patients who meet one of the following three criteria despite optimization of MV ($FiO_2 \geq 0.80$, tidal volume 6 ml/kg (ideal weight), PEEP $\geq$ 10 $cmH_2O$) for longer than 7 days:

1. $PaO_2$: $FiO_2$ <50mmHg> 3 hours.
2. $PaO_2$: $FiO_2$ <80 mmHg> 6 hours.
3. pH <7.25 and $PaCO_2 \geq$ 60mmHg> 6 hours; respiratory frequency increased to 35 per minute, plateau pressure 32 $cmH_2O$ (Brodie *et al*, 2019).

## Sepsis and COVID-19

In many research, supranormal levels of inflammatory cytokines have been associated with grave outcomes in patients with COVID-19. a cytokine storm (CS) is common in patients with COVID-19, exhibiting severe-to-critical symptoms. Concurrently, lymphocytes and natural killer (NK) cell counts are sharply reduced, along with high levels of D-dimer, C-reactive protein (CRP), ferritin, and procalcitonin (Chen, 2020). Consequences of a lethal CS exhibit diffuse alveolar damage characterized by hyaline membrane formation and infiltration of interstitial lymphocytes. The collateral tissue damage, organ failure, and poor outcomes of people with COVID-19 and its accompanying uncontrolled inflammatory responses share similarities with SARS and MERS.

Conceptual model of aberrant activation of leukocytes and cytokine production contributing to a CS and pathology attributed to severe SARS-CoV-2 infection was illustrated in Fig. (**11**).

In a study comparing levels of inflammatory markers in sera of hospitalized severe and critically ill COVID-19 patients, with those of patients with ARDS or sepsis, Wilson *et al*, reported no statistically significant differences in baseline levels of IL-1β, IL-1RA, IL-6, IL-8, IL-18, and TNF-α between patients with COVID-19 and critically ill controls with ARDS or sepsis (Wilson *et al*, 2020). Levels of inflammatory cytokines were not higher in severe COVID-19 patients than in moderate COVID-19 or critically ill patients with ARDS or sepsis. Among the other 67 cytokines, no significant differences were found between the 4 groups, which suggests that none of these cytokine levels were dramatically increased in patients with COVID-19 compared with critically ill patients with ARDS or sepsis. The data from these additional cytokines suggest that a "cytokine storm" in COVID-19 that is distinct from other critical illnesses (*e.g.*, sepsis and ARDS) is unlikely.

**Is it just CS or immunity failure?** Two divergent hypotheses have been proposed: hyperinflammatory CS; and failure of host protective immunity that results in unrestrained viral dissemination and organ injury. Remy *et al*, applied ELISpot, a highly sensitive, functional immunoassay, in 27 patients with COVID-19, 51 patients with sepsis, 18 critically ill nonseptic (CINS) patients, and 27 healthy control volunteers to evaluate adaptive and innate immune status by quantitating T cell IFN-ɣ and monocyte TFN-α production (Remy, 2020). They have reported that circulating T cell subsets were profoundly reduced in COVID-19 patients. These findings support the hypothesis that COVID-19 suppresses host functional adaptive and innate immunity.

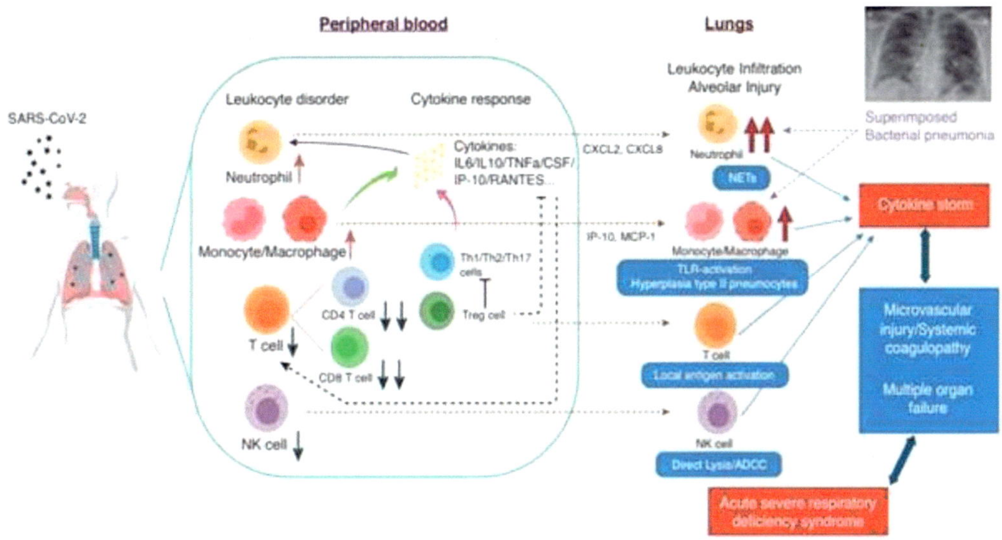


**Fig. (11).** Severe SARS-CoV-2 infection: summary of aberrant activation of leukocytes and cytokine production contributing to a CS and pathology. Conceptual model of observations associated with severe SARS-CoV-2 infection. The activation of monocytes/macrophages and lymphocyte subsets in blood are likely to be major sources of cytokine release, together with the infiltration of leukocytes into lung tissue (Adapted from Wang, 2020).

## ANTICOAGULANT TREATMENT WITH HEPARIN IN COVID-19

Thrombotic events in the lungs and different tissues have been reported in COVID-19 patients with relevant clinical symptoms, as well as laboratory and radiological findings (Zhang *et al*, 2020; Cattaneo *et al*, 2020). Perfusion abnormalities in the lungs have been identified in thoracic CT angiograms (CTPA) of the patients (Lang *et al*, 2020). In addition, there is pathological evidence of the presence of thrombi in small arterial vessels in lung tissues of patients dying from COVID-19 (Carsana *et al*, 2020).

In the largest multi-center study investigating the coagulation status in COVID-19 patients, heparin was given in addition to the treatment of 1734 patients who were being treated for COVID-19 in 17 different hospitals in Spain between 1 March and 20 April 2020 (Ayerbe *et al*, 2020). In this study, additional heparin therapy was not administered to 285 patients. 242 (14%) of those who were given heparin, 44 (15%) of those who were not given died. Therefore, heparin administration was associated with lower mortality in patients presenting with COVID-19, when compared to those not receiving this treatment. The relationship between heparin and survival demonstrated in this study is also consistent with the findings of an observational study that the mortality of 99 patients who received heparin and had a sepsis-induced coagulopathy (SIC) index> 4 was significantly lower than the other patients (Tang N, Bai *et al*, 2020). Although the nature of lung hypoperfusion in COVID-19 patients is still not fully understood, these and other studies support a thrombotic component contributing to the development of respiratory distress for these patients (Cattaneo *et al*, 2020; Lang *et al*, 2020).

**Histopathological findings:** Distinctive vascular characteristics have been visualized in the lungs of COVID-19 patients, consisting of severe endothelial damage along with the presence of intracellular virus and distorted cellular membranes. Diffuse thrombosis with microangiopathy was observed in the histological analysis of the pulmonary vascular structures. It has been reported that alveolar capillary microthrombi are 9 times more common ($p < 0.001$) in patients with COVID-19 compared to patients with influenza. Endothelitis developing in COVID-19 patients may be related to these physiopathological findings detected after death (Varga *et al*, , 2020).

In a study comparing the lung autopsy reports of 14 patients who died of ARDS due to COVID-19 and influenza A (H1N1) infection (7 patients in each group), histological examinations of both groups of patients exhibited perivascular T-cell infiltration in the periphery of the lung tissue associated with extensive alveolar damage (Ackermann *et al*, , 2020).

In a postmortem study conducted on 12 patients with COVID-19, thrombosis was found in 58% of the cases, and this condition was reported to be responsible for 25% of deaths (Wichmann *et al*, , 2020). Examinations of patients with large vessel occlusion stroke with COVID-19, including those younger than 50 years of age, also indicate hypercoagulability (Oxley *et al*, , 2020).

**Value of D-dimer:** During COVID-19 infection, serum D-dimer levels increase as a result of desquamation, endothelial inflammation and thrombosis in the vessels (The 3/4/2020 Chinese Health and Public Health Ministry Guideline on Novel Coronavirus Disease (COVID-19) Diagnosis and Treatment (Revision # 6); Diagnosis and Treatment Protocol for Novel Coronavirus Pneumonia. Trial Version 7. Released by National Health Commission & State Administration of Traditional Chinese Medicine on March 3, 2020; She *et al*, 2020).

Although developing coagulopathy is associated with high mortality, elevated D-dimer levels are also an important marker for developing coagulopathy (Tang N, Li *et al*, 2020). Therefore, low molecular weight heparin (LMWH) should be used for prophylactic purposes. In order to reduce the incidence of VTE, it should be administered to patients with severe conditions and who are dependent on mechanical ventilation. Mechanical prophylaxis (intermittent pneumatic compression devices) is warranted for those with contraindications (The 3/4/2020 Chinese Health and Public Health Ministry Guideline on Novel Coronavirus Disease (COVID-19) Diagnosis and Treatment (Revision # 6)).

**LMWH and anticoagulant therapy and mortality:** The use of LMWH and anticoagulant therapy has been shown to reduce mortality in COVID-19 (Tang N, Bai *et al*, 2020). The importance of anticoagulant therapy comes to the fore especially when patients with sepsis-induced coagulopathy (SIC) score <4 points are compared with those with scores ≥4 points. The scoring system for SIC is shown in Table **6**. It has been reported that heparin treatment in those with elevated levels of D-dimer ( *i.e.*, more than six times the upper limit of normal) was associated with an approximately 20% reduction in mortality (Tang N, Bai *et al*, 2020; Iba *et al*, 2017). Prophylactic dose LMWH should be considered in patients with significantly elevated D-dimers or high SIC scores.

**Table 6. Diagnostic scoring of "Sepsis Induced Coagulopathy" (SIC).**

| Category | Variable | 0 | 1 | 2 |
|---|---|---|---|---|
| Prothrombin time | INR | ≤1,2 | >1,2 | >1,4 |
| Coagulation | Platelet count ($x10^9/L$) | ≥150 | <150 | <100 |
| SOFA (4 criteria) | Respiration ($PaO_2$ / $FiO_2$)<br>Liver (Total Bilirubin)<br>Mean Arterial Pressure<br>-Creatinine / urine output (daily) | 0 | 1 | ≥2 |

The analysis of 2,773 patients with COVID-19 in the Mount Sinai Health System is one of the largest studies evaluating the efficacy of anticoagulation (Paranipe *et al*, 2020). This study enrolled patients who received invasive mechanical ventilation support and the authors reported that in-hospital mortality rate was 29.1% in those who received anticoagulation, while 62.7% of patients who did not receive anticoagulation died.

It has been reported that the risk of venous thromboembolism (VTE) is increased in patients admitted to hospitals in Italy due to COVID-19. Prophylactic LMWH will benefit patients at high risk of VTE. But there are other benefits with LMWH in COVID-19 patients. It has been suggested that severe pulmonary inflammation and impaired gas exchange in COVID-19 is due to the elevation of proinflammatory cytokines (Xiong *et al*, 2020). The significant increase in D-dimer values is also due to this severe inflammation that stimulates intrinsic fibrinolysis in the lungs and is caused by release into the blood (Idell, 2003). Based on the immuno-thrombosis model that emphasizes the bidirectional relationship between the immune system and thrombin production, blocking of thrombin by heparin may reduce the inflammatory response (Gaertner *et al*, 2016) (Fig. **12**).

However, the anti-inflammatory function of heparin, one of the more well-known non-anticoagulant properties, may also be fitting in this situation. Several publications have demonstrated this non-anticoagulant property, and some of the mechanisms described include binding to inflammatory cytokines, inhibiting neutrophil chemotaxis and leukocyte migration, neutralizing positively charged peptide complement factor C5a, and sequestration of acute phase proteins (Young, 2008; Li *et al*, 2009; Esmon, 2014; Poterucha *et al*, 2017). It was concluded that heparin may reduce the levels of inflammatory biomarkers, but this should be confirmed by larger studies clinically (Mousavi *et al*, 2015).

**Acute respiratory distress syndrome (ARDS)** is one of the most common complications of COVID-19 infection. Coagulation system activation is significant in ARDS pathogenesis. Ozolina *et al*, showed that the median plasma tissue factor and plasminogen activator inhibitor-1 (PAI-1) concentrations in patients with ARDS were significantly higher than those without ARDS (Ozolina *et al*, 2016). These mechanisms contributing to lung coagulopathy are the inhibition of bronchoalveolar plasminogen activator-mediated fibrinolysis through the production of thrombin *via* localized tissue factor and the increase of PAI-1 (Ozolina *et al*, 2016; Glas *et al*, 2013). Hence, treatment with heparin may be helpful in reducing this pulmonary coagulopathy. In a meta-analysis study, it was stated that adjuvant treatment with LMWH at the beginning of the first seven days of ARDS significantly improved the $PaO_2$ / $FiO_2$ ratio but reduced the 7-day mortality risk by 48% and the 28-day mortality risk by 37%. Improvement is especially significant in the subgroup receiving high-dose LMWH with 5000 units / day (Li *et al*, 2018).

In another study, oxygenation was reported to be improved following heparin treatment in 27 patients with COVID-19 (Negri *et al*, , 2020).

## Can we Administer Nebulized Anticoagulation?

Provided that coagulopathy in ARDS may have started in the lungs, the use of nebulized anticoagulation is in the trial phase (Camprubí-Rimblas *et al*, 2020). It has been reported that the nebulized route of heparin administration will be suitable not only for prophylaxis, but also for patients under mechanical ventilation, and the anticoagulant activity does not pose a problem (Mycroft-West *et al*, 2020).

Vascular endothelial cells are usually affected by pathogenic invasion and organ failure develops as a result of endothelial dysfunction. In addition to the pathogen, histones released from damaged cells can also cause endothelial damage (Xu *et al*, 2009). Heparin can antagonize histones and thus protect endothelial tissue (Iba *et al*, 2015; Zhu *et al*, 2019). This protective function can be extended to endothelial tight junctions as shown in a sepsis model. Here, unfractionated heparin (UFH) can reduce pulmonary edema and vascular leakage following lipopolysaccharide-induced injury. Another mechanism is due to histone methylation and its effects on mitogen activated protein kinase and Nuclear factor-kB signaling pathways. Thus, heparin may affect microcirculation dysfunction and possibly reduce organ damage (Liu *et al*, 2019; Ma *et al*, 2015).

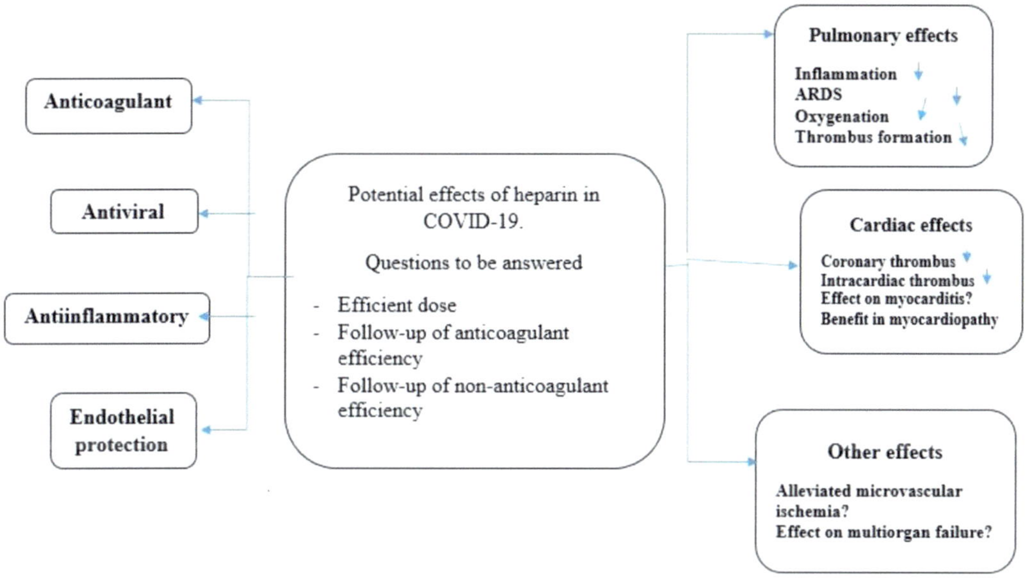


**Fig. (12).** Potential effects of heparin in COVID-19.

Endothelial dysfunction also contributes to cardiac effects, another important complication of the coronavirus (Xiong *et al*, 2020). Heparin may also be useful against microvascular dysfunction in heart failure, assuming that ischemic hypoxia in the subendocardial layer may cause loss of its natural anticoagulant properties (Wojnicz *et al*, 2006). In an article published in the 90's, it was reported that heparin can reduce myocardial inflammation and reduce collagen deposition in an animal model of myocarditis (Frizelle *et al*, 1992).

## Does It Also Have An Anti-inflammatory And Antiviral Effect?

Heparin is thought to have direct SARS-CoV-2 antiviral activity in addition to anticoagulation effects in COVID-19 patients.

The antiviral effect of heparin is under investigation with experimental studies. Due to the polyanionic nature of heparin, it can bind to several proteins and thus act as an effective inhibitor of viral binding. For example, in the case of herpes simplex virus (HSV) infections, heparin competes with the virus to limit infection by host cell surface glycoproteins, and it prevents virus-induced cell death of human neural progenitor cells in Zika virus infection (Shukla *et al*, 2001; Ghezzi *et al*, 2017). In a study from Italy, the use of heparin at a concentration of 100 mcg / ml halved the infection in experimental vero cells injected with sputum from a patient with SARS-CoV pneumonia (Vicenzi *et al*, 2004).

Heparan sulfate is postulated to interact with the spike protein as an adhesion receptor, which could be the first step in facilitating the interference of the SARS-CoV and ACE2 receptor (Milewska *et al*, 2018). It was recently disclosed that the SARS-CoV-2 spike protein interacts with heparan sulfate with higher affinity than the SARS-CoV or MERS-CoV spike proteins (Kim *et al*, , 2020). In this study, it was reported that the SARS-CoV-2 spike protein showed extremely strong and almost irreversible binding to heparin using surface plasmon resonance. The results of this study showed that heparin can bind the SARS-CoV-2 spike protein and reduce infectivity by acting as a competitive inhibitor for viral entry.

In a retrospective study conducted to compare and evaluate the effect of LMWH treatment on the progression of COVID-19 disease, 42 COVID-19 patients were examined (Shi *et al*, 2020). LMWH was added to the treatment of 21 of these patients, and it was not added to the other 21, which were the control group. Changes in lymphocyte ratios before and after LMWH addition were found to be significant from those in the control group ($p=0.011$). Similarly, changes in D-dimer and fibrinogen levels before and after LMWH addition were found to be significant ($p=0.035$) from those in the control group. Remarkably, IL-6 levels also decreased significantly after LMWH was added to the treatment ($p=0.006$). This indicates that LMWH has an anti-inflammatory effect and can partially alleviate the cytokine storm caused by the virus, which also supports its use as a potential therapeutic drug in the treatment of COVID-19.

Studies have reported that heparin can be beneficial in COVID through various mechanisms. The dosage of LMWH is also subject to debate. Although the prophylactic dose is sufficient in most patients, a higher dose should be considered in obese patients with high body mass index. The route and dose of administration, antidotes, contraindications, side effects and drug interactions of some LMWH molecules are listed in Table **7**.

## The Role of Antiplatelet Drugs in COVID-19 Treatment

### *Phosphodieasterase Inhibitors (PDEI): Dipyridamole*

Dipyridamole (DIP), which acts by inhibiting the phosphodiesterase enzyme, is the precursor of these drugs. DIP is used as an antiplatelet agent by inhibiting platelet aggregation and thrombus formation. DIP has effects such as inhibition of vascular smooth muscle cell proliferation, prevention of endothelial-leukocyte interactions, increasing antithrombotic properties of endothelial cells, interaction of leukocytes with endothelium, increased NO production stimulated by smooth muscle cells, and inhibition of inflammatory gene expression in platelet-monocyte aggregates. DIP also enhances extracellular adenosine, which reduces superoxide anion formation by human neutrophils and scavenges oxygen and hydroxyl radicals directly. It also has a direct antioxidant effect (Gresele *et al*, 2011; Kim *et al*, 2008). Previous clinical trials have shown that DIP has a broad-spectrum antiviral activity, particularly effective against positive strand RNA viruses (Fata-Hartley *et al*, 2005). It has also been claimed that DIP can prevent acute injury and progressive fibrosis of the lung, heart, liver, and kidney, suppresses inflammation, and supports mucosal healing (Insel *et al*, 2012; Huang *et al*, 2019).

In a clinical study conducted to evaluate the antiviral therapeutic effect of DIP in COVID-19 disease and its potential to reduce the risk of coagulation, DIP (3x50mg / day P.O. for 14 days), in addition to the usual treatments (ribavirin, glucocorticoids and $O_2$ therapy) administered to 14 of 31 patients with COVID-19 and compared with a control group of 17 patients who were given the same regimen without DIP (Liu *et al*, 2020). As a result of this study.

1. D-dimer concentrations were supranormal in 50% (4/8) of patients in the group with DIP added to their treatment and in 42% (5/12) of severe patients in the control group.
2. A total of 7 (87.5%) of 8 severe patients in the group treated with DIP were discharged after clinical recovery; whilst the remaining 1 patient (12.5%) was in clinical remission. On the other hand, only four (33.3%) of 12 severe patients in the control group were discharged, 2 (16.7%) were in remission, and 2 patients (16.7%) died. It was concluded that DIP add-on therapy was significantly associated with clinical improvement and remission rates (odds ratio 23.75, p: 0.06).
3. According to the qualitative RT-PCR results, the mean virus clearance time was shortened by 1.6 days for patients in the group with DIP added to their treatment compared to the control group.
4. Absolute lymphocyte and platelet counts were increased consistently in patients

who received DIP treatment compared to control patients, albeit not statistically significant.

5. Chest CT scans of all patients revealed typical irregular ground glass images in the lungs with various degrees of absorption after the treatment with DIP, while only one out of 12 severe patients in the control group showed radiological improvement.

**Table 7. Method of administration and dosage, antidote, contraindications, side effects and drug interactions of some LMWH molecules.**

| | Dosing | Route | Notes | Side/ Adverse Effects | Drug Interactions |
|---|---|---|---|---|---|
| **1.Enoksaparin (Clexane®)** | 1 mg/kg/12 h or 1,5 mg/kg/24 h (not to exceed 180 mg/d) | Once Daily or BID; SC | • Its antidote is protamine sulphate, (1 mg protamine for 100 anti-Xa units) • It is contraindicated in cases of peptic ulcer, ulcerative colitis, those with bleeding risk, coagulation disorder, septic endocarditis, eye, ear and CNS injuries, severe HT, abortion. | Hemorrhage, bruising at the injection site, allergic reactions, thrombocytopenia | • It should not be used with acetaminophen, AscA, ASA, Atorvastatin, Celecoxib, cholecalciferol, cyanocobalamin, Duloxetine, Esomeprazole, Furosemide. |
| **2. Dalteparin (Fragmin®)** | 100IU/kg/12 h or 200 IU/kg/24 h (not to exceed 18000 IU/day) | Once Daily or BID; SC / İM | • Its antidote is protamine sulphate, (1 mg protamine for 100 anti-Xa units) • It is contraindicated in peptic ulcer, ulcerative colitis, conditions with bleeding risk, coagulation disorder, septic endocarditis, eye, ear, and CNS injuries. | Hemorrhage, bruising at the injection site, allergic reactions, thrombocytopenia, elevated liver enzymes, alopecia | • It should not be used with AscA, ASA, K vit. antagonists dipyridamol, dextran, phenylbutazone, indomethacine, ethacrynic acid, antihistaminics, digitalis glucosides, tetracycline |

*(Table 7) cont.....*

| | Dosing | Route | Notes | Side/ Adverse Effects | Drug Interactions |
|---|---|---|---|---|---|
| **3. Nadroparin (Fraxiparine®)** | 85,5 IU/kg/12 h or 171 IU/kg/24 h (not to exceed 17100 IU/ day) | Once Daily or BID; SC / IV | • Its antidote is protamine sulphate, (1 mg protamine for 100 anti-Xa units)<br>• It is contraindicated in cases of peptic ulcer, ulcerative colitis, those with bleeding risk, coagulation disorder, septic endocarditis, eye, ear and CNS injuries, severe HT, abortion, and severe liver dysfunction. | Hemorrhage, bruising at the injection site, allergic reactions, thrombocytopenia, elevated liver enzymes, hypoaldesteronism | • Should not be used together with NSAID, K vit. antagonists, dipyridamole, dextran, phenylbutazone, probenecid, ethacrynic acid, antihistamines, digitoxin, tetracycline, AscA. |
| **4. Tinzaparin** | 175 IU/kg/24 h | Once daily, SC/IV | • Its antidote is protamine sulphate, (1 mg protamine for 100 anti-Xa units)<br>• It is contraindicated in cases of peptic ulcer, ulcerative colitis, those with bleeding risk, coagulation disorder, septic endocarditis, eye, ear and CNS injuries, severe HT, abortion and spinal or epidural anesthesia. | Hemorrhage, bruising at the injection site, allergic reactions, thrombocytopenia | Should not be used with ASA and other NSAID, thrombolytic agents, K vit. antagonists, activated protein C, direct factor Xa and IIa inhibitors. |

*(Table 7) cont.....*

| | Dosing | Route | Notes | Side/ Adverse Effects | Drug Interactions |
|---|---|---|---|---|---|
| **5. Fondaparinux (Arixtra®)** | 5 mg/d if <50 kg. 7,5 mg/d between 50 and 100 kg. 10 mg/d if >100 kg | Once daily, SC | • It can be used instead of heparin as an anticoagulant in **heparin-induced thrombocytopenia (HIT).** • It is contraindicated in cases of peptic ulcer, ulcerative colitis, those with bleeding risk, coagulation disorder, septic endocarditis, eye, ear and CNS injuries, severe HT, abortion. **Note: It has no antidote.** | Hemorrhage (this risk is higher than other LMWHs), bruising at the injection site, allergic reactions Note: It does not cause thrombocytopenia since it does not interact with Platelet Factor 4 (PF4). | • Oral anticoagulants (warfarin), platelet inhibitors (ASA), NSAIDs (piroxicam) and digoxin did not interact with the pharmacokinetics of fondaparinux. • Fondaparinux did not affect the INR activity of warfarin, bleeding time while on ASA or piroxicam treatment, or the pharmacokinetics of stable digoxin level. |

This study showed that prophylactic anticoagulation therapy with DIP may be considered in COVID-19 patients to reduce the risk of hypercoagulation and multiorgan damage (Fig. **13**).

All articles published on DIP activity since 1977 were reviewed and the authors pointed out that DIP could substantially improve the clinical outcomes of COVID-19 due to its antiplatelet activity, besides its antiviral, anti-inflammatory and antioxidant effects (Aliter *et al*, 2020).

In brief, DIP is a safe, well tolerated, widely available and inexpensive drug that could be helpful in prophylactic anticoagulation therapy in COVID-19. It can be added to the regimen within a few days after symptom onset.

### *Thienopyridines: Ticlopidine & Clopidogrel*

Both drugs inhibit ADP-mediated stimulation of platelets. Thienopyridines irreversibly inhibit P2Y12, receptors on the platelet surface. Their effectiveness is not bound to arachidonic acid and is independent of the mechanism of action of aspirin. Ticlopidine was previously used as an alternative to aspirin to prevent recurrent cerebral ischemia and strokes. However, its use is currently restricted due to the fatal side effects it causes (*e.g.*, severe neutropenia and thrombotic thrombocytopenic purpura).

Clopidogrel was developed as an alternative to ticlopidine and is now the outstanding member of this group. Clopidogrel is rapidly absorbed after oral intake and metabolized in the liver, with a half-life 8 hours. Following a 400 mg oral loading dose, nearly 40% of platelets are inhibited within 2 hours. 75 mg is recommended for the daily dose. Although ticlopidine-like side effects are not observed, thrombotic thrombocytopenic purpura has been reported rarely, especially at loading doses (Bennett *et al*, 2000).

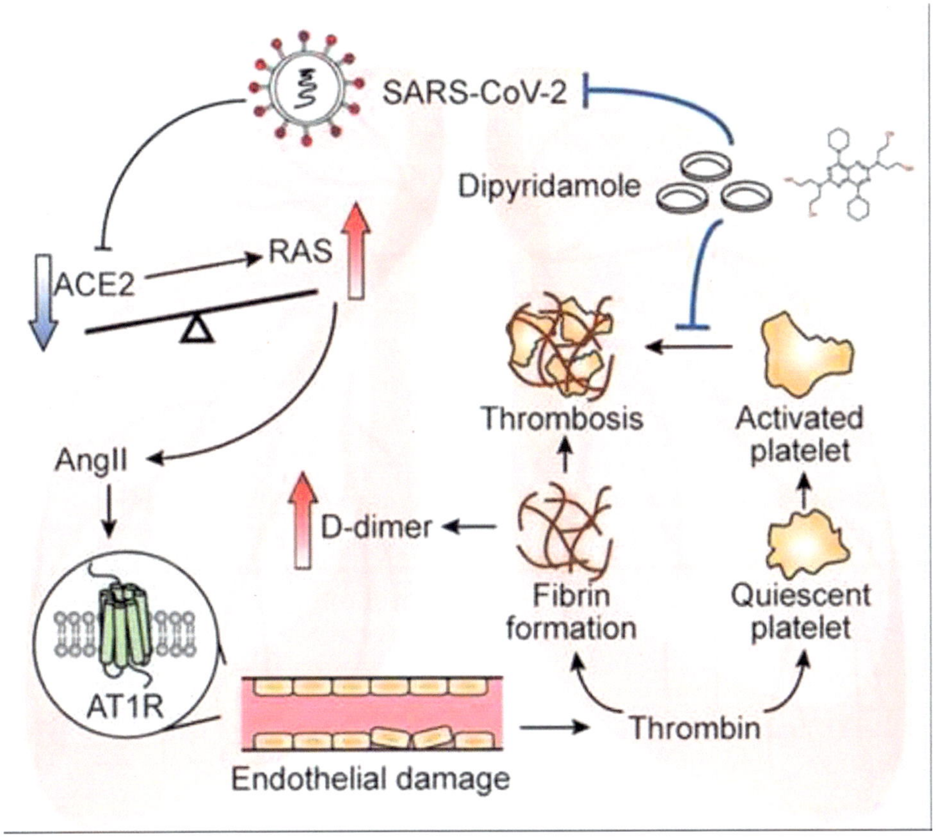


**Fig. (13).** Thromboinflammatory process in COVID-19 pathogenesis and the mechanism of action of DIP on platelets.

To investigate the effects of antiplatelet therapy on arterial oxygenation and clinical outcomes in patients with COVID-19, a study was conducted in which five patients with severe respiratory failure requiring CPAP, bilateral pulmonary infiltration, and a D-dimer level higher than 3 times the upper limit of the normal range was included and a control group was formed from five patients with similar conditions (Viecca *et al*, 2020). The study group received standard maintenance therapy plus 250 mg acetylsalicylic acid (ASA) infusion and 300 mg clopidogrel orally, followed by 25 µg / kg tirofiban bolus infusion for 3 minutes, followed by a continuous infusion of 0.15 μg / kg / min for 48 hours. Then, clopidogrel was administered to both groups at a daily dose of 75 mg / day for 30 days. In addition, 2.5 mg / day Fondaparinux SC was given during the hospital stay. When compared to controls, antiplatelet-treated patients had consistent significant reductions in the mean A-a $O_2$ gradient at 24, 48 hours and 7 days after treatment (mean -32.6 mmHg, -52.4 mmHg, and -151.1 mmHg, respectively). Moreover, $PaO_2$ / $FiO_2$ ratio increased by an average of 52 mmHg, 64 mmHg and 112 mmHg after 24, 48 hours and 7 days, respectively (Fig. **14**). All patients except one were successfully weaned from CPAP 3 days later, but the patients in the control group were reported to be unable to leave CPAP. No significant adverse effects were recorded in the patient group. The researchers concluded that antiplatelet therapy may be effective in improving the ventilation / perfusion (V / Q) ratio in COVID-19 patients with severe respiratory failure.

In conclusion, thienopyridines can be alternative antiplatelet agents in the treatment of COVID-19, but this should be supported by broad, multi-centric and well-designed studies.

### *Glycoprotein IIb / IIIa Inhibitors*

When platelets are activated, the number of GP IIb / IIIa receptors increases on their surface. Antiaggregant effect occurs by inhibiting GP IIb / IIIa receptors by these agents which also inhibit the binding of fibrinogen with GP IIb / IIIa receptors. This mechanism is employed to prevent thromboembolic events that may occur in acute coronary syndrome and interventional cardiology (Behan *et al*, 2004).

**Abciximab, eptifibatide and tirofiban**, are parenterally used GP IIb / IIIa inhibitors. Orofiban, cybrafiban, xemilofiban and lotrafiban are orally used.

**COVID-19 and STEMI:** In a study of 115 patients with ST segment elevation myocardial infarction (STEMI) concurrent with COVID-19 treated with primary percutaneous coronary intervention (PCI), these patients were found to have higher thrombus rates, more frequent thrombosis of coronary vessels or stents, more common use of glycoprotein IIb / IIIa inhibitors and thrombus aspiration rates were higher, while left ventricular functions were significantly lower than non-COVID-19 patients with STEMI (Choudry *et al*, 2020). In addition, it has been reported that these patients stayed in the hospital for longer periods and the rate of admission to ICU is higher than the others.

**What should we use after revascularization in STEMI patients with COVID-19?** In another study, it is suggested that primary PCI is the first option for revascularization in STEMI patients with COVID-19. In addition, the importance of using clopidogrel together with GPIIb / IIIa inhibitors to achieve more favorable outcomes after stent implantation is emphasized (Seif *et al*, 2020).

In conclusion, a large number of studies with broad participation are needed to recommend the use of GPIIb / IIIa inhibitors in STEMI patients with COVID-19. No articles evaluating the use of these drugs as an alternative antithrombotic agent in the treatment of COVID-19 were found in the literature reviews.

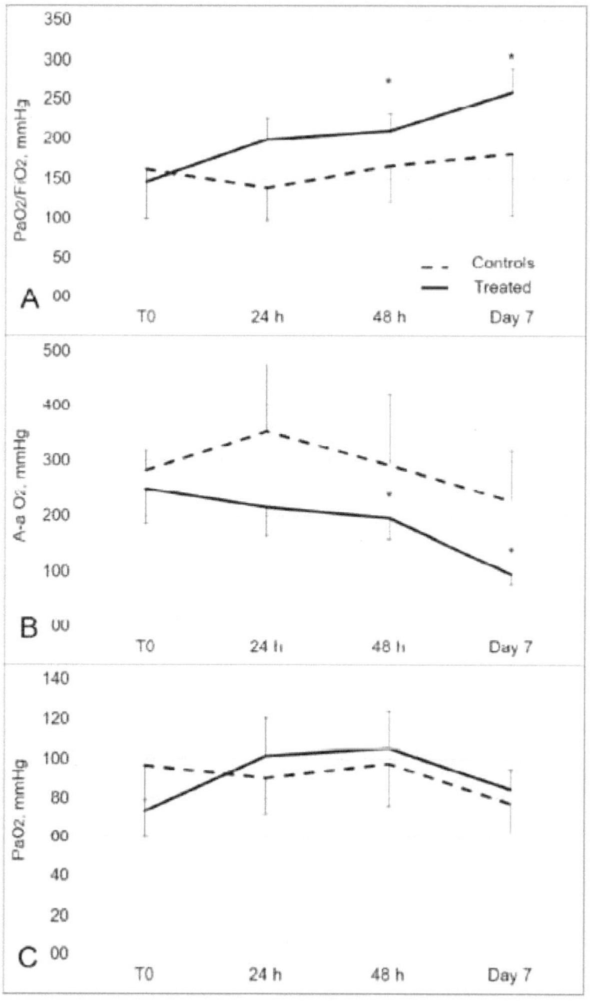


**Fig. (14).** Changes in $PaO_2$ / $FiO_2$ ratio (A), A-a $O_2$ gradient (B) and $PaO_2$ level (C) within 7 days in patients treated with antiplatelets and controls (Viecca *et al*, 2020).

## COVID-19 PLASMA TREATMENT: THE CURRENT SITUATION, DREAMS, AND REALITY

### Passive Antibody Treatment (Convalescent / Immune Plasma Treatment)

**Plasma:** It is the yellow-colored liquid that remains on top after the separation (precipitation) of red blood cells, white blood cells and other cells in the blood. 55% of the blood is plasma which mainly contains water, salt, antibodies, enzymes. Many functions related to blood coagulation and immunity are processed within plasma (Fig. **15**).

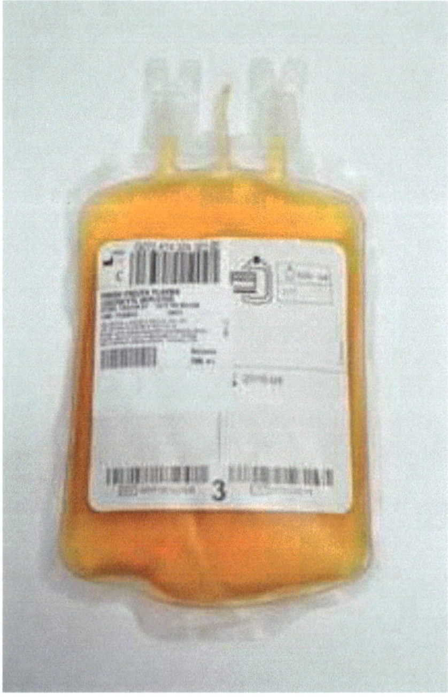


**Fig. (15).** Appearance of plasma in its bag.

**In the plasmapheresis process,** the plasma of the blood taken from the healthy person is separated and subjected to fractionation. Thus, any part (such as immune globulin, coagulation factor) can be purified and administered to a patient.

**Passive antibody therapy, also called therapeutic plasma exchange,** includes convalescent (immune) plasma therapy (CPT), which involves administering to a susceptible person to prevent infection by a microorganism or to treat patients who are inflicted already and exhibit symptoms of varying severity.

The purpose of CPT is to use neutralizing antibodies (NEA) produced against the virus by individuals who have had the disease to protect patients against the virus.

In addition, it is valuable for vaccination and drug studies to identify which NEAs are expressed against the virus in individuals with the disease.

The increasing number of patients recovered and discharged after being diagnosed with COVID-19 represents an opportunity to treat other patients *via* CPT. Passive antibody therapy is to expect antibodies against a specific agent given to a susuceptible individual to fight the viruses. Active vaccination is to give the agent with (mostly attenuated) virulence, that is, the microbe, to the body and expect it to generate antibodies, which is a time-consuming process. Therefore, passive immunization may be the only practical method for expedient immunization (Casadevall, 2004).

First of all, this treatment is referred to as "Investigational COVID-19 Convalescent Plasma" in contemporary medical literature. As the name suggests, it is still under investigation.

## Do People Who Have Experienced COVID-19 Have IgG?

After 6 months of the epidemic, in Nature, Robbiani *et al*, published on examination of CP samples from 149 people and their NEA levels (Robbiani, 2020). NEA levels were measured in CPs taken 39 days after the onset of symptoms, and it was observed that it changed from person to person. It has been found that antibodies against the SARS-CoV-2 spike (S) protein and especially the receptor binding region of S are at high levels. When CP samples are used in the counter neutralization tests of SARS-CoV-2 S protein, NEA levels are less than 1:50 in 33% of them; less than 1: 1000 in 79% and less than 1: 5000 in 1%. In summary, NEA titrations in CP samples are quite lower than expected.

## Mechanism of Action

Experience with other CoV viruses such as SARS-CoV-1 from previous outbreaks shows that such CPs contain NEA against the relevant virus (Zhang, 2005). CP obtained from recovered COVID-19 patients who have developed humoral immunity to the virus contains a large amount of NEA that can neutralize SARS-CoV-2 and destroy the pathogen from the bloodstream and pulmonary tissues. Antibodies derived from CP can neutralize the virus by blocking replication (eg, through complement activation or phagocytosis) or by binding without interfering with replication (van Erp, 2019). The therapeutic effect of CP on COVID-19 is determined by the level of the SARS-CoV-2 NEA titer. In a study on SARS, it was found that specific immunoglobulin (Ig) G antibodies started to increase in the $3^{rd}$ week after the onset of the disease and peaked at the $12^{th}$ week (Li, 2003). Anti-COVID-19 IgM and IgG were thought to directly neutralize the virus and their anti-inflammatory activity could prevent cytokine storm. It should be kept in mind that CP is most effective when given prophylactically or when used in the early period (cytokine storm) of the disease (Casadevall, 2003).

Pearl: In the review published in JAMA in April 2020, Sanders *et al*, stated that antibody replacement by plasma infusion may be beneficial in the first 7-10 days of the disease, when the virus load is high and antibody response has not yet occurred and will not be useful outside this period (Sanders, 2020).

## Preparation of CP

CP taken from the donor should be given to the patient recipient in the first 6 hours. Patients may receive an initial dose of 200-500 ml (4-5 ml / kg) followed by one or two additional doses 48 hours apart, depending on the patient's weight, disease severity, and tolerance of the infusions. It is very important to ensure ABO compatibility between donor and recipient (National Health Commission of the People's Republic of China, 2020, Chen, 2020). Apheresis is recommended to optimize CP efficiency. Approximately 400-800 ml of plasma is obtained from a single apheresis donation, and then 2-4 U CP is provided for transfusion (Bloch, 2020). Plasma can be taken from a donor up to 3 times and within a period of 1 month. CPT application method and dose are shown in the Table **8**.

**Table 8. The Characteristics Of The Cp Donor and The Patients Who Will Be Transfused Are Shown.**

| Donation criteria for CPT |
|---|
| • Lab evidence that you have had COVID-19 |
| - By diagnostic test (PCR with nasopharyngeal swab) |
| Or |
| - With positive serological test for SARS-CoV-2 antibodies after recovery |
| Or: |
| • With one of the following: |
| - Complete resolution of symptoms at least 28 days prior to donation of CP |
| - |
| - Complete resolution of symptoms at least 28 days before giving plasma + (-) PCR test with blood or swab |
| • Women not being pregnant and having antibodies (-) to human leukocyte anti-HLA after birth |
| • High SARS-CoV-2 NEA titers (> 1:80) |

Eligible donors should have a COVID-19 NA titer above 1: 640 (Bloch, 2020). It has been reported that the SARS-CoV-specific NEA level gradually decreased 4 months after the disease process, and IgG antibodies declined to undetectable levels in 16.1% of patients at 36 months after the disease state. In a study conducted by MERS-CoV infected patients and exposed healthcare workers, it was shown that the prevalence of MERS-CoV IgG seroreactivity was very low (2.7%) and the antibody titer decreased rapidly within 3 months (Arabi, 2016).

Mostly, the dose chosen was based on previous experience with the use of CPT in SARS, and 5 ml / kg plasma at a titer of 1: 160 was used (Cheng, 2005). Given the first order linear proportionality, 3.125 ml / kg plasma with titer > 1:64 will provide an Ig level equivalent to 5 ml / kg plasma with a titer of 1: 160. For an approximately 80 kg patient, this will produce approximately 250 ml of plasma (3.125 ml / kg x 80 kg = 250 ml, titre > 1:64), which is the volume of a standard plasma unit in the USA.

Since there are currently no vaccines, monoclonal antibodies or drugs for COVID-19, CP may be considered as an option for the prevention and treatment of COVID-19 disease in the presence of a sufficient number of people who have recovered and can donate Ig-containing plasma. It has been shown that patients treated with CP have a shorter hospital stay and lower mortality rates compared to other patients (Abolghasemi, 2020).

Sera of the Persons Recovering From COVID-19 Infection Can Be Used in The Prophylaxis Or Treatment Of COVID-19 Infection (Casadevall, 2020).

Before commencement of this treatment, the following six conditions must be met:

1. The existence of a donor population who have recovered from COVID-19 infection and can donate their sera,

2. Availability of a blood bank equipped to process serum donations,

3. The presence of assays, including serological analyzes to detect COVID-19 in serum, and virological assays to measure viral neutralization,

4. Support of the virology laboratory for performing these tests,

5. Prophylactic and therapeutic protocols, which should ideally include randomized clinical trials to assess the effectiveness of any intervention and measure immune responses.

6. Regulatory compliance, including institutional review board approval, which may vary depending on location.

## Who Can Be Treated With CPT?

The FDA has also recently approved the use of CP in the COVID-19 pandemic. CP obtained from patients recovering from viral infections can be used in the treatment before severe adverse events occur. Therefore, it may be useful to test the safety and efficacy of CP transfusion in patients infected with COVID-19 (Chen, 2020).

**The criteria for applying to the FDA for patients who are considered to warrant CPT in the USA (National Expanded Access Treatment Protocol)** (Tanne, 2020)**:**

1.Lab tests showing the diagnosis of COVID-19
2.Severe / life-threatening COVID-19:
a) Patients carrying one or more of the following:
> Shortness of breath / dyspnea,
> Respiratory rate per minute> 30,
> Blood oxygen saturation $\leq$ 93%,
> $PaO_2$ / $FiO_2$ <300,
> 50% increase in lung infiltration (24-48 hours)
2. Life-threatening disease (one of the following):
> Respiratory failure,
> Septic shock, and / or
> multiple organ failure
3. Informed consent

## Side Effects

Physicians performing CPT should closely monitor the adverse effects of plasma transfusion before, during and after the procedure, and record any adverse effects that may ensue. They also need to be able to manage any possible adverse occurrences. The risks to recipients of CP are likely to be no different from those receiving standard plasma. CPT carry the risks that may occur during or after normal plasma transfusion, such as common adverse transfusion reactions, anaphylactic reactions, transfusion-related circulatory overload, acute lung injury, dyspnoea, allergic hypotension, non-hemolytic febrile reaction, acute haemolytic transfusion reactions and delayed haemolytic transfusion reactions, and infection transmission. The donor is tested for transfusion-transmitted infections such as HIV, hepatitis B and C viruses, and syphilis. As a result of the tests, plasma units are harvested only from donors who do not have any contagious diseases. There is an HLA antibody-mediated relationship between pregnancy and transfusion-related acute lung injury (TRALI) in women, and plasma use should be preferred from non-pregnant women including abortion or male donors to avoid this side effect. This precaution reduces the likelihood that antibodies against the HLA or granulocyte antigens that cause TRALI are found in the plasma. TRALI occurs within 6 hours after transfusion of the associated plasma and can have serious consequences (Bloch 2020, Toy, 2019).

The specific risks associated with CP include transfusion-transmitted COVID-19 infection. However, this situation is largely theoretical. Because the recipient is already infected. In addition, there are no reports published so far that a respiratory virus is transmitted by blood transfusion. Therefore, COVID-19 is thought not to be transmitted by transfusion. Table **9** shows the indications, method, dosage, and side effects of CPT.

**Table 9. CP donor and patients to be transfused, method of CPT procedure, dose, and side effects.**

| Who Can Donate CP? | Who Can Receive CPT? |
|---|---|
| 1. COVID-19 antibody positivity proven by PCR test or by serological tests after recovery<br>2.Complete resolution of symptoms at least 28 days before giving CP, or PCR test (-) with blood or swab.<br>3. Women not being pregnant and having postpartum HLA antibodies (-)<br>4.High titers of SARS-CoV-2 NEA (at least 1: 640)<br>• ABO compatibility must be ensured between donor and recipient.<br>• Approximately 400 to 800 ml of plasma is harvested from a single apheresis donation.<br>• Plasma can be taken from a donor at most 3 times and within 1 month. | 1. Prophylaxis<br>2. Presence of laboratory tests showing the diagnosis of COVID-19<br>3.Severe / life-threatening COVID-19:<br>• Patients with at least one of the following conditions:<br>• Shortness of breath / dyspnea,<br>• Respiratory rate> 30 bpm<br>• Oxygen saturation ≤93%<br>• $PaO_2$ / $FiO_2$ <300,<br>• > 50% increase in lung infiltration (in 24 to 48 hours)<br>• Presence of at least one of the following life-threatening conditions:<br>• -Respiratory Failure<br>• Septic shock<br>• -Multipl organ failure |
| **Procedure, route, and Dosage** | **Side / Adverse Effects** |
| • 4-5ml / kg IV is given in 30 minutes<br>• If necessary, one or two additional doses may be given at 48-hour intervals, depending on the patient's weight, disease severity and infusion tolerance. | Anaphylactic reactions<br>Transfusion-related circulatory overload<br>Dyspnea<br>Acute lung injury<br>Hypotension<br>Non-hemolytic febrile reaction,<br>Acute / delayed hemolytic transfusion reactions<br>• Infectious transfusion reactions (such as HIV, hepatitis B and C, syphilis, *etc*) |

PCR: Polymerase Chain Reaction, HLA: Human Leukocyte Antigen, HIV: Human Immmunodeficiency Virus

# CONCLUSION

CPT is one of the most important treatment options that can be used in pandemic COVID-19 infection. Since there are currently no vaccines, monoclonal antibodies or drugs for COVID-19, CPT is an important option for the prevention and treatment of COVID-19 disease in the presence of a sufficient number of people who have recovered and can donate Ig-containing plasma. This treatment method is the only way to immediately immunize susceptible people and is an alternative to vaccination. Patients treated with CP have a shorter hospital stay and lower mortality rates than other patients.

## REFERENCES

Abolghasemi, H, Eshghi, P & Cheraghali, AM (2020) *Clinical efficacy of convalescent plasma for treatment of COVID-19 infections: Results of a multicenter clinical study* Transfus Apher Sci 102875.

Abroug, F, Ouanes-Besbes, L, Dachraoui, F, Ouanes, I & Brochard, L (2011) An updated study-level meta-analysis of randomised controlled trials on proning in ARDS and acute lung injury. *Crit Care,* 15, R6. [http://dx.doi.org/10.1186/cc9403] [PMID: 21211010]

Ackermann, M, Verleden, SE, Kuehnel, M, Haverich, A, Welte, T, Laenger, F, Vanstapel, A, Werlein, C, Stark, H, Tzankov, A, Li, WW, Li, VW, Mentzer, SJ & Jonigk, D (2020) Pulmonary vascular endothelialitis, thrombosis, and angiogenesis in COVID-19. *N Engl J Med,* 383, 120-8. [http://dx.doi.org/10.1056/NEJMoa2015432] [PMID: 32437596]

Aliter, KF & Al-Horani, RA (2020) Potential Therapeutic Benefits of Dipyridamole in COVID-19 Patients. *Curr Pharm Des* [http://dx.doi.org/10.2174/1381612826666201001125604] [PMID: 33001004]

Arabi, YM, Hajeer, AH, Luke, T, Raviprakash, K, Balkhy, H, Johani, S, Al-Dawood, A, Al-Qahtani, S, Al-Omari, A, Al-Hameed, F, Hayden, FG, Fowler, R, Bouchama, A, Shindo, N, Al-Khairy, K, Carson, G, Taha, Y, Sadat, M & Alahmadi, M (2016) Feasibility of using convalescent plasma immunotherapy for MERS-CoV infection, Saudi Arabia. *Emerg Infect Dis,* 22, 1554-61. [http://dx.doi.org/10.3201/eid2209.151164] [PMID: 27532807]

Ayerbe, L, Risco, C & Ayis, S (2020) The association between treatment with heparin and survival in patients with COVID-19. *J Thromb Thrombolysis,* 50, 298-301. [http://dx.doi.org/10.1007/s11239-020-02162-z] [PMID: 32476080]

Barker, J, Koeckerling, D & West, R (2020) A need for prone position CPR guidance for intubated and non-intubated patients during the COVID-19 pandemic. *Resuscitation,* 151, 135-6. [http://dx.doi.org/10.1016/j.resuscitation.2020.04.029] [PMID: 32371028]

Beck, BR, Shin, B, Choi, Y, Park, S & Kang, K (2020) Predicting commercially available antiviral drugs that may act on the novel coronavirus (SARS-CoV-2) through a drug-target interaction deep learning model. *Comput Struct Biotechnol J,* 18, 784-90. [http://dx.doi.org/10.1016/j.csbj.2020.03.025] [PMID: 32280433]

Behan, MW & Storey, RF (2004) Antiplatelet therapy in cardiovascular disease. *Postgrad Med J,* 80, 155-64. [http://dx.doi.org/10.1136/pgmj.2003.007062] [PMID: 15016937]

Bennett, CL, Connors, JM, Carwile, JM, Moake, JL, Bell, WR, Tarantolo, SR, McCarthy, LJ, Sarode, R, Hatfield, AJ, Feldman, MD, Davidson, CJ & Tsai, HM (2000) Thrombotic thrombocytopenic purpura associated with clopidogrel. *N Engl J Med,* 342, 1773-7. [http://dx.doi.org/10.1056/NEJM200006153422402] [PMID: 10852999]

Bessière, F, Roccia, H, Delinière, A, Charrière, R, Chevalier, P, Argaud, L & Cour, M (2020) Assessment of QT Intervals in a Case Series of Patients With Coronavirus Disease 2019 (COVID-19) Infection Treated

With Hydroxychloroquine Alone or in Combination With Azithromycin in an Intensive Care Unit. *JAMA Cardiol,* 5, 1067-9.
[http://dx.doi.org/10.1001/jamacardio.2020.1787] [PMID: 32936266]

Bloch, EM, Shoham, S, Casadevall, A, Sachais, BS, Shaz, B, Winters, JL, van Buskirk, C, Grossman, BJ, Joyner, M, Henderson, JP, Pekosz, A, Lau, B, Wesolowski, A, Katz, L, Shan, H, Auwaerter, PG, Thomas, D, Sullivan, DJ, Paneth, N, Gehrie, E, Spitalnik, S, Hod, EA, Pollack, L, Nicholson, WT, Pirofski, LA, Bailey, JA & Tobian, AA (2020) Deployment of convalescent plasma for the prevention and treatment of COVID-19. *J Clin Invest,* 130, 2757-65.
[http://dx.doi.org/10.1172/JCI138745] [PMID: 32254064]

Brewster, DJ, Chrimes, N, Do, TB, Fraser, K, Groombridge, CJ, Higgs, A, Humar, MJ, Leeuwenburg, TJ, McGloughlin, S, Newman, FG, Nickson, CP, Rehak, A, Vokes, D & Gatward, JJ (2020) Consensus statement: Safe Airway Society principles of airway management and tracheal intubation specific to the COVID-19 adult patient group. *Med J Aust,* 212, 472-81.
[http://dx.doi.org/10.5694/mja2.50598] [PMID: 32356900]

Brodie, D & Bacchetta, M (2011) Extracorporeal membrane oxygenation for ARDS in adults. *N Engl J Med,* 365, 1905-14.
[http://dx.doi.org/10.1056/NEJMct1103720] [PMID: 22087681]

Brodie, D, Slutsky, AS & Combes, A (2019) Extracorporeal Life Support for Adults With Respiratory Failure and Related Indications: A Review. *JAMA,* 322, 557-68.
[http://dx.doi.org/10.1001/jama.2019.9302] [PMID: 31408142]

Brown, J, Rogers, J & Soar, J (2001) Cardiac arrest during surgery and ventilation in the prone position: a case report and systematic review. *Resuscitation,* 50, 233-8.
[http://dx.doi.org/10.1016/S0300-9572(01)00362-8] [PMID: 11719152]

Camprubí-Rimblas, M, Tantinyà, N, Guillamat-Prats, R, Bringué, J, Puig, F, Gómez, MN, Blanch, L & Artigas, A (2020) Effects of nebulized antithrombin and heparin on inflammatory and coagulation alterations in an acute lung injury model in rats. *J Thromb Haemost,* 18, 571-83.
[http://dx.doi.org/10.1111/jth.14685] [PMID: 31755229]

Carsana, L, Sonzogni, A & Nasr, A (2020) Pulmonary post-mortem findings in a large series of COVID-19 cases from Northern Italy. *Lancet Infect Dis,* 20, 1135-40.
[http://dx.doi.org/10.1016/S1473-3099(20)30434-5] [PMID: 32526193]

Casadevall, A, Dadachova, E & Pirofski, LA (2004) Passive antibody therapy for infectious diseases. *Nat Rev Microbiol,* 2, 695-703.
[http://dx.doi.org/10.1038/nrmicro974] [PMID: 15372080]

Casadevall, A & Pirofski, LA (2003) Antibody-mediated regulation of cellular immunity and the inflammatory response. *Trends Immunol,* 24, 474-8.
[http://dx.doi.org/10.1016/S1471-4906(03)00228-X] [PMID: 12967670]

Casadevall, A & Pirofski, LA (2020) The convalescent sera option for containing COVID-19. *J Clin Invest,* 130, 1545-8.
[http://dx.doi.org/10.1172/JCI138003] [PMID: 32167489]

Cattaneo, M, Bertinato, EM, Birocchi, S, Brizio, C, Malavolta, D, Manzoni, M, Muscarella, G & Orlandi, M (2020) Pulmonary embolism or pulmonary thrombosis in COVID-19? Is the recommendation to use high-dose heparin for thromboprophylaxis justified? *Thromb Haemost,* 120, 1230-2.
[http://dx.doi.org/10.1055/s-0040-1712097] [PMID: 32349132]

Chen, L, Xiong, J, Bao, L & Shi, Y (2020) Convalescent plasma as a potential therapy for COVID-19. *Lancet Infect Dis,* 20, 398-400.
[http://dx.doi.org/10.1016/S1473-3099(20)30141-9] [PMID: 32113510]

Chen, N, Zhou, M, Dong, X, Qu, J, Gong, F, Han, Y, Qiu, Y, Wang, J, Liu, Y, Wei, Y, Xia, J, Yu, T, Zhang, X & Zhang, L (2020) Epidemiological and clinical characteristics of 99 cases of 2019 novel coronavirus pneumonia in Wuhan, China: a descriptive study. *Lancet,* 395, 507-13.

[http://dx.doi.org/10.1016/S0140-6736(20)30211-7] [PMID: 32007143]

Chen, N, Zhou, M, Dong, X, Qu, J, Gong, F, Han, Y, Qiu, Y, Wang, J, Liu, Y, Wei, Y, Xia, J, Yu, T, Zhang, X & Zhang, L (2020) Epidemiological and clinical characteristics of 99 cases of 2019 novel coronavirus pneumonia in Wuhan, China: a descriptive study. *Lancet,* 395, 507-13.
[http://dx.doi.org/10.1016/S0140-6736(20)30211-7] [PMID: 32007143]

Cheng, Y, Wong, R, Soo, YO, Wong, WS, Lee, CK, Ng, MH, Chan, P, Wong, KC, Leung, CB & Cheng, G (2005) Use of convalescent plasma therapy in SARS patients in Hong Kong. *Eur J Clin Microbiol Infect Dis,* 24, 44-6.
[http://dx.doi.org/10.1007/s10096-004-1271-9] [PMID: 15616839]

Cho, JW, Jung, H & Lee, MJ (2020) Preparedness of personal protective equipment and implementation of new CPR strategies for patients with out-of-hospital cardiac arrest in the COVID-19 era. *Resuscitation Plus,* 3100015
[http://dx.doi.org/10.1016/j.resplu.2020.100015]

Choudhury, R, Barrett, CD, Moore, HB, Moore, EE, McIntyre, RC, Moore, PK, Talmor, DS, Nydam, TL & Yaffe, MB (2020) Salvage use of tissue plasminogen activator (tPA) in the setting of acute respiratory distress syndrome (ARDS) due to COVID-19 in the USA: a Markov decision analysis. *World J Emerg Surg,* 15, 29.
[http://dx.doi.org/10.1186/s13017-020-00305-4] [PMID: 32312290]

Choudry, FA, Hamshere, SM, Rathod, KS, Akhtar, MM, Archbold, RA, Guttmann, OP, Woldman, S, Jain, AK, Knight, CJ, Baumbach, A, Mathur, A & Jones, DA (2020) High Thrombus Burden in Patients With COVID-19 Presenting With ST-Segment Elevation Myocardial Infarction. *J Am Coll Cardiol,* 76, 1168-76.
[http://dx.doi.org/10.1016/j.jacc.2020.07.022] [PMID: 32679155]

Chung, M, Bernheim, A, Mei, X, Zhang, N, Huang, M, Zeng, X, Cui, J, Xu, W, Yang, Y, Fayad, ZA, Jacobi, A, Li, K, Li, S & Shan, H (2020) CT imaging features of 2019 novel coronavirus (2019-nCoV). *Radiology,* 295, 202-7.
[http://dx.doi.org/10.1148/radiol.2020200230] [PMID: 32017661]

Combes, A, Bacchetta, M, Brodie, D, Müller, T & Pellegrino, V (2012) Extracorporeal membrane oxygenation for respiratory failure in adults. *Curr Opin Crit Care,* 18, 99-104.
[http://dx.doi.org/10.1097/MCC.0b013e32834ef412] [PMID: 22186218]

Craig, S, Cubitt, M, Jaison, A, Troupakis, S, Hood, N, Fong, C, Bilgrami, A, Leman, P, Ascencio-Lane, JC, Nagaraj, G, Bonning, J, Blecher, G, Mitchell, R, Burkett, E, McCarthy, SM, Rojek, AM, Hansen, K, Psihogios, H, Allely, P, Judkins, S, Foong, LH, Bernard, S & Cameron, PA (2020) Management of adult cardiac arrest in the COVID-19 era: consensus statement from the Australasian College for Emergency Medicine. *Med J Aust,* 213, 126-33.
[http://dx.doi.org/10.5694/mja2.50699] [PMID: 32656798]

Dargent, A, Chatelain, E, Kreitmann, L, Quenot, JP, Cour, M & Argaud, L (2020) Lung ultrasound score to monitor COVID-19 pneumonia progression in patients with ARDS. *PLoS One,* 15e0236312
[http://dx.doi.org/10.1371/journal.pone.0236312] [PMID: 32692769]

de Lange, DW, Sikma, MA & Meulenbelt, J (2013) Extracorporeal membrane oxygenation in the treatment of poisoned patients. *Clin Toxicol (Phila),* 51, 385-93.
[http://dx.doi.org/10.3109/15563650.2013.800876] [PMID: 23697460]

Diagnosis and Treatment Protocol for Novel Coronavirus Pneumonia (2020)

Diagnosis and Treatment Protocol for Novel Coronavirus Pneumonia (2020)

Dreher, M, Kersten, A, Bickenbach, J, Balfanz, P, Hartmann, B, Cornelissen, C, Daher, A, Stöhr, R, Kleines, M, Lemmen, SW, Brokmann, JC, Müller, T, Müller-Wieland, D, Marx, G & Marx, N (2020) The Characteristics of 50 Hospitalized COVID-19 Patients With and Without ARDS. *Dtsch Arztebl Int,* 117, 271-8.

[http://dx.doi.org/10.3238/arztebl.2020.0271] [PMID: 32519944]

Edelson, DP, Sasson, C, Chan, PS, Atkins, DL, Aziz, K, Becker, LB, Berg, RA, Bradley, SM, Brooks, SC, Cheng, A, Escobedo, M, Flores, GE, Girotra, S, Hsu, A, Kamath-Rayne, BD, Lee, HC, Lehotsky, RE, Mancini, ME, Merchant, RM, Nadkarni, VM, Panchal, AR, Peberdy, MAR, Raymond, TT, Walsh, B, Wang, DS, Zelop, CM & Topjian, AA (2020) Interim Guidance for Basic and Advanced Life Support in Adults, Children, and Neonates With Suspected or Confirmed COVID-19: From the Emergency Cardiovascular Care Committee and Get With The Guidelines-Resuscitation Adult and Pediatric Task Forces of the American Heart Association. *Circulation,* 141, e933-43.
[http://dx.doi.org/10.1161/CIRCULATIONAHA.120.047463] [PMID: 32270695]

Esmon, CT (2014) Targeting factor Xa and thrombin: impact on coagulation and beyond. *Thromb Haemost,* 111, 625-33.
[http://dx.doi.org/10.1160/TH13-09-0730] [PMID: 24336942]

Fata-Hartley, CL & Palmenberg, AC (2005) Dipyridamole reversibly inhibits mengovirus RNA replication. *J Virol,* 79, 11062-70.
[http://dx.doi.org/10.1128/JVI.79.17.11062-11070.2005] [PMID: 16103157]

Frizelle, S, Schwarz, J, Huber, SA & Leslie, K (1992) Evaluation of the effects of low molecular weight heparin on inflammation and collagen deposition in chronic coxsackievirus B3-induced myocarditis in A/J mice. *Am J Pathol,* 141, 203-9.
[PMID: 1321562]

Gaertner, F & Massberg, S (2016) Blood coagulation in immunothrombosis-At the frontline of intravascular immunity. *Semin Immunol,* 28, 561-9.
[http://dx.doi.org/10.1016/j.smim.2016.10.010] [PMID: 27866916]

Gao, J, Tian, Z & Yang, X (2020) Breakthrough: Chloroquine phosphate has shown apparent efficacy in treatment of COVID-19 associated pneumonia in clinical studies. *Biosci Trends,* 14, 72-3.
[http://dx.doi.org/10.5582/bst.2020.01047] [PMID: 32074550]

Gattinoni, L, Carlesso, E, Taccone, P, Polli, F, Guérin, C & Mancebo, J (2010) Prone positioning improves survival in severe ARDS: a pathophysiologic review and individual patient meta-analysis. *Minerva Anestesiol,* 76, 448-54.
[PMID: 20473258]

Gautret, P, Lagier, JC, Parola, P, Hoang, VT, Meddeb, L, Mailhe, M, Doudier, B, Courjon, J, Giordanengo, V, Vieira, VE, Tissot Dupont, H, Honoré, S, Colson, P, Chabrière, E, La Scola, B, Rolain, JM, Brouqui, P & Raoult, D (2020) Hydroxychloroquine and azithromycin as a treatment of COVID-19: results of an open-label non-randomized clinical trial. *Int J Antimicrob Agents,* 56105949
[http://dx.doi.org/10.1016/j.ijantimicag.2020.105949] [PMID: 32205204]

Ghezzi, S, Cooper, L, Rubio, A, Pagani, I, Capobianchi, MR, Ippolito, G, Pelletier, J, Meneghetti, MCZ, Lima, MA, Skidmore, MA, Broccoli, V, Yates, EA & Vicenzi, E (2017) Heparin prevents Zika virus induced-cytopathic effects in human neural progenitor cells. *Antiviral Res,* 140, 13-7.
[http://dx.doi.org/10.1016/j.antiviral.2016.12.023] [PMID: 28063994]

Glas, GJ, Van Der Sluijs, KF, Schultz, MJ, Hofstra, JJ, Van Der Poll, T & Levi, M (2013) Bronchoalveolar hemostasis in lung injury and acute respiratory distress syndrome. *J Thromb Haemost,* 11, 17-25.
[http://dx.doi.org/10.1111/jth.12047] [PMID: 23114008]

Gresele, P, Momi, S & Falcinelli, E (2011) Anti-platelet therapy: phosphodiesterase inhibitors. *Br J Clin Pharmacol,* 72, 634-46.
[http://dx.doi.org/10.1111/j.1365-2125.2011.04034.x] [PMID: 21649691]

Guan, WJ, Ni, ZY, Hu, Y, Liang, WH, Ou, CQ, He, JX, Liu, L, Shan, H, Lei, CL, Hui, DSC, Du, B, Li, LJ, Zeng, G, Yuen, KY, Chen, RC, Tang, CL, Wang, T, Chen, PY, Xiang, J, Li, SY, Wang, JL, Liang, ZJ, Peng, YX, Wei, L, Liu, Y, Hu, YH, Peng, P, Wang, JM, Liu, JY, Chen, Z, Li, G, Zheng, ZJ, Qiu, SQ, Luo, J, Ye, CJ, Zhu, SY & Zhong, NS (2020) Clinical characteristics of coronavirus disease 2019 in China. *N Engl J Med,* 382, 1708-20.

[http://dx.doi.org/10.1056/NEJMoa2002032] [PMID: 32109013]

Guérin, C, Reignier, J, Richard, JC, Beuret, P, Gacouin, A, Boulain, T, Mercier, E, Badet, M, Mercat, A, Baudin, O, Clavel, M, Chatellier, D, Jaber, S, Rosselli, S, Mancebo, J, Sirodot, M, Hilbert, G, Bengler, C, Richecoeur, J, Gainnier, M, Bayle, F, Bourdin, G, Leray, V, Girard, R, Baboi, L & Ayzac, L (2013) Prone positioning in severe acute respiratory distress syndrome. *N Engl J Med,* 368, 2159-68.
[http://dx.doi.org/10.1056/NEJMoa1214103] [PMID: 23688302]

Huang, B, Chen, Z, Geng, L, Wang, J, Liang, H, Cao, Y, Chen, H, Huang, W, Su, M, Wang, H, Xu, Y, Liu, Y, Lu, B, Xian, H, Li, H, Li, H, Ren, L, Xie, J, Ye, L, Wang, H, Zhao, J, Chen, P, Zhang, L, Zhao, S, Zhang, T, Xu, B, Che, D, Si, W, Gu, X, Zeng, L, Wang, Y, Li, D, Zhan, Y, Delfouneso, D, Lew, AM, Cui, J, Tang, WH, Zhang, Y, Gong, S, Bai, F, Yang, M & Zhang, Y (2019) Mucosal profiling of pediatric-onset colitis and IBD reveals common pathogenics and therapeutic pathways. *Cell,* 179, 1160-1176.e24.
[http://dx.doi.org/10.1016/j.cell.2019.10.027] [PMID: 31730855]

Huang, C, Wang, Y, Li, X, Ren, L, Zhao, J, Hu, Y, Zhang, L, Fan, G, Xu, J, Gu, X, Cheng, Z, Yu, T, Xia, J, Wei, Y, Wu, W, Xie, X, Yin, W, Li, H, Liu, M, Xiao, Y, Gao, H, Guo, L, Xie, J, Wang, G, Jiang, R, Gao, Z, Jin, Q, Wang, J & Cao, B (2020) Clinical features of patients infected with 2019 novel coronavirus in Wuhan, China. *Lancet,* 395, 497-506.
[http://dx.doi.org/10.1016/S0140-6736(20)30183-5] [PMID: 31986264]

Iba, T, Hashiguchi, N, Nagaoka, I, Tabe, Y, Kadota, K & Sato, K (2015) Heparins attenuated histone-mediated cytotoxicity *in vitro* and improved the survival in a rat model of histone-induced organ dysfunction. *Intensive Care Med Exp,* 3, 36.
[http://dx.doi.org/10.1186/s40635-015-0072-z] [PMID: 26715580]

Iba, T, Nisio, MD, Levy, JH, Kitamura, N & Thachil, J (2017) New criteria for sepsis-induced coagulopathy (SIC) following the revised sepsis definition: a retrospective analysis of a nationwide survey. *BMJ Open,* 7e017046
[http://dx.doi.org/10.1136/bmjopen-2017-017046] [PMID: 28963294]

Idell, S (2003) Coagulation, fibrinolysis, and fibrin deposition in acute lung injury. *Crit Care Med,* 31 (Suppl.), S213-20.
[http://dx.doi.org/10.1097/01.CCM.0000057846.21303.AB] [PMID: 12682443]

Insel, PA, Murray, F, Yokoyama, U, Romano, S, Yun, H, Brown, L, Snead, A, Lu, D & Aroonsakool, N (2012) cAMP and Epac in the regulation of tissue fibrosis. *Br J Pharmacol,* 166, 447-56.
[http://dx.doi.org/10.1111/j.1476-5381.2012.01847.x] [PMID: 22233238]

Interim Clinical Guidance For Patients Suspected of / Confirmed With COVID-19 in Belgium (2020)

Izmirly, PM, Costedoat-Chalumeau, N, Pisoni, CN, Khamashta, MA, Kim, MY, Saxena, A, Friedman, D, Llanos, C, Piette, JC & Buyon, JP (2012) Maternal use of hydroxychloroquine is associated with a reduced risk of recurrent anti-SSA/Ro-antibody-associated cardiac manifestations of neonatal lupus. *Circulation,* 126, 76-82.
[http://dx.doi.org/10.1161/CIRCULATIONAHA.111.089268] [PMID: 22626746]

Jain, S, Workman, V, Ganeshan, R, Obasare, ER, Burr, A, DeBiasi, RM, Freeman, JV, Akar, J, Lampert, R & Rosenfeld, LE (2020) Enhanced electrocardiographic monitoring of patients with Coronavirus Disease 2019. *Heart Rhythm,* 17, 1417-22.
[http://dx.doi.org/10.1016/j.hrthm.2020.04.047] [PMID: 32387247]

Kim, HH & Liao, JK (2008) Translational therapeutics of dipyridamole. *Arterioscler Thromb Vasc Biol,* 28, s39-42.
[http://dx.doi.org/10.1161/ATVBAHA.107.160226] [PMID: 18174451]

Kim, SY, Jin, W & Sood, A (2020) Kim SY, Jin W, Sood A, et al. Preprint from bioRxiv 2020. doi:10.1101/2020.04.14.041459. Glycosaminoglycan binding motif at S1/S2 proteolytic cleavage site on spike glycoprotein may facilitate novel coronavirus (SARS-CoV-2) host cell entry. *Preprint from bioRxiv.*
[http://dx.doi.org/10.1101/2020.04.14.041459]

Kinney, B & Slama, R (2020) Rapid outdoor non-compression intubation (RONCI) of cardiac arrests to mitigate COVID-19 exposure to emergency department staff. *Am J Emerg Med,* 38, 2760.e1-3. [http://dx.doi.org/10.1016/j.ajem.2020.05.080] [PMID: 32507572]

Lai, PH, Lancet, EA, Weiden, MD, Webber, MP, Zeig-Owens, R, Hall, CB & Prezant, DJ (2020) Characteristics Associated With Out-of-Hospital Cardiac Arrests and Resuscitations During the Novel Coronavirus Disease 2019 Pandemic in New York City. *JAMA Cardiol,* e202488 [http://dx.doi.org/10.1001/jamacardio.2020.2488] [PMID: 32558876]

Lamontagne, F, Meade, MO, Hébert, PC, Asfar, P, Lauzier, F, Seely, AJE, Day, AG, Mehta, S, Muscedere, J, Bagshaw, SM, Ferguson, ND, Cook, DJ, Kanji, S, Turgeon, AF, Herridge, MS, Subramanian, S, Lacroix, J, Adhikari, NKJ, Scales, DC, Fox-Robichaud, A, Skrobik, Y, Whitlock, RP, Green, RS, Koo, KKY, Tanguay, T, Magder, S & Heyland, DK (2016) Higher *versus* lower blood pressure targets for vasopressor therapy in shock: a multicentre pilot randomized controlled trial. *Intensive Care Med,* 42, 542-50. [http://dx.doi.org/10.1007/s00134-016-4237-3] [PMID: 26891677]

Lang, M, Som, A, Mendoza, DP, Flores, EJ, Reid, N, Carey, D, Li, MD, Witkin, A, Rodriguez-Lopez, JM, Shepard, JO & Little, BP (2020) Hypoxaemia related to COVID-19: vascular and perfusion abnormalities on dual-energy CT. *Lancet Infect Dis,* 20, 1365-6. [http://dx.doi.org/10.1016/S1473-3099(20)30367-4] [PMID: 32359410]

Levy, MM, Evans, LE & Rhodes, A (2018) The Surviving Sepsis Campaign Bundle: 2018 update. *Intensive Care Med,* 44, 925-8. [http://dx.doi.org/10.1007/s00134-018-5085-0] [PMID: 29675566]

Li, G, Chen, X & Xu, A (2003) Profile of specific antibodies to the SARS-associated coronavirus. *N Engl J Med,* 349, 508-9. [http://dx.doi.org/10.1056/NEJM200307313490520] [PMID: 12890855]

Li, J, Li, Y & Yang, B (2018) Low-molecular-weight heparin treatment for acute lung injury/acute respiratory distress syndrome: a meta-analysis of randomized controlled trials. *Int J Clin Exp Med,* 11, 414-22.

Li, JP & Vlodavsky, I (2009) Heparin, heparan sulfate and heparanase in inflammatory reactions. *Thromb Haemost,* 102, 823-8. [PMID: 19888515]

Li, X & Ma, X (2020) Acute respiratory failure in COVID-19: is it "typical" ARDS? *Crit Care,* 24, 198. [http://dx.doi.org/10.1186/s13054-020-02911-9] [PMID: 32375845]

Lisney, AR, Szelinski, F, Reiter, K, Burmester, GR, Rose, T & Dörner, T (2017) High maternal expression of SIGLEC1 on monocytes as a surrogate marker of a type I interferon signature is a risk factor for the development of autoimmune congenital heart block. *Ann Rheum Dis,* 76, 1476-80. [http://dx.doi.org/10.1136/annrheumdis-2016-210927] [PMID: 28501799]

Liu, X, Li, Z, Liu, S, Sun, J, Chen, Z, Jiang, M, Zhang, Q, Wei, Y, Wang, X, Huang, YY, Shi, Y, Xu, Y, Xian, H, Bai, F, Ou, C, Xiong, B, Lew, AM, Cui, J, Fang, R, Huang, H, Zhao, J, Hong, X, Zhang, Y, Zhou, F & Luo, HB (2020) Potential therapeutic effects of dipyridamole in the severely ill patients with COVID-19. *Acta Pharm Sin B,* 10, 1205-15. [http://dx.doi.org/10.1016/j.apsb.2020.04.008] [PMID: 32318327]

Liu, Y, Mu, S, Li, X, Liang, Y, Wang, L & Ma, X (2019) Unfractionated Heparin Alleviates Sepsis-Induced Acute Lung Injury by Protecting Tight Junctions. *J Surg Res,* 238, 175-85. [http://dx.doi.org/10.1016/j.jss.2019.01.020] [PMID: 30771687]

Loubani, OM & Green, RS (2015) A systematic review of extravasation and local tissue injury from administration of vasopressors through peripheral intravenous catheters and central venous catheters. *J Crit Care,* 30, 653. e9-17

Ma, J & Bai, J (2015) Protective effects of heparin on endothelial cells in sepsis. *Int J Clin Exp Med,* 8, 5547-52. [PMID: 26131136]

Martinez, MA (2020) Compounds with therapeutic potential against novel respiratory 2019 coronavirus. *Antimicrob Agents Chemother,* 64, e00399-20.https://doi.org/10 .1128/AAC.00399-20
[http://dx.doi.org/10.1128/AAC.00399-20] [PMID: 32152082]

Mazer, SP, Weisfeldt, M, Bai, D, Cardinale, C, Arora, R, Ma, C, Sciacca, RR, Chong, D & Rabbani, LE (2003) Reverse CPR: a pilot study of CPR in the prone position. *Resuscitation,* 57, 279-85.
[http://dx.doi.org/10.1016/S0300-9572(03)00037-6] [PMID: 12804805]

Meduri, GU, Siemieniuk, RAC, Ness, RA & Seyler, SJ (2018) Prolonged low-dose methylprednisolone treatment is highly effective in reducing duration of mechanical ventilation and mortality in patients with ARDS. *J Intensive Care,* 6, 53.
[http://dx.doi.org/10.1186/s40560-018-0321-9] [PMID: 30155260]

Milewska, A, Nowak, P, Owczarek, K, Szczepanski, A, Zarebski, M, Hoang, A, Berniak, K, Wojarski, J, Zeglen, S, Baster, Z, Rajfur, Z & Pyrc, K (2018) Entry of human coronavirus NL63 into the cell. *J Virol,* 92e01933
[PMID: 29142129]

Mousavi, S, Moradi, M, Khorshidahmad, T & Motamedi, M (2015) Anti-Inflammatory Effects of Heparin and Its Derivatives: A Systematic Review. *Adv Pharmacol Sci,* 2015507151
[http://dx.doi.org/10.1155/2015/507151] [PMID: 26064103]

Mycroft-West, C, Su, D & Elli, S (2020) The 2019 coronavirus (SARS-CoV-2) surface protein (Spike) S1 Receptor Binding Domain undergoes conformational change upon heparin binding. *bioRxiv.*
[http://dx.doi.org/10.1101/2020.02.29.971093]

National Health Commission of the People's Republic of China The clinical guidance of convalescent plasma therapy (trial version 3). http://www.nhc.gov.cn/yzygj/s7658/202003/61d608 a7e8bf49fca418a6074c2 bf5a2.shtml

Negri, EM, Piloto, B & Morinaga, LK (2020) Heparin therapy improving hypoxia in COVID-19 patients: a case series. *medRxiv.*
[http://dx.doi.org/10.1101/2020.04.15.20067017]

Ou, X, Hua, Y, Liu, J, Gong, C & Zhao, W (2017) Effect of high-flow nasal cannula oxygen therapy in adults with acute hypoxemic respiratory failure: a meta-analysis of randomized controlled trials. *CMAJ,* 189, E260-7.
[http://dx.doi.org/10.1503/cmaj.160570] [PMID: 28246239]

Oxley, TJ, Mocco, J, Majidi, S, Kellner, CP, Shoirah, H, Singh, IP, De Leacy, RA, Shigematsu, T, Ladner, TR, Yaeger, KA, Skliut, M, Weinberger, J, Dangayach, NS, Bederson, JB, Tuhrim, S & Fifi, JT (2020) Large-vessel stroke as a presenting feature of COVID-19 in the young. *N Engl J Med,* 382e60
[http://dx.doi.org/10.1056/NEJMc2009787] [PMID: 32343504]

Ozolina, A, Sarkele, M, Sabelnikovs, O, Skesters, A, Jaunalksne, I, Serova, J, Ievins, T, Bjertnaes, LJ & Vanags, I (2016) Activation of coagulation and fibrinolysis in acute respiratory distress syndrome: a prospective pilot study. *Front Med (Lausanne),* 3, 64.
[http://dx.doi.org/10.3389/fmed.2016.00064] [PMID: 27965960]

Paranjpe, I, Fuster, V, Lala, A, Russak, AJ, Glicksberg, BS, Levin, MA, Charney, AW, Narula, J, Fayad, ZA, Bagiella, E, Zhao, S & Nadkarni, GN (2020) Association of treatment dose anticoagulation with in-hospital survival among hospitalized patients with COVID-19. *J Am Coll Cardiol,* 76, 122-4.
[http://dx.doi.org/10.1016/j.jacc.2020.05.001] [PMID: 32387623]

Poterucha, TJ, Libby, P & Goldhaber, SZ (2017) More than an anticoagulant: Do heparins have direct anti-inflammatory effects? *Thromb Haemost,* 117, 437-44.
[http://dx.doi.org/10.1160/TH16-08-0620] [PMID: 27975101]

Remy, KE, Mazer, M, Striker, DA, Ellebedy, AH, Walton, AH, Unsinger, J, Blood, TM, Mudd, PA, Yi, DJ, Mannion, DA, Osborne, DF, Martin, RS, Anand, NJ, Bosanquet, JP, Blood, J, Drewry, AM, Caldwell, CC, Turnbull, IR, Brakenridge, SC, Moldwawer, LL & Hotchkiss, RS (2020) Severe immunosuppression and not a cytokine storm characterizes COVID-19 infections. *JCI Insight,* 5140329 [http://dx.doi.org/10.1172/jci.insight.140329] [PMID: 32687484]

Rhodes, A, Evans, LE, Alhazzani, W, Levy, MM, Antonelli, M, Ferrer, R, Kumar, A, Sevransky, JE, Sprung, CL, Nunnally, ME, Rochwerg, B, Rubenfeld, GD, Angus, DC, Annane, D, Beale, RJ, Bellinghan, GJ, Bernard, GR, Chiche, JD, Coopersmith, C, De Backer, DP, French, CJ, Fujishima, S, Gerlach, H, Hidalgo, JL, Hollenberg, SM, Jones, AE, Karnad, DR, Kleinpell, RM, Koh, Y, Lisboa, TC, Machado, FR, Marini, JJ, Marshall, JC, Mazuski, JE, McIntyre, LA, McLean, AS, Mehta, S, Moreno, RP, Myburgh, J, Navalesi, P, Nishida, O, Osborn, TM, Perner, A, Plunkett, CM, Ranieri, M, Schorr, CA, Seckel, MA, Seymour, CW, Shieh, L, Shukri, KA, Simpson, SQ, Singer, M, Thompson, BT, Townsend, SR, Van der Poll, T, Vincent, JL, Wiersinga, WJ, Zimmerman, JL & Dellinger, RP (2017) Surviving Sepsis Campaign: International Guidelines for Management of Sepsis and Septic Shock: 2016. *Intensive Care Med,* 43, 304-77. [http://dx.doi.org/10.1007/s00134-017-4683-6] [PMID: 28101605]

Robbiani, DF, Gaebler, C, Muecksch, F, Lorenzi, JCC, Wang, Z, Cho, A, Agudelo, M, Barnes, CO, Gazumyan, A, Finkin, S, Hägglöf, T, Oliveira, TY, Viant, C, Hurley, A, Hoffmann, HH, Millard, KG, Kost, RG, Cipolla, M, Gordon, K, Bianchini, F, Chen, ST, Ramos, V, Patel, R, Dizon, J, Shimeliovich, I, Mendoza, P, Hartweger, H, Nogueira, L, Pack, M, Horowitz, J, Schmidt, F, Weisblum, Y, Michailidis, E, Ashbrook, AW, Waltari, E, Pak, JE, Huey-Tubman, KE, Koranda, N, Hoffman, PR, West, AP, Jr, Rice, CM, Hatziioannou, T, Bjorkman, PJ, Bieniasz, PD, Caskey, M & Nussenzweig, MC (2020) Convergent antibody responses to SARS-CoV-2 in convalescent individuals. *Nature,* 584, 437-42. [http://dx.doi.org/10.1038/s41586-020-2456-9] [PMID: 32555388]

Rosenberg, ES, Dufort, EM, Udo, T, Wilberschied, LA, Kumar, J, Tesoriero, J, Weinberg, P, Kirkwood, J, Muse, A, DeHovitz, J, Blog, DS, Hutton, B, Holtgrave, DR & Zucker, HA (2020) Association of Treatment With Hydroxychloroquine or Azithromycin With In-Hospital Mortality in Patients With COVID-19 in New York State. *JAMA,* 323, 2493-502. [http://dx.doi.org/10.1001/jama.2020.8630] [PMID: 32392282]

Ruan, Q, Yang, K, Wang, W, Jiang, L & Song, J (2020) Clinical predictors of mortality due to COVID-19 based on an analysis of data of 150 patients from Wuhan, China. *Intensive Care Med* Epub ahead of print [http://dx.doi.org/10.1007/s00134–020–05991-x]

Ruiz-Irastorza, G, Ramos-Casals, M, Brito-Zeron, P & Khamashta, MA (2010) Clinical efficacy and side effects of antimalarials in systemic lupus erythematosus: a systematic review. *Ann Rheum Dis,* 69, 20-8. [http://dx.doi.org/10.1136/ard.2008.101766] [PMID: 19103632]

Sanders, JM, Monogue, ML, Jodlowski, TZ & Cutrell, JB (2020) Pharmacologic Treatments for Coronavirus Disease 2019 (COVID-19): A Review. *JAMA,* 323, 1824-36. [PMID: 32282022]

Scholten, EL, Beitler, JR, Prisk, GK & Malhotra, A (2017) Treatment of ARDS With Prone Positioning. *Chest,* 151, 215-24. [http://dx.doi.org/10.1016/j.chest.2016.06.032] [PMID: 27400909]

Schrezenmeier, E & Dörner, T (2020) Mechanisms of action of hydroxychloroquine and chloroquine: implications for rheumatology. *Nat Rev Rheumatol,* 16, 155-66. [http://dx.doi.org/10.1038/s41584-020-0372-x] [PMID: 32034323]

Seif, S, Ayuna, A, Kumar, A & Macdonald, J (2020) Massive coronary thrombosis caused primary percutaneous coronary intervention to fail in a COVID-19 patient with ST-elevation myocardial infarction. *Catheter Cardiovasc Interv,* 1-3 [http://dx.doi.org/10.1002/ccd.29050] [PMID: 32473051]

She, J, Jiang, J, Ye, L, Hu, L, Bai, C & Song, Y (2020) 2019 novel coronavirus of pneumonia in Wuhan, China: emerging attack and management strategies. *Clin Transl Med,* 9, 19. [http://dx.doi.org/10.1186/s40169-020-00271-z] [PMID: 32078069]

Shi, C, Wang, C, Wang, H, Yang, C, Cai, F, Zeng, F, Cheng, F, Liu, Y, Zhou, T, Deng, B, Vlodavsky, I, Li, JP & Zhang, Y (2020) The Potential of Low Molecular Weight Heparin to Mitigate Cytokine Storm in Severe COVID-19 Patients: A Retrospective Cohort Study. *Clin Transl Sci,* 13, 1087-95.

[http://dx.doi.org/10.1111/cts.12880] [PMID: 32881340]

Shukla, D & Spear, PG (2001) Herpesviruses and heparan sulfate: an intimate relationship in aid of viral entry. *J Clin Invest,* 108, 503-10.
[http://dx.doi.org/10.1172/JCI200113799] [PMID: 11518721]

Soar, J, Lott, C & Böttiger, BW (2020) European Resuscitation Council COVID-19 Guidelines Section 3 Advanced Life Support in Adults.

Sud, S, Friedrich, JO, Taccone, P, Polli, F, Adhikari, NK, Latini, R, Pesenti, A, Guérin, C, Mancebo, J, Curley, MA, Fernandez, R, Chan, MC, Beuret, P, Voggenreiter, G, Sud, M, Tognoni, G & Gattinoni, L (2010) Prone ventilation reduces mortality in patients with acute respiratory failure and severe hypoxemia: systematic review and meta-analysis. *Intensive Care Med,* 36, 585-99.
[http://dx.doi.org/10.1007/s00134-009-1748-1] [PMID: 20130832]

Tang, N, Bai, H, Chen, X, Gong, J, Li, D & Sun, Z (2020) Anticoagulant treatment is associated with decreased mortality in severe coronavirus disease 2019 patients with coagulopathy. *J Thromb Haemost,* 18, 1094-9.
[http://dx.doi.org/10.1111/jth.14817] [PMID: 32220112]

Tang, N, Li, D, Wang, X & Sun, Z (2020) Abnormal coagulation parameters are associated with poor prognosis in patients with novel coronavirus pneumonia. *J Thromb Haemost,* 18, 844-7.
[http://dx.doi.org/10.1111/jth.14768] [PMID: 32073213]

Tanne, JH (2020) COVID-19: FDA approves use of convalescent plasma to treat critically ill patients. *BMJ,* 368, m1256.
[http://dx.doi.org/10.1136/bmj.m1256] [PMID: 32217555]

The 3/4/2020 Chinese Health and Public Health Ministry Guideline on Novel Coronavirus Disease (COVID-19) Diagnosis and Treatment (Revision #6)

The 3/4/2020 Chinese Health and Public Health Ministry Guideline on Novel Coronavirus Disease (COVID-19) Diagnosis and Treatment (Revision #6)

Tisdale, JE, Jaynes, HA, Kingery, JR, Mourad, NA, Trujillo, TN, Overholser, BR & Kovacs, RJ (2013) Development and validation of a risk score to predict QT interval prolongation in hospitalized patients. *Circ Cardiovasc Qual Outcomes,* 6, 479-87.
[http://dx.doi.org/10.1161/CIRCOUTCOMES.113.000152] [PMID: 23716032]

Toy, P (2019) Update on transfusion-related acute lung injury. *Clin Adv Hematol Oncol,* 17, 378-81.
[PMID: 31449502]

van Erp, EA, Luytjes, W, Ferwerda, G & van Kasteren, PB (2019) Fc-mediated antibody effector functions during respiratory syncytial virus infection and disease. *Front Immunol,* 10, 548.
[http://dx.doi.org/10.3389/fimmu.2019.00548] [PMID: 30967872]

Varga, Z, Flammer, AJ, Steiger, P, Haberecker, M, Andermatt, R, Zinkernagel, AS, Mehra, MR, Schuepbach, RA, Ruschitzka, F & Moch, H (2020) Endothelial cell infection and endotheliitis in COVID-19. *Lancet,* 395, 1417-8.
[http://dx.doi.org/10.1016/S0140-6736(20)30937-5] [PMID: 32325026]

Vicenzi, E, Canducci, F, Pinna, D, Mancini, N, Carletti, S, Lazzarin, A, Bordignon, C, Poli, G & Clementi, M (2004) Coronaviridae and SARS-associated coronavirus strain HSR1. *Emerg Infect Dis,* 10, 413-8.
[http://dx.doi.org/10.3201/eid1003.030683] [PMID: 15109406]

Viecca, M, Radovanovic, D, Forleo, GB & Santus, P (2020) Enhanced platelet inhibition treatment improves hypoxemia in patients with severe COVID-19 and hypercoagulability. A case control, proof of concept study. *Pharmacol Res,* 158104950
[http://dx.doi.org/10.1016/j.phrs.2020.104950] [PMID: 32450344]

Vincent, MJ, Bergeron, E, Benjannet, S, Erickson, BR, Rollin, PE, Ksiazek, TG, Seidah, NG & Nichol, ST (2005) Chloroquine is a potent inhibitor of SARS coronavirus infection and spread. *Virol J,* 2, 69.

[http://dx.doi.org/10.1186/1743-422X-2-69] [PMID: 16115318]

Wang, D, Hu, B, Hu, C, Zhu, F, Liu, X, Zhang, J, Wang, B, Xiang, H, Cheng, Z, Xiong, Y, Zhao, Y, Li, Y, Wang, X & Peng, Z (2020) Clinical characteristics of 138 hospitalized patients with 2019 novel coronavirus-infected pneumonia in Wuhan, China. *JAMA,* 323, 1061-9.
[http://dx.doi.org/10.1001/jama.2020.1585] [PMID: 32031570]

Wang, J, Jiang, M, Chen, X & Montaner, LJ (2020) Cytokine storm and leukocyte changes in mild *versus* severe SARS-CoV-2 infection: Review of 3939 COVID-19 patients in China and emerging pathogenesis and therapy concepts. *J Leukoc Biol,* 108, 17-41.
[http://dx.doi.org/10.1002/JLB.3COVR0520-272R] [PMID: 32534467]

Wang, J, Ma, Q, Zhang, H, Liu, S & Zheng, Y (2018) Predictors of survival and neurologic outcome for adults with extracorporeal cardiopulmonary resuscitation: A systemic review and meta-analysis. *Medicine (Baltimore),* 97e13257
[http://dx.doi.org/10.1097/MD.0000000000013257] [PMID: 30508912]

Wang, M, Cao, R, Zhang, L, Yang, X, Liu, J, Xu, M, Shi, Z, Hu, Z, Zhong, W & Xiao, G (2020) Remdesivir and chloroquine effectively inhibit the recently emerged novel coronavirus (2019-nCoV) *in vitro*. *Cell Res,* 30, 269-71.
[http://dx.doi.org/10.1038/s41422-020-0282-0] [PMID: 32020029]

Wei, J, Tung, D, Sue, SH, Wu, SV, Chuang, YC & Chang, CY (2006) Cardiopulmonary resuscitation in prone position: a simplified method for outpatients. *J Chin Med Assoc,* 69, 202-6.
[http://dx.doi.org/10.1016/S1726-4901(09)70219-9] [PMID: 16835981]

WHO. Clinical management of severe acute respiratory infection when novel coronavirus (nCoV) infection is suspected. (2020) https://www.who.int/docs/default-source/coronaviruse/clinical-management-of-n-vel-cov.pdf

Wichmann, D, Sperhake, JP, Lütgehetmann, M, Steurer, S, Edler, C, Heinemann, A, Heinrich, F, Mushumba, H, Kniep, I, Schröder, AS, Burdelski, C, de Heer, G, Nierhaus, A, Frings, D, Pfefferle, S, Becker, H, Bredereke-Wiedling, H, de Weerth, A, Paschen, HR, Sheikhzadeh-Eggers, S, Stang, A, Schmiedel, S, Bokemeyer, C, Addo, MM, Aepfelbacher, M, Püschel, K & Kluge, S (2020) Autopsy findings and venous thromboembolism in patients with COVID-19: a prospective cohort study. *Ann Intern Med,* 173, 268-77.
[http://dx.doi.org/10.7326/M20-2003] [PMID: 32374815]

Wilson, JG, Simpson, LJ, Ferreira, AM, Rustagi, A, Roque, J, Asuni, A, Ranganath, T, Grant, PM, Subramanian, A, Rosenberg-Hasson, Y, Maecker, HT, Holmes, SP, Levitt, JE, Blish, CA & Rogers, AJ (2020) Cytokine profile in plasma of severe COVID-19 does not differ from ARDS and sepsis. *JCI Insight,* 5140289
[http://dx.doi.org/10.1172/jci.insight.140289] [PMID: 32706339]

Wojnicz, R, Nowak, J, Szyguła-Jurkiewicz, B, Wilczek, K, Lekston, A, Trzeciak, P, Nowalany-Kozielska, E, Zembala, M, Wodniecki, J & Poloński, L (2006) Adjunctive therapy with low-molecular-weight heparin in patients with chronic heart failure secondary to dilated cardiomyopathy: one-year follow-up results of the randomized trial. *Am Heart J,* 152, 713.e1-7.
[http://dx.doi.org/10.1016/j.ahj.2006.06.028] [PMID: 16996844]

World Health Organization. (2020) . Clinical management of severe acute respiratory infection when novel coronavirus (2019-nCoV) infection is suspected: interim guidance, 28 January 2020. World Health Organization. (2020) https://apps.who.int/iris/handle/10665/330893

Wu, Z & McGoogan, JM (2020) Characteristics of and important lessons from the coronavirus disease 2019 (COVID-19) outbreak in China: summary of a report of 72 314 cases from the Chinese Center for Disease Control and Prevention. *JAMA,* 323, 1239-42.
[http://dx.doi.org/10.1001/jama.2020.2648] [PMID: 32091533]

Xiong, TY, Redwood, S, Prendergast, B & Chen, M (2020) Coronaviruses and the cardiovascular system: acute and long-term implications. *Eur Heart J,* 41, 1798-800.
[http://dx.doi.org/10.1093/eurheartj/ehaa231] [PMID: 32186331]

Xu, J, Zhang, X, Pelayo, R, Monestier, M, Ammollo, CT, Semeraro, F, Taylor, FB, Esmon, NL, Lupu, F & Esmon, CT (2009) Extracellular histones are major mediators of death in sepsis. *Nat Med,* 15, 1318-21. [http://dx.doi.org/10.1038/nm.2053] [PMID: 19855397]

Ye, Z, Wang, Y, Colunga-Lozano, LE, Prasad, M, Tangamornsuksan, W, Rochwerg, B, Yao, L, Motaghi, S, Couban, RJ, Ghadimi, M, Bala, MM, Gomaa, H, Fang, F, Xiao, Y & Guyatt, GH (2020) Efficacy and safety of corticosteroids in COVID-19 based on evidence for COVID-19, other coronavirus infections, influenza, community-acquired pneumonia and acute respiratory distress syndrome: a systematic review and meta-analysis. *CMAJ,* 192, E756-67.
[http://dx.doi.org/10.1503/cmaj.200645] [PMID: 32409522]

Young, E (2008) The anti-inflammatory effects of heparin and related compounds. *Thromb Res,* 122, 743-52. [http://dx.doi.org/10.1016/j.thromres.2006.10.026] [PMID: 17727922]

Zhang, JS, Chen, JT, Liu, YX, Zhang, ZS, Gao, H, Liu, Y, Wang, X, Ning, Y, Liu, YF, Gao, Q, Xu, JG, Qin, C, Dong, XP & Yin, WD (2005) A serological survey on neutralizing antibody titer of SARS convalescent sera. *J Med Virol,* 77, 147-50.
[http://dx.doi.org/10.1002/jmv.20431] [PMID: 16121363]

Zhang, Y, Xiao, M, Zhang, S, Xia, P, Cao, W, Jiang, W, Chen, H, Ding, X, Zhao, H, Zhang, H, Wang, C, Zhao, J, Sun, X, Tian, R, Wu, W, Wu, D, Ma, J, Chen, Y, Zhang, D, Xie, J, Yan, X, Zhou, X, Liu, Z, Wang, J, Du, B, Qin, Y, Gao, P, Qin, X, Xu, Y, Zhang, W, Li, T, Zhang, F, Zhao, Y, Li, Y & Zhang, S (2020) Coagulopathy and antiphospholipid antibodies in patients with COVID-19. *N Engl J Med,* 382e38 [http://dx.doi.org/10.1056/NEJMc2007575] [PMID: 32268022]

Zhou, D, Dai, SM & Tong, Q (2020) COVID-19: a recommendation to examine the effect of hydroxychloroquine in preventing infection and progression. *J Antimicrob Chemother,* 75, 1667-70. [http://dx.doi.org/10.1093/jac/dkaa114] [PMID: 32196083]

Zhou, F, Yu, T, Du, R, Fan, G, Liu, Y, Liu, Z, Xiang, J, Wang, Y, Song, B, Gu, X, Guan, L, Wei, Y, Li, H, Wu, X, Xu, J, Tu, S, Zhang, Y, Chen, H & Cao, B (2020) Clinical course and risk factors for mortality of adult inpatients with COVID-19 in Wuhan, China: a retrospective cohort study. *Lancet,* 395, 1054-62. [http://dx.doi.org/10.1016/S0140-6736(20)30566-3] [PMID: 32171076]

Zhu, C, Liang, Y, Li, X, Chen, N & Ma, X (2019) Unfractionated heparin attenuates histone-mediated cytotoxicity *in vitro* and prevents intestinal microcirculatory dysfunction in histone-infused rats. *J Trauma Acute Care Surg,* 87, 614-22.
[http://dx.doi.org/10.1097/TA.0000000000002387] [PMID: 31454337]

# CHAPTER 16

# Principles of Vaccination: Will it be the Definitive Solution?

**Abstract:** Vaccination immunity is vital to prevent widespread viral infection and reduce morbidity and mortality. Patients with COVID-19 infection develop a polyclonal active immune response to viral antigens. Antibodies that develop as a result of this polyclonal immunity can neutralize the virus and prevent further infection in the recovered host. The magnitude and duration of protection of a vaccine administered to humans in society cannot be the same for every individual. The acquisition of immunity depends on the functioning of the person's own immune system. Therefore, a vaccine in the population is never 100 % protective. There are expectations that the COVID-19 vaccine should have at least a 50% protection rate. Vaccine development stages also require a process that can take years; therefore, the public will probably hardly reach a vaccine that is safe and economical for public use in the near future. The global medical community should search for effective ways to provide vaccination be easily reached by vulnerable groups all over the world in order to secure healthy new generations.

**Keywords:** COVID-19, Management, Vaccination, Vaccination immunity.

## IS VACCINATION THE DEFINITIVE SOLUTION TO PANDEMICS?

Mostly yes. COVID-19 poses a major threat to public health around the world. It is highly contagious, and most individuals in the community are susceptible to infection. For the prevention, control, and critical management of this severe epidemic, strict precautions should be taken along with updated treatment guidelines. The most important of these measures is to provide vaccine immunity. Vaccination immunity is vital to prevent widespread viral infection and reduce morbidity and mortality. Patients with COVID-19 infection develop a polyclonal active immune response to viral antigens. Antibodies that develop as a result of this polyclonal immunity can neutralize the virus and prevent further infection in the recovered host (Chan *et al.*, 2020). The magnitude and duration of protection of a vaccine administered to humans in society cannot be the same for every individual. Acquisition of immunity depends on the functioning of the person's own immune system. Therefore, a vaccine in the population is never 100 percent

**Ozgur KARCIOGLU, Selman YENIOCAK and Mandana HOSSEINZADEH**

protective. There are expectations that the COVID-19 vaccine should have at least a 50% protection rate (FDA).

## DOES IT TAKE LONG TO DEVELOP THE COVID-19 VACCINE?

Yes, it takes years to develop the simplest vaccine and make it ready for use. For example, a long period of 14 to 16 years has passed from the first trial to the end of the licensing phase for HPV and rotavirus vaccines (Douglas *et al.*, 2018).

An examination of the history of vaccine development depicts that even in diseases afflicting populations *en masse*, vaccines were found after many years, and they were never found in many important diseases such as AIDS, Ebolavirus, SARS, and MERS. (Strugnell *et al.*, 2011).

Currently, no vaccine that can provide immunity against the COVID-19 pandemic has yet been developed. Worldwide studies in this field continue at a great pace. Thanks to the fact that the vaccine development studies initiated for the SARS epidemic, which was also a coronavirus in 2003, could be quickly adapted to COVID-19, it was possible to go from the preclinical stage to the first trial in humans in a record few months in COVID-19 vaccine studies (Kim *et al.*, 2020). Vaccine development stages also require a process that can continue for years. The stages of vaccine development are depicted in Table **1** (Dandan *et al.*, 2017).

## AGAINST WHICH PART OF THE SARS-COV-2 STRUCTURE ARE VACCINES DEVELOPED?

In Stage I, which is the first stage in the vaccine development process, the essential step is to recognize the structure of the virus in an in-vitro environment in order to determine which part of the CoV vaccine should be developed during the experimental laboratory studies. Similar to other microorganisms, it is necessary to obtain strains that will damage or change their antigenic structures while developing vaccines against SARS-CoV-2 (Dandan *et al.*, 2017).

### Structure of CoV

The virion particle of SARS-CoV-2, which is a β CoV and whose subgroup members are also present, is typically round or polymorphous, with a diameter of 60-140 nm and a single-stranded RNA genome (Zhou *et al.*, 2020). Along with the Spike (S) protein, which is a common feature of CoVs, their genomes encode three additional structural proteins, including Membrane (M) protein, Envelope (E) protein, and Nucleocapsid (N) protein. The binding of the SARS-CoV-2 S protein to the cell surface receptor via ACE2 initiates viral entry into lung type II pneumocytes (Li, 2016). This is why the S protein plays a central role in the initial transmission and ongoing infection of COVID-19. The CoV S protein contains two main domains: The S1 domain at the N-terminus of the protein mediates binding to ACE2. The C-terminal S2 domain supports the fusion of the virus membrane with the cellular membrane of the host cell. Therefore, vaccines based on S protein can induce antibodies to block virus binding and fusion, thereby neutralizing virus infection (Huang *et al.*, 2020; Ji *et al.*, 2020). The S protein is one of the most important antigenic components of coronavirus structural proteins as it can induce both host immune responses and neutralizing antibodies. Therefore, it has been chosen as a promising target for the vaccine (He *et al.*, 2005).

**Table 1. Stages of vaccine development.**

| | | | |
|---|---|---|---|
| **Stage I** (Experimental laboratory studies, viral recognition, in-vitro tests) | | It is the stage of production of strains and antigens that can be used in vaccine production against the targeted agent. By using vaccine formulations, strains, and antigens to be used in vaccines are produced in accordance with international standards. | 2 years |
| **Stage II** (Animal experiments, pre-clinical analyses) These studies are conducted with the permission of animal ethics committees. | | Pre-clinical animal experiments are conducted. If positive data are obtained in this phase, the studies are continued with Phase I studies. | 1-2 years |
| **Stage III** These studies are carried out with the permission of the Ministry of Health and human ethics committees. | **Phase I** | In this phase, the reliability and immunity status of the vaccine are assessed. | Several months-1 year |
| | **Phase II** | In addition to Phase I, the effectiveness and optimal dose of the vaccine are evaluated. | 1–2 years |
| | **Phase III** | In addition to Phase II, the efficacy of the vaccine against the disease is determined. | 3–5 years |
| **Permit and Licensing** | | Formal procedures vary with the countries and states. | |
| **Post-Marketing evaluations (Phase IV)** | | Once vaccines are licensed and launched on the market, surveillance studies are conducted to monitor vaccine safety and efficacy in larger populations. | No predefined period |

Although COVID-19 is lower than SARS around 10% and MERS with a case fatality rate of approximately 3% to 4%, its pandemic severity is much higher; It has 3 and 10-times higher contagiousness than SARS-CoV and MERS, respectively (WHO, 2020). Droplet and direct contact are the main routes of transmission of SARS-CoV-2 from person to person. Aerosol and fecal-oral transmissions are other potential routes of transmission that have not yet been confirmed (GONHC of the PRC, Version 5, 2020).

## POTENTIAL VACCINE INITIATIVES THAT CAN BE DEVELOPED AGAINST COVID-19

Vaccines are typically divided into different types: inactivated, live attenuated, vectored, nucleic acid-based and recombinant subunit vaccines (Gao *et al.*, 2019). Live attenuated vaccines are derived from microbial agents attenuated by physical, chemical, or biological means under laboratory conditions (Badgett *et al.*, 2002). Codagenix (USA) has formed a collaboration with the Serum Institute of India to develop a rationally designed live attenuated vaccine synthesized by viral codon deoptimization against SARS-CoV-2 (Chen *et al.*, 2020).

Vectored vaccines are those that use other viruses as vectors for SARS-CoV-2 proteins. Scientists from Rocky Mountain Laboratories (USA) and Oxford University (England) are collaborating to develop a chimpanzee adenovirus vectored vaccine against SARS-CoV-2. Similarly, Zydus Cadila, an India-based pharmaceutical company, launched a program to develop a vectored vaccine for the novel coronavirus SARS-CoV-2 using live attenuated recombinant measles virus (rMV) (Shi *et al.*, 2020).

Injection of nucleic acid constructs capable of expressing viral or bacterial genes can cause activation of both humoral and cellular immune responses. Clover Biopharmaceuticals (Chengdu, China) initiated the development of a recombinant subunit vaccine for SARS-CoV-2 using S protein subunit trimer antigens (Salvatori *et al.*, 2020). Zydus Cadila has a program to develop a DNA vaccine against the main viral membrane S protein responsible for cell entry of SARS-CoV-2. After plasmid DNA is introduced into host cells, it will be translated into viral protein and elicit immune responses. This provides protection from infection and can lead to viral clearance. (Shi *et al.*, 2020). Inovio Pharmaceuticals (USA) is currently collaborating with Beijing Advaccine Biotechnology Company (China) to advance the development of INO-4800 as a vaccine candidate targeting SARS-CoV-2. This vaccine is currently in phase I and is undergoing pre-clinical testing (Chen *et al.*, 2020). The subsidiary of Applied DNA Sciences (New York, USA), LineaRx (New York, USA) and Takis Biotech (Rome, Italy) are developing a linear DNA vaccine for SARS-CoV-2 using PCR-based DNA generation technology. In addition, Moderna (USA) is developing a messenger RNA (mRNA) vaccine against SARS-CoV-2, which encodes the viral S protein in collaboration with the National Institutes of Health (USA) (Shi *et al.*, 2020).

### Recombinant DNA Approaches to Vaccine Antigens:

Protein antigens are produced using recombinant DNA technology, where the DNA sequence coding for the antigenic protein is inserted into an expression system that is then able to produce large quantities of that specific antigen in vitro or following administration to the host, *e.g.*, using a DNA plasmid or a live vaccine vector (panel C) as the expression system. (Adapted from Strugnell *et al.*, 2011).

Some centers are currently trying to develop various types of vaccines against SARS-CoV-2 and some features of these vaccine types are shown in Table **2**.

**Table 2. Advantages and disadvantages of vaccines to be developed against the COVID-19 pandemic.**

| Vaccine | Advantages | Disadvantages |
|---|---|---|
| **Live attenuated vaccine** | • It has a unique ability to stimulate the immune system by inducing toll-like receptors (TLR) such as TLR 3, TLR 7/8 and TLR 9 of the innate immune system, which includes B cells, CD4 and CD8 T cells.<br>• It can be derived from cold-adapted virus strains, reclassifiers and reverse genetics. | • Live attenuated vaccines require extensive accessory testing to ensure safety and efficacy.<br>• During viral replication, there is a possibility of substituting nucleotides, resulting in post-vaccination recombinants. |
| **Inactive Virus vaccines** | • It is more stable and safer than live attenuated vaccines.<br>• The technology and infrastructure required for its development is already present.<br>• Tested for SARS-CoV and a variety of other diseases.<br>• Can be used with adjuvants to increase their immunogenicity. | Additional vaccinations (rapel) are required to maintain immunity status.<br>• Large quantities of viruses must be processed, and the integrity of immunogenic particles should be preserved. |
| **Recombinant vaccines** | • No exposure to any live elements of the viral particles.<br>• It is safe with less side effects. | • Future responses and efficacy are unknown. |
| **Viral vector-based vaccines** | • It shows a highly specific gene transfer to the host cell with a strong immune response.<br>• It prevents the transport of any infectious particles and has been widely used for MERS-CoV with favorable results from studies. | • The host may have immunity to the vector due to prior exposure, which reduces efficiency.<br>• Can trigger carcinogenesis due to integration of the viral genome into the host genome. |

*(Table 2) cont.....*

| Vaccine | | Advantages | Disadvantages |
|---|---|---|---|
| **Nucleic acid-based vaccines** | **DNA vaccines** | • Synthetic DNA is temperature-resistant and free of cold chains<br>• It can be developed at an accelerated time.<br>• Does not require processing of infectious viral particle. | • Although it provides both cellular and humoral immunity, the titers may remain low.<br>• Insertion of foreign DNA into the host genome may cause abnormalities in the cell.<br>• May cause antibody production against itself. |
| | **RNA vaccines** | • Translation of mRNA occurs in the cytosol of the host cell and avoids any risk of integration into the host genome. | • Safety issues related to reactogenicity have been reported for a variety of RNA-based vaccines. |

Different types and rates of vaccines that are being developed against COVID-19 are shown in Fig. (**1**).

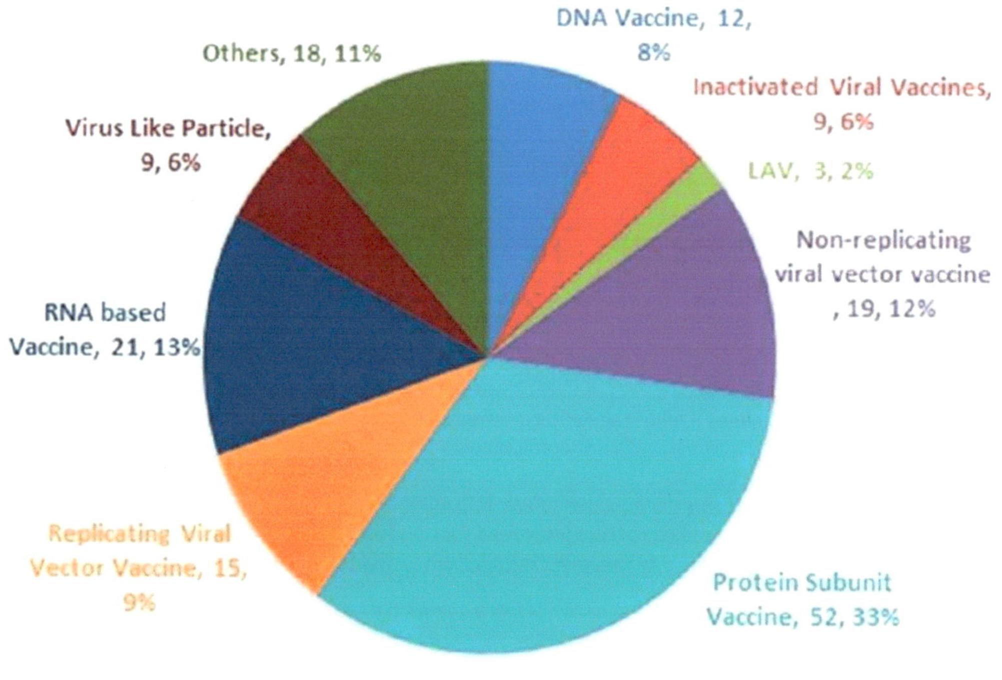


**Fig. (1).** The percentages of the COVID-19 vaccines that are in the stage of development in accord with their biological structures (Kaur *et al.*, 2020).

Immunotherapy appears to be an effective method for the prophylaxis and treatment of various infectious diseases and cancers, which includes artificial triggering of the immune system to elicit the immune response (Masihi *et al.*,

2001). The latest developments as of September 2020 in the status of some vaccines that are being developed to provide active immunity in COVID-19 pandemic immunotherapy and are close to the end are shown in Table **3**.

**Table 3. Recent developments in the status of some vaccines that are being developed and are nearing completion for the COVID-19 outbreak.**

| Vaccine | Producer | Evaluation - Notes | Stages of Clinical Trials |
|---|---|---|---|
| BNT162 (Kaur *et al.*, 2020) | BioNTech / Fosun Pharma / Pfizer | BNT162b1, the mRNA-based vaccine, induced high dose-dependent nAb titers along with RBD-binding IgG concentrations after the second dose. This was accompanied by CD4 + and CD8 + T cell responses. Vaccine administration precipitated nonsevere adverse effects such as fatigue, fever, chills, muscle pain *etc.* | Phase 3: NCT04368728 |
| ChAdOx1 (Folegatti *et al.*, 2020) | Oxford University / AstraZeneca | Preliminary reports of phase 1-2, single-blind, randomized controlled trials of the ChAdOx1 vaccine showed spike-specific T cell responses with anti-spike IgG response in 91% of participants. The neutralization assay (MNA80), a plaque reduction neutralization assay (PRNT50) showed 100% response after a single dose. However, antibodies were seen in all participants who had a significant correlation with the neutralizing antibody titers measured by ELISA. Volunteers reported local and systemic reactions which were minimized by paracetamol administration. Therefore, the vaccine candidate demonstrated an adequate safety and immunogenicity profile in phase 1 and 2 clinical trials. | Phase 3: ISRCTN89951424 |
| mRNA-1273 (Jackson *et al.*, 2020) | Moderna / NIAID | The geometric mean of RBD-specific antibody titers increased rapidly in all participants. Seroconversion was observed after 15 days and the median magnitude of antibody responses was similar to those in recovering sera. However, the pseudovirus neutralizing activity was not adequate prior to the administration of the second dose, which indicated the need for a two-dose vaccination schedule. In addition, serum neutralizing activity, which is a generally accepted functional biomarker of in vivo humoral response to respiratory viruses, has not been determined at this time. | Phase 3: NCT04470427 |

*(Table 3) cont.....*

| Vaccine | Producer | Evaluation - Notes | Stages of Clinical Trials |
|---|---|---|---|
| PiCoVacc (Kaur *et al.*, 2020) | Sinovac | Phase 1-2 clinical trials of the inactivated viral vaccine PiCoVacc showed that the vaccine induced neutralizing antibodies with a seroconversion rate of 90% on a 0-14-day schedule. Preliminary results confirmed that there were no adverse systemic or local events post-vaccination.<br>Phase 2 clinical trials are expected to be completed by the end of 2020. The company obtained permission to conduct phase 3 clinical trials in Brazil in collaboration with Instituto Bhutantan. Moreover, it is expected to gain further approvals for phase 3 clinical trials in Bangladesh. | Phase 3: NCT04456595 |
| Adenovirus Type 5 Vector / nonreplicable viral vaccine (Zhu *et al.*, 2020) | CanSino Biological Inc. / Beijing Institute of Biotechnology | Randomized, double-blind, placebo-controlled phase 2 clinical trials of recombinant Ad5-vectored vaccine proved a positive cellular response in $5 \times 10^{10}$ viral particles with seroconversion of the humoral immune response. Severe adverse events were reported in 9% of individuals in the $1 \times 10^{11}$ viral particles dose group, and 1% of the volunteers exhibited these side effects in the $5 \times 10^{10}$ viral particles dose group. | Phase 2: ChiCTR2000031781 |
| BBV152 (AC) (Myupchar, 2020) | Bharat Biotech/ ICMR/ NIV | It is a fully virion-inactivated experimental vaccine under Phase 1-2 clinical trials. These trials are expected to highlight safety and reactogenicity, tolerability and immunogenicity in healthy volunteers. The inactivated vaccine will be administered intramuscularly in two doses on day 0 and day 14, and 1125 volunteers will be observed for the next 6 months and evaluated for immune responses after vaccination. For vaccine development, the viral strain was isolated by the ICMR and transferred to Bharat Biotech, where the inactivation process was conducted at a BSL-3 facility. | Phase 1-2: NCT04471519 |
| ZyCoV-D (CTRI/ 2020/07/026352, 2020; Myupchar, 2020) | Zydus Cadila | ZyCoV-D is a genetically engineered DNA plasmid-based vaccine that encodes the membrane proteins of the virus. In clinical studies designed to examine the immunogenicity and safety of the vaccine, 1048 individuals will receive three doses at 28-day intervals. | Phase 1-2: CTRI / 2020/07/026352 |

## SOME TYPES OF VACCINES BEING DEVELOPED AGAINST SARS-COV-2

### 1. Protein Subunit (Subunit) Vaccines

It is a type of vaccine based on synthetic peptides or recombinant antigenic proteins required to provide long-term protective and / or therapeutic immunity (Ning *et al.*, 2020). These vaccines trigger low immunogenicity and require the support of an adjuvant to potentiate the vaccine-induced immune reactions. An adjuvant can increase the biological half-life of the antigenic material or improve the immunomodulatory cytokine response. Therefore, the addition of an adjuvant helps to overcome the deficiencies of protein subunit vaccines (Cao *et al.*, 2018).

Consisting of S1 and S2 subunits of SARS-CoV-2, the S protein is the most suitable antigen to induce neutralizing antibodies against the pathogen (Ou *et al.*, 2020). SARS-CoV-2 binds to the ACE2 receptor through the spike (S) protein and enters the cell through endocytosis. Therefore, the S protein and its antigenic fragments are the main targets of protein subunit vaccines (Ning *et al.*, 2020). S glycoprotein is a dynamic protein with pre- and post-fusion states. Therefore, the antigen must preserve the surface chemistry and the original prefusion S protein profile to preserve epitopes to fire good quality antibody responses (Graham *et al.*, 2020).

**NVX-CoV2373 (Novavax, Inc. | Emergent BioSolutions):** NVX-CoV2373 is a nanoparticle-based immunogenic vaccine based on recombinant expression of the stable pre-fusion CoV S-protein (Coleman *et al.*, 2020). The manufacturer plans to use Matrix-M adjuvant to increase the immune response to the SARS-CoV-2 S protein through induction of high levels of neutralizing antibodies. In animal models, a single vaccination has been reported to produce high levels of anti-S protein antibodies that block the human ACE2 receptor binding site and can elicit SARS-CoV-2 neutralizing antibodies (Novavax covid 19 vaccine trial, 2020).

**Molecular Clamp Stabilized S protein vaccine:** It is developed by Queensland University in collaboration with GSK and Dynavax. The University stated that it is believed to be able to access the vaccine adjuvant platform technology (AS03 Adjuvant system), enhance the vaccine response and minimize the amount of vaccine required per dose (Lee, 2020). The university reported that it is developing a stabilized prefusion, recombinant viral protein subunit vaccine based on Molecular Clamp technology, and this technology has proven to induce neutralizing antibody production (Tu *et al.*, 2020).

**PittCoVacc (University of Pittsburgh):** It is a "Microneedle Array (MNA)" based recombinant SARS-CoV-2 vaccine that involves administration of recombinant immunogens rSARS-CoV-2 S1 and rSARS-CoV-2-S1fRS09. A significant increase in antigen-specific antibodies with statistical significance was observed in pre-clinical trials at the end of two weeks in mouse models. Statistically significant antibody titers in the early stages, as well as prior to augmentation, have been cited to support applicability of the MNA-SARS-CoV-2 vaccine (Kim, 2020).

**Triple Antigen Vaccine (Premas Biotech, India):** It is a multiple antigenic VLP vaccine prototype in which the recombinant spike tip, membrane and envelope protein of SARS-CoV-2 are co-expressed in a predesigned Saccharomyces cerevisiae expression platform (D-Crypt ™). This prototype is thought to have the potential to enter pre-clinical trials as a vaccine candidate after further research and development and is considered safe and easy to mass-produce in a cost-effective manner (Arora *et al.*, 2020).

**2. Viral Vectored Vaccines**

It consists of non-pathogenic or genetically modified viruses that can express one or more protective genes of a different virus. They provide effective immunity with a high reliability by stimulating the humoral and cellular response for a long time. These vaccines are highly specific in delivering genes to target cells. It is highly effective in gene transduction and strongly induces the immune response (Ura *et al.*, 2014). Due to their long-term and high level of antigenic protein expression, these vaccines have been reported to induce cytotoxic T cells (CTL) leading to the elimination of virus-infected cells and have considerable potential for prophylactic use (Le *et al.*, 2020).

**Ad5-nCoV (CanSino Biologics Inc / Beijing Institute of Biotechnology):** The S protein recombinant of SARS-CoV-2 is a replication-defective adenovirus type-5 vector (Ad5). The plasminogen activator signal in the Ad5 vector lacking the E1 and E3 genes was prepared by cloning an optimized full-length gene of the S protein together with the peptide gene. Phase I clinical trials elicited a positive antibody response. A four-fold increase in NEA for neutralizing antibodies specific for RBD and S protein was noted within 14 days after inoculation and peaked on day 28 post-vaccination. In addition, CD4 + T cells and CD8 + T cells response peaked on day 14 post inoculation. However, pre-existing anti-Ad5 immunity partially limited both antibody and T cell responses (Zhu *et al.*, 2020). The study reported that, with follow-up 3 and 6 months after vaccination, it will further evaluate antibody response in recipients aged 18 to 60 years and receiving one of three study doses (Kaur *et al.*, 2020).

**Coroflu (University of Wisconsin-Madison / FluGen / Bharat Biotech):** It is a M2SR vaccine, a self-limiting version of the influenza virus modified by the addition of the SARS-CoV-2 gene sequence of the S protein. This vaccine also expresses the hemagglutinin protein of the influenza virus; thus, inducing an immune response against both viruses. M2SR is self-limited and does not replicate as it lacks the M2 gene. It enters the cell and triggers immunity against the virus. It is planned to be administered into the nose to mimic the natural path of viral infection. The intranasal route of administration activates various modes of the immune system and has higher immunogenicity compared to intramuscular injections (Kaur *et al.*, 2020).

**LV-SMENP-DC (Shenzhen Geno-Immune Medical Institute):** It is prepared by engineering dendritic cells (DC) with a lentiviral vector expressing conserved domains of SARS-CoV-2 structural proteins and protease using SMENP minigenes. SC administration of the vaccine presents antigens on antigen presenting cells (APCs), and ultimately activates cytotoxic T cells and generates an immune response (Le *et al.*, 2020).

**ChAdOx1 (Oxford University):** The ChAdOx1 recombinant adenovirus vaccine was developed using the codon-optimized S glycoprotein and synthesized with the tissue plasminogen activator (tPA) leader sequence at the 5' end. The SARS-CoV-2 coding sequence for amino acids and the tPA leader was amplified in the shuttle plasmid. This shuttle plasmid is responsible for encoding the major early genes of human cytomegalovirus (CMV) together with the polyadenylation signal from bovine growth hormone (BGH) between the tetracycline operator (TetO) regions and the Gateway® recombination cloning site. The adenovirus vector genome is created in the Bacterial Artificial Chromosome by inserting the SARS-CoV-2 S gene into the E1 locus of the ChAdOx1 adenovirus genome. The virus was then allowed to grow in T-Rex 293 HEK (Human Embryonic Kidney 293) cell lines and purified by CsCl gradient ultracentrifugation. In preclinical studies, the absence of any sub-genomic RNA (sgRNA) in intramuscularly vaccinated animals is indicative of increased immunity to the virus (Doremalen *et al.*, 2020). The vaccine has entered phase II clinical trials where it will be evaluated in a large sample of the population (Kaur *et al.*, 2020).

## 3. MRNA Vaccines

In recent months, some work has been done on non-replicating RNA and virus derived self-replicating RNAs. In these studies, the immunogenicity of mRNA can be minimized, and changes can be made to increase the stability of these vaccines. Also, since mRNA is the minimal immunogenic genetic vector, it allows repeated administration of the vaccine, so anti-vector immunity is avoided (Cuiling *et al.*, 2020) . This platform has strengthened the rapid vaccine development program due to its flexibility and ability to mimic the antigen structure and expression seen during a natural infection (Mulligan *et al.*, 2020).

**mRNA-1273 (Moderna TX, Inc):** It is a vaccine consisting of synthetic mRNA encapsulated in Lipid nanoparticle (LNP) encoding the full-length, pre-fusion stabilized S protein of SARS-CoV-2. It has the potential to elicit a potent antiviral response specific to the S-protein. It is considered to be relatively safe since it does not use any of the inactivated pathogen or subunits of the living pathogen in its construction (Tu *et al.*, 2020). The vaccine received rapid approval from the FDA to run phase II studies (Kaur *et al.*, 2020). The manufacturer published phase I interim data on antibodies of 8 participants who received various doses, and participants of the 25 μg dose group exhibited comparable results with healing sera. Meanwhile, NEA for nAb levels of participants receiving the 100 μg dose, exceeded the levels found in healing sera. While the vaccine appeared to be predominantly safe and well tolerated in the 25 μg and 100 μg dose cohorts, three participants were reported to experience “grade 3 systemic symptoms” after administration of the second shots of 250 μg dose levels (Kaur *et al.*, 2020).

**BNT162b1 (BioNTech / FosunPharma / Pfizer):** BNT162b1 is a codon-optimized mRNA vaccine encoding trimerized SARS-CoV-2 RBD, a critical target of the nAb virus. The vaccine exhibits increased immunogenicity due to the addition of the T4 fibritin-derived foldon trimerization domain to the RBD antigen. The mRNA is encapsulated in 80 nm ionizable cationic lipid nanoparticles that ensure its efficient transmission. Phase 1-2 clinical trials revealed that high RBD-specific IgG antibody levels were as high as 8 to 46.3 times the geometric mean concentration of the recovery serum. Whereas the geometric mean titers of SARS-CoV-2 neutralizing antibodies were found to be 1.8 to 2.8 times the healing serum panel. No serious side effects were seen; however, transient local reactions and systemic events have been observed (Mulligan *et al.*, 2020).

## 4. DNA Vaccines

The most innovative approach to vaccination is the introduction of a DNA vaccine encoding the antigen and an adjuvant that induces an adaptive immune response. Transfected cells express the transgene that provides transgene-specific proteins that are highly similar to the live virus. The antigenic material is taken up by endocytosis by immature dendritic cells that ultimately present the antigen to CD4 + and CD8 + T cells in conjunction with MHC-2 and MHC-1 antigens on the cell surface. Thus, it stimulates effective humoral and cellular immune responses (Hobernik *et al.*, 2018).

**INO-4800 (Inovio Pharmaceuticals):** It is a prophylactic DNA vaccine against SARS-CoV-2 (Kaur *et al.*, 2020). It uses the codon-optimized S protein sequence to which the IgE leader sequence of SARS-CoV-2 is attached. SARS-CoV-2 IgE-spike sequence was synthesized and digested using BamHI and XhoI. Digested DNA was incorporated into expression plasmid pGX0001 under the direction of the IE CMV and BGH polyadenylation signal. The presence of functional antibodies and T cell reaction in preclinical studies suggest that the vaccine can produce an effective immune response within 7 days after vaccination (Smith *et al.*, 2020). The vaccine entered Phase I clinical trials (Phase I: CT04336410). Participants received 1.0 mg of INO-4800 by electroporation using the CELLECTRA® 2000 device per dosing visit. At the end of the trial period, the immunological profile, safety, and tolerability of the vaccine candidate on intradermal injection and electroporation in healthy adults will be evaluated (Kaur *et al.*, 2020).

## 5. Attenuated Live Vaccines

It is produced by reducing the ability of viruses to cause disease without changing their immune ability. These vaccines stimulate the immune system (lymphoid and myeloid cells) in the body. It is derived from microbial agents attenuated by physical, chemical, or biological means under laboratory conditions (Badgett *et al.*, 2002).

**DelNS1-SARS-CoV2-RBD (University of Hong Kong):** This vaccine is an influenza-based vaccine strain with a deletion in the NS1 gene. It is rearranged to express the RBD domain of the SARS-CoV-2 S protein on its surface and grown in chick embryo and / or Madin Darby Canine Kidney Cells (MDCK) cells. It is potentially more immunogenic than natural-type influenza virus and can be administered as a nasal spray (Kaur *et al.*, 2020).

## 6. Other Vaccines

The uncovering of the structure and genome of SARS-CoV-2 has led to the rapid development of various vaccine candidates with potential immunogenicity as well as adverse reactogenicity. Various biotechnology initiatives are used to develop vaccines. British and American Tobacco Company (BAT) has recently developed the COVID-19 vaccine using the new and fast-growing tobacco plant technology, and Tianjin University produced an oral vaccine which successfully uses Saccharomyces cerevisiae (Kaur *et al.*, 2020).

**Self-Assembling Vaccine (HaloVax):** The vaccine uses a heat shock protein (HSP) to activate the immune system. It consists of a fusion protein sandwiched between a HSP and Avidin. Biotinated immunogenic peptides can also be added to customize the vaccine (Voltron Therapeutics, Inc, 2020)

## PUBLISHED INTERIM RESULTS OF PHASE 3 CLINICAL STUDIES OF SOME VACCINES DEVELOPED AGAINST SARS-COV-2

### 1. BNT162b2 mRNA COVID-19 Vaccine Phase 3 Safety and Efficacy Analysis Results

Phase 3 safety and efficacy analysis of BNT162b2 mRNA Covid-19 vaccine was erformed via an ongoing multinational, placebo-controlled, observer-blind trial with, 43,548 participants aged 16 and over (randomized at a 1: 1 ratio). In this study, two doses of 30 μg each dose were administered 21 days apart, the control group was given a placebo injection, and the BNT162b2 vaccine was administered to the vaccine group, and the data obtained were shared with the public (Polack *et al.*, 2020). Within the scope of the study, 9 COVID-19 cases were identified among the vaccine group participants, one of which started one day after the first dose, 8 started at least 7 days after the second dose; and 171 among the control group participants; 9 started after the first dose and 162 at least 7 days after the second dose. The BNT162b2 vaccine was found to be 95% effective in preventing COVID-19 (95% Cl; 90.3 – 97.6). Similar vaccine efficacy (usually 90 to 100%) was observed in subgroups defined by age, sex, race, ethnicity, baseline body mass index, and presence of comorbid diseases. The incidence of serious side effects was found to be low and similar in vaccine and control groups. The safety profile of the BNT162b2 vaccine has been characterized by short duration, mild / moderate pain at the injection site, fatigue, and headache.

In brief, a two-dose BNT162b2 vaccine has been reported to provide 95% protection against COVID-19 in individuals aged 16 and over, its safety for an average of two months, similar to other viral vaccines.

### 2. Results of Phase 3 Safety and Efficacy Analysis of ChAdOx1 nCoV-19 Vaccine

Phase 3 safety and efficacy analysis of the ChAdOx1 nCoV-19 vaccine includes data from four ongoing single-blind, randomized, controlled trials in the United Kingdom, Brazil, and South Africa (Folegatti *et al.*, 2020). Participants aged 18 and over were randomized to the vaccine and control group with a 1: 1 ratio (meningococcal group A, C, W, and Y conjugated vaccine or saline). Participants in the vaccine group received two doses containing 5 x 10 μl of viral particles (standard dose; SD / SD cohort). A subset in the UK trial received a standard dose with their first dose as half dose (low dose) and second doses (LD / SD cohort). The primary efficacy analysis included nucleic acid amplification test positive symptomatic COVID-19 in seronegative participants 14 days after a second dose of vaccine. Participants were analyzed for treatment received up to the data cut-off date on November 4, 2020. Vaccine efficacy was calculated as 1− relative risk derived from a strong age-adjusted Poisson regression model.

A total of 23848 participants were enrolled in the study between 23 April and 4 November 2020, and 11636 participants (7548 in the UK, 4088 in Brazil) were included in the interim primary efficacy analysis. The vaccine efficacy was 62.1% in participants who received two standard doses, and 90.0% in participants who received the low dose and then the standard dose (the overall vaccine efficiency was 70.4%). 21 days after the first dose, 10 in the control group were hospitalized due to COVID-19; 2 are classified as severe COVID-19, and one patient died. 175 serious side effects were observed in a month in 168 participants; 84 of which occurred in the vaccine group and 91 in the control group.

This interim analysis of ongoing clinical trials concluded that the ChAdOx1 nCoV-19 vaccine has an effective and acceptable safety profile against COVID-19.

## WILL THE SARS-COV-2 VIRUS VACCINE BE ABLE TO EFFECTIVELY PROTECT US AGAINST THE EPIDEMIC? IF SO, HOW LONG WILL IT PROTECT?

It is still unclear whether infection with SARS-CoV-2 in humans protects from reinfection and how long it will protect it if it does.

Protection for any viral infection usually relies on a certain level of antibodies acquired through vaccination or natural infection, which significantly reduces the risk of reinfection. For example, a hemagglutination inhibition titer of 1:40 for influenza virus reduces the risk of infection by 50% (Krammer *et al.*, 2020). Similar titers have been established for measles virus (an ID 50 titer of 1: 120), hepatitis A virus, hepatitis B virus, and others (Plotkin *et al.*, 2010). These titers guided and facilitated vaccine development. For some viruses and vaccines, the kinetics of the antibody response is also highlighted and allows a precise prediction of how long protection will last (Herc *et al.*, 2001).

In studies on COVID-19 patients, it is proven that neutralizing antibodies are induced, and these antibodies can last for years and can protect against re-infection or alleviate the disease in case of reinfection (Huang *et al.*, 2020). In primate models, infection with SARS-CoV-2 protects from reinfection, at least for some time (Deng *et al.*, 2020; Chandrashekar *et al.*, 2020). In addition, an experimental study showed that transferring animal serum infected with SARS-CoV-2 and recovered to non-infected animals can be protective and significantly reduces viral replication in case of infection with this virus (Imai *et al.*, 2020).

In a study conducted in New York, based on a dataset of 30,082 people screened at Mount Sinai Health System, the vast majority of infected individuals with mild to moderate COVID-19 developed strong IgG antibodies to the viral S protein for at least about 5 months. (Wajnberg *et al.*, 2020). The data of this study disclosed that over 90% of seroconverters elicit detectable neutralizing antibody responses. These titers remained relatively constant over several months after infection.

## CONCLUSION

In conclusion, developing a vaccine is both a very demanding process, and it also requires long-term evaluation at some clinical stages. In this regard, organized efforts continue in various centers around the world. In order to safely get rid of this pandemic disease threat, it is necessary to develop the vaccines with due safety profile and put into use quickly by announcing the effects and side effects recorded in the phase trials with the public. Openness, accountability, and transparency are of utmost importance both for the regression of possible vaccine opposition and also for gaining access to vaccines by everyone, especially by vulnerable groups and labor class. Therefore, providing free access to vaccines with a social state approach is vital.

## REFERENCES

Arora, K, Rastogi, R & Arora, NM (2020) Multi-Antigenic Virus-like Particle of SARS CoV-2 produced in Saccharomyces cerevisiae as a vaccine candidate. *bioRxiv.* https://www.biorxiv.org/content/10.1101/2020.05.18.099234v1 .abstract

Badgett, MR, Auer, A, Carmichael, LE, Parrish, CR & Bull, JJ (2002) Evolutionary dynamics of viral attenuation. *J Virol,* 76, 10524-9.
[http://dx.doi.org/10.1128/JVI.76.20.10524-10529.2002] [PMID: 12239331]

Badgett, MR, Auer, A, Carmichael, LE, Parrish, CR & Bull, JJ (2002) Evolutionary dynamics of viral attenuation. *J Virol,* 76, 10524-9.
[http://dx.doi.org/10.1128/JVI.76.20.10524-10529.2002] [PMID: 12239331]

Cao, Y, Zhu, X, Hossen, MN, Kakar, P, Zhao, Y & Chen, X (2018) Augmentation of vaccine-induced humoral and cellular immunity by a physical radiofrequency adjuvant. *Nat Commun,* 9, 3695.
[http://dx.doi.org/10.1038/s41467-018-06151-y] [PMID: 30209303]

Chan, JF, Kok, KH, Zhu, Z, Chu, H, To, KK, Yuan, S & Yuen, KY (2020) Genomic characterization of the 2019 novel human-pathogenic coronavirus isolated from a patient with atypical pneumonia after visiting Wuhan. *Emerg Microbes Infect,* 9, 221-36.
[http://dx.doi.org/10.1080/22221751.2020.1719902] [PMID: 31987001]

Chandrashekar, A, Liu, J, Martinot, AJ, McMahan, K, Mercado, NB, Peter, L, Tostanoski, LH, Yu, J, Maliga, Z, Nekorchuk, M, Busman-Sahay, K, Terry, M, Wrijil, LM, Ducat, S, Martinez, DR, Atyeo, C, Fischinger, S,

Burke, JS, Slein, MD, Pessaint, L, Van Ry, A, Greenhouse, J, Taylor, T, Blade, K, Cook, A, Finneyfrock, B, Brown, R, Teow, E, Velasco, J, Zahn, R, Wegmann, F, Abbink, P, Bondzie, EA, Dagotto, G, Gebre, MS, He, X, Jacob-Dolan, C, Kordana, N, Li, Z, Lifton, MA, Mahrokhian, SH, Maxfield, LF, Nityanandam, R, Nkolola, JP, Schmidt, AG, Miller, AD, Baric, RS, Alter, G, Sorger, PK, Estes, JD, Andersen, H, Lewis, MG & Barouch, DH (2020) SARS-CoV-2 infection protects against rechallenge in rhesus macaques. *Science,* 369, 812-7.
[http://dx.doi.org/10.1126/science.abc4776] [PMID: 32434946]

Chen, WH, Strych, U, Hotez, PJ & Bottazzi, ME (2020) The SARS-CoV-2 Vaccine Pipeline: an Overview. *Curr Trop Med Rep,* 1-4, 1-4.
[http://dx.doi.org/10.1007/s40475-020-00201-6] [PMID: 32219057]

Coleman, CM, Liu, YV, Mu, H, Taylor, JK, Massare, M, Flyer, DC, Smith, GE & Frieman, MB (2014) Purified coronavirus spike protein nanoparticles induce coronavirus neutralizing antibodies in mice. *Vaccine,* 32, 3169-74.
[http://dx.doi.org/10.1016/j.vaccine.2014.04.016] [PMID: 24736006]

*CTRI/2020/07/026352.*
http://ctri.nic.in/Clinicaltrials/showallp.php?mid1=45306&EncHid=&userName=Zydus

Cuiling, Z, Giulietta, M & Hu, S (2019) *Advances in mRNA Vaccines for Infectious Diseases Frontiers in Immunology,* 10, 594.

Dandan, RH & Brunton, LL (2017) *Goodman ve Gilman's Pharmacology and Treatment Handbook* Güneş Medical Bookstores, Istanbul 4-7.

Deng, W, Bao, L, Liu, J, Xiao, C, Liu, J, Xue, J, Lv, Q, Qi, F, Gao, H, Yu, P, Xu, Y, Qu, Y, Li, F, Xiang, Z, Yu, H, Gong, S, Liu, M, Wang, G, Wang, S, Song, Z, Liu, Y, Zhao, W, Han, Y, Zhao, L, Liu, X, Wei, Q & Qin, C (2020) Primary exposure to SARS-CoV-2 protects against reinfection in rhesus macaques. *Science,* 369, 818-23.
[http://dx.doi.org/10.1126/science.abc5343] [PMID: 32616673]

van Doremalen, N, Lambe, T, Spencer, A, Belij-Rammerstorfer, S, Purushotham, JN, Port, JR, Avanzato, VA, Bushmaker, T, Flaxman, A, Ulaszewska, M, Feldmann, F, Allen, ER, Sharpe, H, Schulz, J, Holbrook, M, Okumura, A, Meade-White, K, Pérez-Pérez, L, Edwards, NJ, Wright, D, Bissett, C, Gilbride, C, Williamson, BN, Rosenke, R, Long, D, Ishwarbhai, A, Kailath, R, Rose, L, Morris, S, Powers, C, Lovaglio, J, Hanley, PW, Scott, D, Saturday, G, de Wit, E, Gilbert, SC & Munster, VJ (2020) ChAdOx1 nCoV-19 vaccine prevents SARS-CoV-2 pneumonia in rhesus macaques. *Nature,* 586, 578-82.
[http://dx.doi.org/10.1038/s41586-020-2608-y] [PMID: 32731258]

Douglas, RG & Samant, VB (2018) *The Vaccine Industry in Plotkin's Vaccines* 43.

Folegatti, PM, Ewer, KJ, Aley, PK, Angus, B, Becker, S, Belij-Rammerstorfer, S, Bellamy, D, Bibi, S, Bittaye, M, Clutterbuck, EA, Dold, C, Faust, SN, Finn, A, Flaxman, AL, Hallis, B, Heath, P, Jenkin, D, Lazarus, R, Makinson, R, Minassian, AM, Pollock, KM, Ramasamy, M, Robinson, H, Snape, M, Tarrant, R, Voysey, M, Green, C, Douglas, AD, Hill, AVS, Lambe, T, Gilbert, SC & Pollard, AJ Oxford COVID Vaccine Trial Group (2020) Safety and immunogenicity of the ChAdOx1 nCoV-19 vaccine against SARS-CoV-2: a preliminary report of a phase 1/2, single-blind, randomised controlled trial. *Lancet,* 396, 467-78.
[http://dx.doi.org/10.1016/S0140-6736(20)31604-4] [PMID: 32702298]

Folegatti, PM, Ewer, KJ, Aley, PK, Angus, B, Becker, S, Belij-Rammerstorfer, S, Bellamy, D, Bibi, S, Bittaye, M, Clutterbuck, EA, Dold, C, Faust, SN, Finn, A, Flaxman, AL, Hallis, B, Heath, P, Jenkin, D, Lazarus, R, Makinson, R, Minassian, AM, Pollock, KM, Ramasamy, M, Robinson, H, Snape, M, Tarrant, R, Voysey, M, Green, C, Douglas, AD, Hill, AVS, Lambe, T, Gilbert, SC & Pollard, AJ Oxford COVID Vaccine Trial Group (2020) Safety and immunogenicity of the ChAdOx1 nCoV-19 vaccine against SARS-CoV-2: a preliminary report of a phase 1/2, single-blind, randomised controlled trial. *Lancet,* 396, 467-78.
[http://dx.doi.org/10.1016/S0140-6736(20)31604-4] [PMID: 32702298]

Gao, S, Song, S & Zhang, L (2019) Recent progress in vaccine development against chikungunya virus. *Front Microbiol,* 10, 2881.

[http://dx.doi.org/10.3389/fmicb.2019.02881] [PMID: 31921059]

General Office of National, Health Commission of the People's Republic of China. (2020) *Diagnosis and treatment for novel coronavirus (Version 5).* http://www.nhc.gov.cn/xcs/zhengcwj/202002/3b09b894ac9b4204a79db5b8912d4440.shtml

Graham, BS (2020) Rapid COVID-19 vaccine development. *Science,* 368, 945-6.
[http://dx.doi.org/10.1126/science.abb8923] [PMID: 32385100]

He, Y & Jiang, S (2005) Vaccine design for severe acute respiratory syndrome coronavirus. *Viral Immunol,* 18, 327-32.
[http://dx.doi.org/10.1089/vim.2005.18.327] [PMID: 16035944]

Van Herck, K & Van Damme, P (2001) Inactivated hepatitis A vaccine-induced antibodies: follow-up and estimates of long-term persistence. *J Med Virol,* 63, 1-7.
[http://dx.doi.org/10.1002/1096-9071(200101)63:1<1::AID-JMV1000>3.0.CO;2-U] [PMID: 11130881]

Hobernik, D & Bros, M (2018) DNA Vaccines-How Far From Clinical Use? *Int J Mol Sci,* 19, 3605.
[http://dx.doi.org/10.3390/ijms19113605] [PMID: 30445702]

Huang, AT, Garcia-Carreras, B, Hitchings, MDT, Yang, B, Katzelnick, LC, Rattigan, SM, Borgert, BA, Moreno, CA, Solomon, BD, Trimmer-Smith, L, Etienne, V, Rodriguez-Barraquer, I, Lessler, J, Salje, H, Burke, DS, Wesolowski, A & Cummings, DAT (2020) A systematic review of antibody mediated immunity to coronaviruses: kinetics, correlates of protection, and association with severity. *Nat Commun,* 11, 4704.
[http://dx.doi.org/10.1038/s41467-020-18450-4] [PMID: 32943637]

Huang, C, Wang, Y, Li, X, Ren, L, Zhao, J, Hu, Y, Zhang, L, Fan, G, Xu, J, Gu, X, Cheng, Z, Yu, T, Xia, J, Wei, Y, Wu, W, Xie, X, Yin, W, Li, H, Liu, M, Xiao, Y, Gao, H, Guo, L, Xie, J, Wang, G, Jiang, R, Gao, Z, Jin, Q, Wang, J & Cao, B (2020) Clinical features of patients infected with 2019 novel coronavirus in Wuhan, China. *Lancet,* 395, 497-506.
[http://dx.doi.org/10.1016/S0140-6736(20)30183-5] [PMID: 31986264]

Imai, M, Iwatsuki-Horimoto, K, Hatta, M, Loeber, S, Halfmann, PJ, Nakajima, N, Watanabe, T, Ujie, M, Takahashi, K, Ito, M, Yamada, S, Fan, S, Chiba, S, Kuroda, M, Guan, L, Takada, K, Armbrust, T, Balogh, A, Furusawa, Y, Okuda, M, Ueki, H, Yasuhara, A, Sakai-Tagawa, Y, Lopes, TJS, Kiso, M, Yamayoshi, S, Kinoshita, N, Ohmagari, N, Hattori, SI, Takeda, M, Mitsuya, H, Krammer, F, Suzuki, T & Kawaoka, Y (2020) Syrian hamsters as a small animal model for SARS-CoV-2 infection and countermeasure development. *Proc Natl Acad Sci USA,* 117, 16587-95.
[http://dx.doi.org/10.1073/pnas.2009799117] [PMID: 32571934]

Jackson, LA, Anderson, EJ, Rouphael, NG, Roberts, PC, Makhene, M, Coler, RN, McCullough, MP, Chappell, JD, Denison, MR, Stevens, LJ, Pruijssers, AJ, McDermott, A, Flach, B, Doria-Rose, NA, Corbett, KS, Morabito, KM, O'Dell, S, Schmidt, SD, Swanson, PA, II, Padilla, M, Mascola, JR, Neuzil, KM, Bennett, H, Sun, W, Peters, E, Makowski, M, Albert, J, Cross, K, Buchanan, W, Pikaart-Tautges, R, Ledgerwood, JE, Graham, BS & Beigel, JH mRNA-1273 Study Group (2020) An mRNA Vaccine against SARS-CoV-2 - Preliminary Report. *N Engl J Med,* 383, 1920-31.
[http://dx.doi.org/10.1056/NEJMoa2022483] [PMID: 32663912]

Ji, W, Wang, W, Zhao, X, Zai, J & Li, X (2020) Cross-species transmission of the newly identified coronavirus 2019-nCoV. *J Med Virol,* 92, 433-40.
[http://dx.doi.org/10.1002/jmv.25682] [PMID: 31967321]

Kaur, SP & Gupta, V (2020) COVID-19 Vaccine: A comprehensive status report. *Virus Res,* 288, 198114.
[http://dx.doi.org/10.1016/j.virusres.2020.198114] [PMID: 32800805]

Kim, E, Erdos, G, Huang, S, Kenniston, TW, Balmert, SC, Carey, CD, Raj, VS, Epperly, MW, Klimstra, WB, Haagmans, BL, Korkmaz, E, Falo, LD, Jr & Gambotto, A (2020) Microneedle array delivered recombinant coronavirus vaccines: Immunogenicity and rapid translational development. *EBioMedicine,* 55, 102743.
[http://dx.doi.org/10.1016/j.ebiom.2020.102743] [PMID: 32249203]

Kim, YC, Dema, B & Reyes-Sandoval, A (2020) COVID-19 vaccines: breaking record times to first-i-

-human trials. *NPJ Vaccines,* 5, 34.
[http://dx.doi.org/10.1038/s41541-020-0188-3]

Krammer, F, Weir, JP, Engelhardt, O, Katz, JM & Cox, RJ (2020) Meeting report and review: Immunological assays and correlates of protection for next-generation influenza vaccines. *Influenza Other Respir Viruses,* 14, 237-43.
[http://dx.doi.org/10.1111/irv.12706] [PMID: 31837101]

Thanh Le, T, Andreadakis, Z, Kumar, A, Gómez Román, R, Tollefsen, S, Saville, M & Mayhew, S (2020) The COVID-19 vaccine development landscape. *Nat Rev Drug Discov,* 19, 305-6.
[http://dx.doi.org/10.1038/d41573-020-00073-5] [PMID: 32273591]

Lee, J (2020) These 23 companies are working on coronavirus treatments or vaccines — here's where things stand. *Market watch.* https://www.marketwatch.com/story/these-nine-companies-are-working -o- -coronavirus-treatments-or-vaccines-heres-where-things-stand-2020-03-06

Li, F (2016) Structure, Function, and Evolution of Coronavirus Spike Proteins. *Annu Rev Virol,* 3, 237-61.
[http://dx.doi.org/10.1146/annurev-virology-110615-042301] [PMID: 27578435]

Masihi, KN (2001) Fighting infection using immunomodulatory agents. *Expert Opin Biol Ther,* 1, 641-53.
[http://dx.doi.org/10.1517/14712598.1.4.641] [PMID: 11727500]

Mulligan, MJ & Lyke, KE Phase 1/2 Study to Describe the Safety and Immunogenicity of a COVID-19 RNA Vaccine Candidate (BNT162b1) in Adults 18 to 55 Years of Age: Interim Report. *medRxiv.*

Myupchar. (2020) *Race for COVID-19 vaccine: Covaxin and ZyCoV-D begin human trials in India*Moderna publishes preliminary data from phase 1. https://www.firstpost.com/health/race-for-covid-19-vac-ine-covaxin-and-zycov-d-begin-human-trials-in-india-moderna-publishes-preliminary-d-ta-from-phase-1-8600211.html/amp

Wang, N, Shang, J, Jiang, S & Du, L (2020) Subunit Vaccines Against Emerging Pathogenic Human Coronaviruses. *Front Microbiol,* 11, 298.
[http://dx.doi.org/10.3389/fmicb.2020.00298] [PMID: 32265848]

Novavax Covid 19 vaccine trial. *Clinical Trials Arena.* https://www.clinicaltrialsarena.com/news/novavax-covid-19-vaccine-trial/

Ou, X, Liu, Y, Lei, X, Li, P, Mi, D, Ren, L, Guo, L, Guo, R, Chen, T, Hu, J, Xiang, Z, Mu, Z, Chen, X, Chen, J, Hu, K, Jin, Q, Wang, J & Qian, Z (2020) Characterization of spike glycoprotein of SARS-CoV-2 on virus entry and its immune cross-reactivity with SARS-CoV. *Nat Commun,* 11, 1620.
[http://dx.doi.org/10.1038/s41467-020-15562-9] [PMID: 32221306]

Plotkin, SA (2010) Correlates of protection induced by vaccination. *Clin Vaccine Immunol,* 17, 1055-65.
[http://dx.doi.org/10.1128/CVI.00131-10] [PMID: 20463105]

Polack, FP, Thomas, SJ, Kitchin, N, Absalon, J, Gurtman, A, Lockhart, S, Perez, JL, Pérez Marc, G, Moreira, ED, Zerbini, C, Bailey, R, Swanson, KA, Roychoudhury, S, Koury, K, Li, P, Kalina, WV, Cooper, D, Frenck, RW, Jr, Hammitt, LL, Türeci, Ö, Nell, H, Schaefer, A, Ünal, S, Tresnan, DB, Mather, S, Dormitzer, PR, Şahin, U, Jansen, KU & Gruber, WC C4591001 Clinical Trial Group (2020) Safety and Efficacy of the BNT162b2 mRNA Covid-19 Vaccine. *N Engl J Med,* 383, 2603-15.
[http://dx.doi.org/10.1056/NEJMoa2034577] [PMID: 33301246]

Salvatori, G, Luberto, L, Maffei, M, Aurisicchio, L, Roscilli, G, Palombo, F & Marra, E (2020) SARS-CoV-2 SPIKE PROTEIN: an optimal immunological target for vaccines. *J Transl Med,* 18, 222.
[http://dx.doi.org/10.1186/s12967-020-02392-y] [PMID: 32493510]

Shi, Y, Wang, G, Cai, XP, Deng, JW, Zheng, L, Zhu, HH, Zheng, M, Yang, B & Chen, Z (2020) An overview of COVID-19. *J Zhejiang Univ Sci B,* 21, 343-60.
[http://dx.doi.org/10.1631/jzus.B2000083] [PMID: 32425000]

Smith, TRF, Patel, A, Ramos, S, Elwood, D, Zhu, X, Yan, J, Gary, EN, Walker, SN, Schultheis, K, Purwar, M, Xu, Z, Walters, J, Bhojnagarwala, P, Yang, M, Chokkalingam, N, Pezzoli, P, Parzych, E, Reuschel, EL, Doan, A, Tursi, N, Vasquez, M, Choi, J, Tello-Ruiz, E, Maricic, I, Bah, MA, Wu, Y, Amante, D, Park, DH,

Dia, Y, Ali, AR, Zaidi, FI, Generotti, A, Kim, KY, Herring, TA, Reeder, S, Andrade, VM, Buttigieg, K, Zhao, G, Wu, JM, Li, D, Bao, L, Liu, J, Deng, W, Qin, C, Brown, AS, Khoshnejad, M, Wang, N, Chu, J, Wrapp, D, McLellan, JS, Muthumani, K, Wang, B, Carroll, MW, Kim, JJ, Boyer, J, Kulp, DW, Humeau, LMPF, Weiner, DB & Broderick, KE (2020) Immunogenicity of a DNA vaccine candidate for COVID-19. *Nat Commun,* 11, 2601.
[http://dx.doi.org/10.1038/s41467-020-16505-0] [PMID: 32433465]

Strugnell, R, Zepp, F & Cunningham, A (2011) Vaccine antigens. *Understanding Modern Vaccines: Perspectives in Vaccinology,* 1, 61e88.
[http://dx.doi.org/10.1016/j.pervac.2011.05.003]

Tu, YF, Chien, CS, Yarmishyn, AA, Lin, YY, Luo, YH, Lin, YT, Lai, WY, Yang, DM, Chou, SJ, Yang, YP, Wang, ML & Chiou, SH (2020) A Review of SARS-CoV-2 and the Ongoing Clinical Trials. *Int J Mol Sci,* 21, 2657.
[http://dx.doi.org/10.3390/ijms21072657] [PMID: 32290293]

Ura, T, Okuda, K & Shimada, M (2014) Developments in Viral Vector-Based Vaccines. *Vaccines (Basel),* 2, 624-41.
[http://dx.doi.org/10.3390/vaccines2030624] [PMID: 26344749]

US Food and Drug Administration (FDA) (2020) Development and Licensure of Vaccines to Prevent COVID-19. *Guidance for Industry.* https://www.fda.gov/media/139638/download https://www.ias.ac.in/public/Resources/News/IASc_Press_Release.pdf

Voltron Therapeutics, Inc. (2020) *Enters into Sponsored Research Agreement with The Vaccine & Immunotherapy Center at the Massachusetts General Hospital to Develop Potential COVID-19 Vaccine.*https://www.prnewswire.com/news-releases/voltron-therapeutics-inc-enters-into-sponsored-r-search-agreement-with-the-vaccine--immunotherapy-center-at-the-massachusetts-genera--hospital-to-develop-potential-covid-19-vaccine-301034225.html

Wajnberg, A, Amanat, F, Firpo, A, Altman, DR, Bailey, MJ, Mansour, M, McMahon, M, Meade, P, Mendu, DR, Muellers, K, Stadlbauer, D, Stone, K, Strohmeier, S, Simon, V, Aberg, J, Reich, DL, Krammer, F & Cordon-Cardo, C (2020) Robust neutralizing antibodies to SARS-CoV-2 infection persist for months. *Science,* 370, 1227-30.
[http://dx.doi.org/10.1126/science.abd7728] [PMID: 33115920]

World Health Organization (2020) Coronavirus disease 2019 (COVID-19). *Situation Report-55.* https://www.who.int/emergencies/diseases/novel-coronavirus-2019/situation-reports

Zhou, P, Yang, XL, Wang, XG, Hu, B, Zhang, L, Zhang, W, Si, HR, Zhu, Y, Li, B, Huang, CL, Chen, HD, Chen, J, Luo, Y, Guo, H, Jiang, RD, Liu, MQ, Chen, Y, Shen, XR, Wang, X, Zheng, XS, Zhao, K, Chen, QJ, Deng, F, Liu, LL, Yan, B, Zhan, FX, Wang, YY, Xiao, GF & Shi, ZL (2020) A pneumonia outbreak associated with a new coronavirus of probable bat origin. *Nature,* 579, 270-3.
[http://dx.doi.org/10.1038/s41586-020-2012-7] [PMID: 32015507]

Zhu, FC, Li, YH, Guan, XH, Hou, LH, Wang, WJ, Li, JX, Wu, SP, Wang, BS, Wang, Z, Wang, L, Jia, SY, Jiang, HD, Wang, L, Jiang, T, Hu, Y, Gou, JB, Xu, SB, Xu, JJ, Wang, XW, Wang, W & Chen, W (2020) Safety, tolerability, and immunogenicity of a recombinant adenovirus type-5 vectored COVID-19 vaccine: a dose-escalation, open-label, non-randomised, first-in-human trial. *Lancet,* 395, 1845-54.
[http://dx.doi.org/10.1016/S0140-6736(20)31208-3] [PMID: 32450106]

# SUBJECT INDEX

## A



## B



Ozgur KARCIOGLU, Selman YENIOCAK and Mandana HOSSEINZADEH

## C

## D

## E



## F

## J



## K



## L

# M

# N



# O



# P

## R

## S

## T



## U



## V

## W



## Y



## Z

Made in the USA
Las Vegas, NV
03 November 2026

57421450R00245